Adults With Developmental Disabilities

Adults With Developmental Disabilities

Current Approaches in Occupational Therapy

Revised Edition

Edited by

Mildred Ross, OTR/L, FAOTA, and
Susan Bachner, MA, OTR/L, FAOTA, CEAC

AOTA
PRESS

The American
Occupational Therapy
Association, Inc.

Mission Statement

The American Occupational Therapy Association advances the quality, availability, use, and support of occupational therapy through standard-setting, advocacy, education, and research on behalf of its members and the public.

AOTA Staff

Karen C. Carey, CAE, Associate Executive Director, Membership, Marketing, and Communications
Audrey Rothstein, Group Leader, Communications

Chris Davis, Managing Editor, Books
Barbara Dickson, Production Editor

Robert A. Sacheli, Manager, Creative Services
Sarah E. Ely, Book Production Coordinator

Marge Wasson, Marketing Manager

The American Occupational Therapy Association, Inc.
4720 Montgomery Lane
PO Box 31220
Bethesda, MD 20824-1220
Phone: 301-652-AOTA (2682)
TDD: 800-377-8555
Fax: 301-652-7711
www.aota.org
To order: 1-877-404-AOTA (2682)

Disclaimers

This publication is designed to provide accurate and authoritative information in regard to the subject matter covered. It is sold or distributed with the understanding that the publisher is not engaged in rendering legal, accounting, or other professional service. If legal advice or other expert assistance is required, the services of a competent professional person should be sought.
—*From the Declaration of Principles jointly adopted by the American Bar Association and
a Committee of Publishers and Associations*

It is the objective of The American Occupational Therapy Association to be a forum for free expression and interchange of ideas. The opinions expressed by the contributors to this work are their own and not necessarily those of either the editors or The American Occupational Therapy Association.

ISBN: 1-56900-190-1

Library of Congress Control Number: 2004104383

Design by Sarah E. Ely
Composition by Electronic Quill, Silver Spring, MD
Printed by Edwards Brothers, Inc., Ann Arbor, MI

Dedications

In honor of

Deborah R. Labovitz, PhD, OTR/L, FAOTA,
an esteemed colleague, mentor, and most important, a dear friend

In honor of

Valnere McLean, MS, OTR/L, FAOTA,
in loving memory of her daughter, Nicole

Contents

List of Tables, Figures, Exhibits, and Chapter Appendixes ix

About the Authors xi

Introduction xvii

Part 1. Core Values

Chapter 1. Advocating for Clients and Legal Issues................................3
Barbara L. Kornblau, JD, OT/L, FAOTA, DAAPM,
and Maria Hinds, JD, MS, OTR/L

Chapter 2. Quality of Life: A Guiding Framework for
Practice With Adults With Developmental Disabilities 20
Rebecca Renwick, PhD, COTA, OTR

Part 2. Profile of Needs

Chapter 3. Clinical Issues Characterizing Adults
With Developmental Disabilities 41
Hollis A. Kellogg, OTR/L

Chapter 4. Using a Sensory Approach for Adults
With Developmental Disabilities 71
Bonnie Hanschu, OTR

Chapter 5. Low-Vision Intervention for Adults
With Developmental Disabilities 114
T. Ann Williams, OTR/L

Part 3. Specific Applications

Chapter 6. Equine-Assisted Therapy for Adults
With Developmental Disabilities 153
Kathryn L. Splinter-Watkins, MOT, OTR/L, FAOTA

Chapter 7. Let's Do Lunch: A Comprehensive,
Nonstandardized Assessment Tool..166
Susan Bachner, MA, OTR/L, FAOTA, CEAC

Chapter 8. Structurally Based Manual Therapy and
Improved Function..206
Lynn D. Simpson, OTR/L

Chapter 9. A Five-Stage Model for Adults
With Developmental Disabilities 250
Mildred Ross, OTR/L, FAOTA

Chapter 10. Groups Are Physical, Social, and
Emotional Therapy—"A Chance to Tell My Story" 268
Mildred Ross, OTR/L, FAOTA

Part 4. Full Participation

Chapter 11. Work *Is* Occupation: What Can I Do as
an Occupational Therapy Practitioner? 291
David J. Wysocki, MS, OTR/L, ATP, and Ann T. Neulicht, PhD, CRC

Chapter 12. Using Supported-Employment Principles to
Develop Self-Employment Opportunities 329
Carol Estes, BS, and David Matheis, BA, ATP

Chapter 13. Adaptive Driver Evaluation and Training 342
Deena Garrison Jones, OTR, CDRS

Index 383

About the Editors 391

List of Tables, Figures, Exhibits, and Chapter Appendixes

Figure 2.1: Three domains of quality of life...28
Figure 2.2: Three domains and nine subdomains of quality of life 29
Figure 2.3: Factors that determine and influence quality of life.................31

Figure 5.1: The fork on the left is much harder to distinguish from
the patterned background of the napkin than is the fork on the
right, which is on a solid-colored napkin...129
Figure 5.2: Examples of head-borne devices and spectacles.....................131
Figure 5.3: Handheld magnifiers in the foreground have built-in
light to illuminate objects being viewed 132
Figure 5.4: Examples of stand magnifiers 133
Figure 5.5: Examples of architect-style lighted magnifiers 133
Figure 5.6: Use of contrast to improve ability to see the level of
liquid in cups..137
Figure 5.7: A large-numbered phone with high-contrast lettering can
make dialing the telephone easier for a person with low vision 139
Appendix 5.A: Resource List 144
Appendix 5.B: Recommended Reading...146
Appendix 5.C: Visual Impairment Checklist of Pertinent Clinical
Observations 147

Figure 6.1: NARHA's four areas of emphasis 155
Figure 6.2: Wil taking part in a hippotherapy treatment session 158
Figure 6.3: Marla taking part in an equine-facilitated mental health
program session 159

Figure 7.1: "Let's Do Lunch" Assessment Tool for Julie...........................184
Figure 7.2: "Let's Do Lunch" Assessment Tool for Steve...........................190
Figure 7.3: "Let's Do Lunch" Assessment Tool for Helen 194
Appendix 7.A: Blank "Let's Do Lunch" Assessment Tool 202

Figure 8.1: The thoracic inlet is vulnerable to neuromusculoskeletal
dysfunction with subsequent problems in, for example,
the circulatory system 208
Figure 8.2(a)(b): Normal posture in which structural alignment in
the coronal plane is assessed 209
Figure 8.2(c): Abnormal posture 210

Figure 8.3: Normal posture in which structural alignment in the
    sagittal plane is assessed by evaluating the degree of deviation
    in the spinal curves...211
Figure 8.4: An example of fascia..215
Figure 8.5: External cranial and facial bones, and some of their
    external articulations..217
Figure 8.6: Protective muscle spasm of the sternocleidomastoid
    muscles can affect the function of the shoulder girdle and the
    respiratory and craniosacral systems...220
Figure 8.7: Protective muscle spasm of the scalene muscles
    can affect the function of the respiratory system, thoracic inlet,
    and head and neck 221
Figure 8.8: An example of leg muscles with their attachments to
    the pelvic girdle and spine...232
Figure 8.9(a): Inferior view of the base of the skull to picture the
    sphenobasilar junction 235
Figure 8.9(b): A sagittal section through the cranium to view the
    sphenobasilar junction 235
Figure 8.10: The bones of the hard palate are the maxillae and
    palatines bilaterally, and the vomer in the midline..............................236

Figure 9.1: Problem solving..254
Figure 9.2: Decision 255
Figure 9.3: Carefully spotting and reaching out for supplies
    without blocking someone else 255
Figure 9.4: Stage V...258
Figure 9.5: Learning to squat, to take care of the back, and
    to coordinate desired movement 260
Figure 9.6: Working together as partners is important while learning
    control of movement, direction with coordination, and focus 261
Figure 9.7: Alternately, the two female adults lead the exercises..............265
Figure 9.8: Alternately, the two female adults lead the exercises..............265

Appendix 11.A: Resources for the Occupational Therapy Practitioner
    in Work and Developmental Disabilities 326

Appendix 13.A: Organizations and Terms...368
Appendix 13.B: Driver Evaluation/Driver Training Checklist....................369
Appendix 13.C: Sample Consent Form..370
Appendix 13.D: Case Studies With Evaluation Reports.............................371
Appendix 13.E: Resources and Suppliers 378

About the Authors

Susan Bachner, MA, OTR/L, FAOTA, CEAC, owner and president of Susan Bachner Consulting, LLC, has almost 40 years of clinical practice with individuals who have developmental disabilities. Susan's numerous articles and book chapters appear in both professional and lay publications. Her universally designed cookbook, *Picture This—An Illustrated Guide to Complete Dinners,* is used extensively by people of all abilities. Evidence of her graduate degree in sociology and anthropology is especially evident in her chapter "Let's Do Lunch," in which she discusses the symbolism of food as it conveys culture, customs, attitudes, and values. Susan became certified as an environmental access consultant in 1999 and now guides the transformation of inaccessible or unsafe residences into supportive environments. In 2003, Susan was awarded Occupational Therapist of the Year 2002–2003 by the Kentucky Occupational Therapy Association.

Carol Estes, BS, has been with the Kentucky Department of Vocational Rehabilitation for 24 years. For 6 years she worked as a counselor in Northern Kentucky, and for the past 18 years she has been involved in various roles in supported employment. She currently serves as the program administrator for Supported Employment Services. She has been instrumental in bringing the concept of "person-centered services" to Kentucky's vocational programs. Carol served as the department's representative on the Kentucky Council on Developmental Disabilities for several years and is a past Board Member of ARC of Kentucky. She is a member of the Kentucky Association for Persons in Supported Employment and the Advisory Council of the Kentucky Autism Training Center. She also serves as the DVR representative on the Kentucky Mental Health Planning Council.

Deena Garrison Jones, OTR, CDRS, founder and manager of Boundless Mobility, has over 16 years' experience working with people with disabilities. She obtained her BS degree in occupational therapy from the Medical College of Virginia in 1986 and her certified driving instructor (CDI) in 1987 from Virginia Commonwealth University. Since that time she has been committed to training people to operate motor vehicles safely and efficiently. She received her certified driver rehabilitation specialist (CDRS) credential as a charter member in 1994. Deena received the Association of Driver Rehabilitation Specialists (ADED) Certificate of Professional Recognition in 1990 and in 1997 was recognized with the Scholar Award from ADED. She received the ADED Achievement award in 2003. Deena has also authored two books and numerous publications for driver rehabilitation and is a frequent presenter at conferences on driver training. She served on the Board of Directors for ADED for 3 years, sat on the board of the Aging Council for the National Department of Transportation, and completed research with the National Highway Traffic Safety Administration.

Bonnie Hanschu, OTR, had 25 years of experience as an occupational therapist and was directing habilitation services at Cambridge Regional Center, a Minnesota ICF-MR facility for adults, when she began devoting her full attention to sensory approaches for people with severe disabilities. Her work directing the Center for Neurodevelopmental Studies in Phoenix, Arizona, solidified her thinking that disordered sensory processing is, for many individuals, a fundamental and primary barrier to their ability to benefit from other services and treatment approaches. Since 1995, she has worked as a consultant and trainer for therapists, psychologists, teachers, and others interested in sensory approaches. Her courses have been presented throughout the United States, and she has served as a consultant to school districts, hospitals, county and state agencies, and private programs for people with developmental disabilities. She coauthored with Judith Reisman *Sensory Integration Inventory for Individuals With Developmental Disabilities* and the companion *User's Guide.*

Maria Hinds, JD, MS, OTR/L, is associate professor and interim director of occupational therapy at Florida A&M University, School of Allied Health Sciences. Maria is a member of the AOTA Model (HuGEM) Project II and author of *Ethical, Legal, and Social Implications of the Human Genome Project: Impact on the Role of the Occupational Therapist* and *Mental Retardation and Corrections: Criminal Defendants Held Hostage.* She has been a member of the Board of Directors of the Florida Advocacy Center for Persons with Disabilities (1998–2002) and Vice President of the Florida Occupational Therapy Association (2001–2003).

Hollis A. Kellogg, OTR/L, received his associate degree as an occupational therapy assistant at Orange County Community College, New York, and has worked in nursing homes and at the Burke Rehabilitation Center, New York. He received his BA in occupational therapy from Dominican College, Blauvelt, New York. He worked in the Orange County Association for the Help of Retarded Citizens for more than 10 years. He also has worked in home care and as a nursing home consultant.

Barbara L. Kornblau, JD, OT/L, FAOTA, DAAPM, is professor of occupational therapy, Public Health and Law, at Nova Southeastern University and a past president of the American Occupational Therapy Association. She has served AOTA as chair of the Commission on Standards and Ethics and of the Work Programs Special Interest Section. In private practice, she provides consulting services to business and industry, attorneys, and others for complying with the Americans With Disabilities Act. A practicing attorney, she specializes in disability discrimination litigation. She is also a certified case manager and a certified disability management specialist and holds board certification in pain management. Barbara has published more than 100 journal articles, books, chapters, and other works and has presented nationally and internationally about creative opportunities for occupational therapy practice in the future.

Dave Matheis, BA, ATP, is a program administrator for the Kentucky Department of Vocational Rehabilitation where, among other things, he manages the department's Rehabilitation Technology Services. He is the department's current representative on the Kentucky Council on Developmental Disabilities and is also on the Board of Directors of the Kentucky Assistive Technology Loan Corporation. He has been certified by RESNA as an assistive technology practitioner. In a career spanning more than 25 years, he has worked at sheltered workshops, a residential facility for individuals with developmental disabilities, a residential treatment center, and a community mental health center. Among his past roles with the Kentucky Department of Vocational Rehabilitation, he was a supported-employment regional consultant.

Ann T. Neulicht, PhD, CRC, earned her doctorate in rehabilitation research and maintains credentials as a certified rehabilitation counselor (CRC), certified vocational evaluator (CVE), certified life care planner (CLCP), certified disability management specialist (CDMS), licensed professional counselor (LPC), and diplomate of the American Board of Vocational Experts. Her consulting practice focuses on life care planning, vocational/earnings capacity assessment, labor market analysis/job placement, case management, and career development facilitator (CDF) training. Ann has over 20 years of experience as a rehabilitation counselor, case manager, supervisor, and university educator. She holds faculty appointments at the University of Florida and East Carolina University and is a frequent speaker at local and national conferences. She was the principal investigator for Project COMPUTE and placement coordinator for Project Techwork, grants that enhanced the employability of individuals with developmental disabilities through computer training. She has also served as chair of the Boards of Directors for the ARCs of Johnson (Kansas) and Wake (North Carolina) counties. The National Rehabilitation Counseling Association honored Ann with the 1996 Distinguished Service Award for her contributions to research and creative activity, dedication to consumers, and commitment to professional organizations.

Rebecca Renwick, PhD, COTA, OTR, is an associate professor in the Graduate Department of Rehabilitation Science and the Department of Occupational Therapy at the University of Toronto. She is also director of the Quality of Life Research Unit, which is jointly sponsored by the Graduate Department of Occupational Therapy and the Centre for Health Promotion, University of Toronto. Her research and publications focus on quality of life for people with and without disabilities as well as related issues, such as coping, social support, independence, and community participation. She is the senior editor of *Quality of Life in Health Promotion and Rehabilitation: Conceptual Approaches, Issues, and Applications* (1996). She was principal investigator on a 5-year study that examined quality of life and related issues for adults with developmental disabilities. A related project studied the quality of life for families that include adult members with developmental disabilities who live at home with biological or chosen families. Currently, she is principal investigator of a research program that is studying quality of life for children with developmental disabilities from a child and family perspective.

Mildred Ross, OTR/L, FAOTA, has practiced as an occupational therapist since her graduation from Columbia University in 1951. Having been engaged in private practice since 1984, she served people with developmental disabilities; worked in home care with dual diagnoses; and held per diem contracts in school settings, in mental health settings, and with nursing facilities. She has provided more than 100 presentations on the Five-Stage Group Model and included this subject, as well as others, in many articles and six books. She is the recipient of several service awards. Her emphasis at present is on the value of movement in the lives of those with and without disabilities.

Lynn D. Simpson, OTR/L, graduated from Quinnipiac College in 1981 with a BS in occupational therapy. She is certified in craniosacral therapy and zero balancing. She worked for the Capitol Region Educational Commission and for Northwest Village School, Plainville, Connecticut, with children with developmental disabilities, behavioral problems, and hearing impairments. For the past 17 years, she has worked for the Connecticut Department of Mental Retardation providing services to group homes for adults with developmental disabilities. In her private practice she works with adults and children. In all her work she focuses on the structural, emotional, and spiritual components of behavioral and movement problems.

Kathryn L. Splinter-Watkins, MOT, OTR/L, FAOTA, is employed at Eastern Kentucky University, Department of Occupational Therapy, Richmond, as associate professor and Level II fieldwork coordinator. She has been an academic fieldwork coordinator for 15 years and served for 3 years as the academic fieldwork coordinator representative on the Commission on Education at AOTA. Besides clinical education, strong interests include hippotherapy and therapeutic horseback riding. She has been involved as volunteer, instructor, therapist, board president, and consultant with various programs of therapeutic horseback riding and hippotherapy since 1982. She is a registered therapeutic riding instructor with the North American Riding for the Handicapped Association (NARHA) and registered therapist with the American Hippotherapy Association (AHA). She has served on the NARHA Health and Education Committee, the Research Sub-Committee, and the AHA Board of Directors. Other professional areas of emphasis include mental health and eating disorders.

T. Ann Williams, OTR/L, is a graduate of the University of Central Arkansas. She has practiced occupational therapy for 10 years and has worked with people with various diagnoses, including those with developmental disabilities. She is a staff therapist at the Eye Foundation of Kansas City, where she helps those with vision loss regain their independence in the home and community. Her interest in computers and their uses for individuals with vision loss has led her to specialize in this area and to pursue certification as a programmer and analyst.

David J. Wysocki, MS, OTR/L, ATP, is a 1994 graduate from the University of North Carolina at Chapel Hill. He has 10 years' experience in the field of developmental disabilities, including community-based occupation and work. He is currently the Therapeutic Healthcare Consultant for UCP of North Carolina, which includes extensive coverage for UCP's diverse vocational and living programs across the state. Prior to UCP, David served as the occupational therapy and assistive technology consultant for Murdoch Center Community Services, performing evaluations and training, while covering diverse community needs in developmental disabilities and brain injury. He is a visiting faculty member and student supervisor for the University of North Carolina and part of the leading team, initiating specialized coursework in developmental disabilities for the university's Department of Allied Health Sciences. David served as the director of a multi-agency grant project to foster computer-based work for adults with severe developmental disabilities. He currently serves on the NCOTA Executive Board and is the OT/PT/SLP Representative on the Council for Allied Health in North Carolina. David is a RESNA-Certified Assistive Technology Practitioner (ATP) with direct experience in computer access, augmentative communication, seating and positioning, and work/home access. He speaks nationally on professional assistive technology applications and developmental disabilities.

Introduction

Several years have passed since the first edition of *Adults With Developmental Disabilities: Current Approaches in Occupational Therapy* was published by the American Occupational Therapy Association (1998). Legislative changes, attitudinal advances in human rights, lessons learned from evidence-based practices and research, and the simple need for additional information on relevant topics have brought this revision to the marketplace. These changing elements, like colors in a kaleidoscope, produce different patterns and images. This edition clearly organizes these contemporary patterns and so has become a more comprehensive guide.

The chapters in Part 1, "Core Values," set the stage. "Advocating for Clients and Legal Issues," by Barbara L. Kornblau and Maria Hinds—both occupational therapists and lawyers—captures the spirit of this book. An updated discussion by Rebecca Renwick, "Quality of Life: A Guiding Framework for Practice With Adults With Developmental Disabilities," commands attention, especially in a client-centered climate.

The chapters in Part 2, "Profile of Needs," discuss clients in various locations along the continuum of abilities. In his chapter, "Clinical Issues Characterizing Adults With Developmental Disabilities," Hollis A. Kellogg describes and intervenes with adults who cope with significant challenges. Bonnie Hanschu's discussion of sensory processing in "Using a Sensory Approach for Adults With Developmental Disabilities" and T. Ann Williams's "Low-Vision Intervention for Adults With Developmental Disabilities" connect all of the other chapters. Each author demonstrates how the sensory systems and, in turn, functioning, are influenced by the registration of sensory stimulation.

In Part 3, "Specific Applications," the chapters shift their focus to the evaluation and guidance arenas. The welcome addition of Kathleen L. Splinter-Watkins's informative and sensitively presented chapter, "Equine-Assisted Therapy for Adults with Developmental Disabilities," has pertinence in both rural or urban locations. Susan Bachner's "Let's Do Lunch: A Comprehensive, Nonstandardized Assessment Tool," Lynn D. Simpson's "Structurally Based Manual Therapy and Improved Function," and Mildred Ross's two chapters, "A Five-Stage Model for Adults With Developmental Disabilities" and "Groups Are Physical, Social, and Emotional Therapy—A Chance to Tell My Story," offer a variety of effective approaches that speak both to occupational assessment and treatment.

Readers will be pleased with the information presented in the entirely new Part 4, "Full Participation." "Work *Is* Occupation: What Can I Do as an Occupational Therapy Practitioner?" by David J. Wysocki and Ann T. Neulicht offers a comprehensive overview of work as a practice area, moving from a description of services from the period of deinstitutionalization in the 1970s to contemporary settings.

Further, we felt it imperative to address emerging self-employment roles—entrepreneurship—as well as to discuss transportation issues for those adults with developmental disabilities who yearn to drive automobiles. These topics represent some of the less common challenges faced by adults with developmental disabilities. However, they are included here because of the recognition that there are adults who, through self-determination, advocacy, and good fortune, are able to assimilate into mainstream society. "Using Supported-Employment Principles to Develop Self-Employment Opportunities," by Carol Estes and David Matheis, and "Adaptive Driver Evaluation and Training," by Deena Garrison Jones, acknowledge the palpable progress in human justice and occupational opportunity. The content in Part 4 is designed to be reproducible by therapists with interests, proper training, and support in these areas.

This revised edition further distinguishes itself because it does not take a disability-specific approach but rather one that is client-centered and aligned with the philosophy of self-determination. It is designed for therapists who work hard to facilitate and support meaningful occupation-based activities. Therefore, *Adults With Developmental Disabilities: Current Approaches in Occupational Therapy, Revised Edition,* is an essential guide.

—*Mildred Ross, OTR/L, FAOTA*
Susan Bachner, MA, OTR/L, FAOTA

PART 1

Core
Values

CHAPTER 1

Advocating for Clients and Legal Issues

Barbara L. Kornblau, JD, OT/L, FAOTA, DAAPM
Maria Hinds, JD, MS, OTR/L

Introduction

One of the earliest efforts to address the needs of individuals with developmental disabilities occurred in 1945, when President Harry S. Truman organized the Committee on Employment of the Physically Handicapped and Mentally Retarded. However, it is over the past decade that substantial changes have occurred in the lives of adults with developmental disabilities. Quality-of-life issues changed from a purely medical model to a quasi-political model. This model reflects correctness of terminology and availability of government funding to provide services for children and adults with developmental disabilities.

The effort, which started as early as 1922 with the establishment of the International Society of Crippled Children, was still in its infancy in 1945. Most individuals with developmental disabilities lived in large institutions or hospitals. During the 1950s and 1960s, the parents' movement came into fruition, spearheaded by John F. Kennedy's visit to Willowbrook (the Staten Island Developmental Center, New York). Deplorable conditions at that institution embarrassed the nation into change. President Kennedy's sister, Eunice Kennedy Shriver, became a visible advocate for the rights of individuals with mental retardation. An effective national movement resulted in changes, such as the closing of Willowbrook. Further, support of training programs for special education teachers by the Office of Education resulted from a study that showed that children with severe forms of mental retardation benefited significantly from early intervention programs.

The 1960s and 1970s were times of great social change and unrest. People with disabilities, their families, and their advocates discovered that their common interests far outweighed their differences. A united disability community emerged, and the concept of empowerment of this community replaced the institutionalized charity/medical model of ministering to passive victims. Disability took on a quasi-minority status, deserving some of the rights and protections granted other minority groups. This new activism spawned the birth of the disability rights movement and promoted the passage of the Rehabilitation Act of 1973 (29 U.S.C. §791)—the Bill of Rights of the 1970s—and the Americans With Disabilities Act (ADA) of 1990 (P.L. 101-336), considered by many the world's most comprehensive legislation on disability rights.

As the civil rights of individuals with developmental disabilities expanded, the role of the occupational therapist changed accordingly. In the 1950s, occupational therapists provided services to children and adults with developmental disabilities within a recreational, activity-oriented model. Like other professionals, occupational therapy practitioners provided these services primarily within large institutions, nursing homes, and hospitals.

Today, the role of the occupational therapist is fundamental. Clinicians provide a variety of services that affect the lives of individuals with developmental disabilities. Their involvement includes, although is not limited to, research, diagnosis, early intervention, employment, and community integration. Occupational therapy takes a total person-centered approach. As such, case management and advocacy are natural parts of the intricate role that occupational therapy clinicians play in the lives of people with developmental disabilities.

Legal Rights in Housing

Laws exist to promote integration of adults with developmental disabilities into the mainstream of society, including housing. Traditionally, society placed individuals with "mental retardation" in large institutions where "people could live protected lives and pose no risk to society" (Mangan, Blake, Prouty, & Lakin, 1993). By the 1960s and early 1970s, advocates for this group realized that people who resided in large institutions missed exposure to a variety of community experiences. This inspired the aggressive movement for deinstitutionalization that resulted in the development of group homes and a variety of residential programs to serve adults and children with developmental disabilities.

However, during the 1980s, advocates still criticized these community residential programs as "small institutions," which merely transferred institutional practices to the community. Individuals remained isolated, segregated,

dependent on paid staff, and without opportunities to become active participants in their communities. Consumer self-advocacy efforts of the mid-1980s
and the Fair Housing Amendments Act of 1988 (42 U.S.C. §2601 *et seq.*)
affected the lives of individuals with developmental disabilities (Shea &
Forrest, 1993). Individuals expressed their opinions about their living environment and level of support services, either themselves or through their families, friends, or advocates. By the end of the 1980s, voices of concern and
advocacy influenced policy and practice at the federal, state, and local levels,
resulting in legislation and funding for the development of a variety of creative community residential options (Mangan et al., 1993):

- *Group homes:* Supervision and training is provided by staff, serving
  one to eight nonrelated people with developmental disabilities.
- *Supervised home or apartment:* Individuals live alone or with roommates in semi-independent units or apartments. Staff may live in a
  separate apartment at the same location.
- *Adult foster care:* One or more individuals live with a family who
  provides care as needed.
- *Personal care home:* Staff provides assistance with personal care but
  provides no training to residents.
- *Board and care home:* Room and board is provided without training or assistance for personal care.

The move into these community-based settings opened a door for the
provision of occupational therapy services. Occupational therapists may
serve as subcontracted service providers, clinical coordinators, qualified mental retardation professionals, legal guardians, or advocates for people who
reside in the community residential facilities referenced above. Clinicians provide individualized services and programs, such as choice making, functional
living skills, adaptive equipment, and purposeful activities that facilitate the
individual's integration into and participation in his or her communities.
Increase of independence and choice-making skills facilitate a shift in power
from professionals to adults with developmental disabilities.

However, this process of integration into communities was not without
opposition. In 1989, the Penhurst longitudinal study identified the NIMBY
syndrome—not in my backyard (Scheffer, 1994). The respondents agreed
with the necessity of a transition out of large institutions for the population
with developmental disabilities. However, most also agreed that those in
charge should establish community-living options anywhere but in their own
neighborhoods. This attitude was common throughout America.

Community concerns included an increase in crime and a decrease in
property values. Interviews of neighbors; real estate agents; and fire, police,
and health officials took place before and after organizers opened the homes.
Virtually everyone interviewed agreed that group homes did not negatively

affect the community. Property values and crime rates remained unaffected (Scheffer, 1994). Despite community opposition, over the past decade the development and expansion of community residential options for those with developmental disabilities increased the quality of life for many individuals, thanks in large part to the Fair Housing Amendments Act (FHAA) of 1988.

The FHAA opened opportunities for individuals with developmental disabilities in the area of housing. The act defines an individual with a handicap as one who has a physical or mental impairment that substantially limits one or more major life activities, has a record of having such an impairment, or is regarded as having an impairment. (Congress has not seen fit to amend this law to substitute the preferred term *disability* for *handicap*.)

The FHAA makes it illegal to discriminate in the sale or rental of dwellings because the buyer, renter, or prospective resident has a handicap (42 U.S.C. §3604{f}{1}). Further, one may not make unavailable or deny a dwelling to a buyer, renter, or prospective resident because of a handicap. Unlawful discrimination includes a refusal to make reasonable accommodations in rules, policies, practices, or services, when such accommodations may be necessary to afford a handicapped person equal use and enjoyment of a dwelling (42 U.S.C. §3604{f}{3}{B}).

In passing the FHAA, Congress recognized that the right to be free from housing discrimination is essential to the goal of independent living (House Report at 18, 1985). The FHAA represents

> a clear pronouncement of a national commitment to end the unnecessary exclusion of persons with handicaps from the American mainstream. It repudiates the use of stereotypes and ignorance, and mandates that persons with handicaps be considered as individuals. Generalized perception about disabilities and unfounded speculations about threats to safety are specifically rejected as grounds to justify exclusion. (House Report at 18, 1985)

In light of the FHAA's broad mandate, many Court decisions have broadly construed its antidiscrimination prescription (e.g., *City of Edmonds v. Oxford House, Inc.,* 1995). Courts have consistently invalidated a wide range of municipal licensing, zoning, and other regulatory practices affecting people with disabilities (e.g., *Potomac Group Homes Corp. v. Montgomery County,* 1983).

In many of these cases, individuals with developmental disabilities found themselves either intentionally discriminated against or in situations in which the government or dwelling owner failed to make a reasonable accommodation. These incidents happen particularly with group homes for adults with developmental disabilities. For example, a town may have an ordinance that requires that "group homes for the mentally or physically handicapped" obtain a special permit. Courts would find this type of ordinance intentionally discriminatory and therefore illegal and in violation of the FHAA (*Bangertner v. Orem City Corp.*, 1995).

The mandate to make reasonable accommodations for individuals with disabilities can affect adults with developmental disabilities in several ways. First, suppose Bridgette, an adult with developmental disabilities, wished to use the swimming pool in her apartment complex on a Sunday. Further, suppose the complex had a policy of "no guests on weekends" and the only way Bridgette could use the pool was with the assistance of her best buddy. The apartment complex would be guilty of failing to reasonably accommodate if it did not make a reasonable accommodation to its rules by allowing the best buddy in the pool. Only with this accommodation could Bridgette have equal enjoyment of the pool facilities. Making a reasonable accommodation "means changing some rule that is generally applicable to everyone to make it less onerous to the handicapped individual" (*Oxford House, Inc., v. Township of Cherry Hill*, 1992).

Another way the reasonable accommodation issue may affect adults with developmental disabilities relates to group home issues. In one case, for example, a city's fire code required that a group home install a fire-warning system and a sprinkler system. The group representing the potential residents asked for a waiver of this requirement as a reasonable accommodation. The city offered no proof that waiving the requirement would threaten the safety of the residents. The residents asserted that the waiver would allow five additional residents to live in the group home. The court found that the city's failure to issue a waiver of the fire code constituted a failure to make a reasonable accommodation under the FHAA (*Alliance for the Mentally Ill et al. v. City of Naperville*, 1996).

There are many similar situations in which city and county regulations place restrictions on group homes for adults with developmental disabilities. For example, cities use local zoning and regulatory restrictions to bar development of community residences for individuals with developmental disabilities. However, court decisions invalidate regulatory and zoning restrictions as discriminatory under the FHAA and a deprivation of the individuals' equal protection under the law.

The FHAA does give cities an exemption for any "reasonable" restriction on the number of individuals permitted to occupy a dwelling. In a suit brought by Oxford House against the City of Edmonds, Washington, the U.S. Supreme Court held "the exemption did not permit cities to close their single family zones to group homes." The restrictions the FHAA exempted were only those that "apply uniformly to all residents of all dwelling units" (*City of Edmonds v. Oxford House, Inc.*, 1995).

In a suit brought by the Cleburne Living Center against the City of Cleburne, Texas, after being denied a special use permit for the operation of a group home for people with mental retardation, the Court held that requiring the permit deprived people with mental retardation of equal protection under the law. The Court said "there was no rational basis for believing that the proposed home would pose a threat to the city" (*City of Cleburne, TX v. Cleburne Living Center*, 1985).

Occupational therapists may ease these community tensions. Clinicians may facilitate the increase of community awareness to promote the total integration and inclusion of individuals with developmental disabilities into communities by coordinating programs and activities that include residents, family, friends, and neighbors.

Legal Issues in Employment

Prior to the enactment of the minimum wage laws of the Fair Labor Standards Act of 1938 as amended (29 U.S.C. §201 *et seq.*), many institutions required adults with developmental disabilities to participate in habilitative labor "therapeutic" program plans, which conferred economic benefits on the institutions without compensation, in accordance with the law (Hasazi, Collins, & Cobb, 1988). In other words, institutions required residents to work under the guise of a therapeutic purpose without being paid. Patient–workers of nonfederal hospitals, homes, and institutions for people with mental retardation brought suit to compel the Secretary of Labor to undertake enforcement of the minimum wage and overtime provisions of the Fair Labor Standards Act (FLSA) to protect the interests of these adults. The court held that the patient–workers were employees within the meaning of the act and had to be paid based on the minimum wage and overtime provisions of the FLSA, notwithstanding the claim that the work was therapeutic (*Nelson Souder et al. v. Secretary of Labor*, 1973).

Therapists should take careful note of the implications of this decision. Therapists cannot engage their clients in activities labeled therapeutic or simulated work, which in reality confer an economic benefit on the institution or agency. Should the work activity include something for which one would normally receive compensation, the law could view this individual as an employee entitled to pay within the meaning of the minimum wage law.

Currently a variety of employment options remain available to adults with developmental disabilities. These include

- *Sheltered workshops and work activity centers.* These are segregated work and vocational skills development programs.
- *Supported employment.* These are paid positions for people with disabilities who need special assistance in learning job requirements and performing the associated tasks. A job coach or a supervisor

who oversees a crew or enclave of people with disabilities working together at a job site provides support for the clients.

- *Competitive employment.* Individuals with developmental disabilities participate in competitive employment opportunities within the community (Hasazi et al., 1988).

Title I Americans With Disabilities Act

Although many view the passage of the ADA as the first real piece of civil rights legislation for individuals with disabilities, in reality, its predecessor, the Rehabilitation Act of 1973 (Rehab Act), holds this distinction. The Rehab Act put into place a system of legal protection meant to give individuals with disabilities, including those with developmental disabilities, the tools they needed to move further into the mainstream of society. As grandfather of the ADA, the Rehab Act prohibited discrimination against individuals with disabilities in employment and programs by agencies of the federal government, nonfederal government entities under contract with the federal government, and nonfederal government concerns that receive or benefit from federal government funds.

The ADA extended the Rehab Act's protections to private entities, whether or not they received federal funds or were under contract with the federal government (29 CFR §1630.2{b}). Like the FHAA, both the Rehab Act and the ADA define a person with a disability as one who has a physical or mental impairment that substantially limits one or more major life activities, has a record of having such an impairment, or is regarded as having an impairment (29 CFR §1630{2}{g}). Three key areas expand the world for individuals with developmental disabilities, thanks to the ADA:

- Employment (with non–state government employers; *University of Alabama v. Garrett*, 2001)
- Access to state and local government services
- Access to places of public accommodations that are privately owned.

The employment provisions of the ADA can facilitate job placement for an individual with developmental disabilities. The following example illustrates this point. Peter, an individual with developmental disabilities, finishes his training program where he learned to work as a janitor. He applies for a job as a janitor with a private school. To do the job, Peter will need an on-site job coach, which the training program will provide at the school until Peter performs to the job standards. The school requires Peter to read all of the cleaning products' labels prior to their use and to check off a chart in the bathroom to indicate which tasks he has done. One problem: Peter does not read well enough to read the labels or the chart.

The ADA introduces into the work area new concepts, such as reasonable accommodations, that can expand opportunities for Peter. Further, the

ADA prevents an employer from not hiring individuals who can do the job merely because they have developmental disabilities. However, occupational therapists need to work with Peter and other individuals to teach them how to exercise their rights under the law.

Under the ADA, employers cannot discriminate against individuals like Peter who can perform a job with or without reasonable accommodations. The ADA further mandates that employers provide, at their own expense, reasonable accommodations for their employees. However, employers must only provide these reasonable accommodations if they know the applicant or worker is a qualified individual with a disability *and* if the applicant or worker requests the accommodation. This means clinicians must work with clients toward a goal of being able to tell employers about their disability and the type of reasonable accommodation they may require to enable their performance.

In Peter's situation, he would need to tell the prospective employer that he has a developmental disability and he needs specific reasonable accommodations to do the job. A representative from Peter's training program could assist him with this. Peter then would need to request the specific accommodations he needs.

The occupational therapist's skills with adaptations come into play here. As part of any training or therapeutic program, occupational therapists need to help clients identify needed reasonable accommodations. Unable to read, Peter needs another way to review the information on the cleaning fluid labels prior to using them.

Instead of reading the labels, the employer could set up, on the cleaning cart, color-coded tape recorders matching the color of the cleaning product labels. Peter could play the tape by color for each cleaning product prior to its use. The chart in the bathrooms could be adapted using pictures instead of words. Peter could use a date stamp to indicate the task he has completed. Though the ADA does not require an employer to provide a job coach at its own expense, the employer could allow the program to provide a job coach as an accommodation. Occupational therapy clinicians, with their training in task analysis and adaptations, will find themselves masters in identifying literally hundreds of other possible reasonable accommodations for Peter and other clients in similar work situations.

Clinicians should provide individualized programs with goals that facilitate choice making, job training and/or advancement and retention, and job-site visits to evaluate the need for assistive technology, retraining, or both. Occupational therapists should also be involved in the ongoing assessment of functional skills as related to the work environment inclusive of ongoing communication with employers to facilitate increased job performance.

Access to Places of Public Accommodations

Title III of the ADA protects individuals with disabilities from discrimination in access to places of public accommodation that are privately owned (28 CFR 36 §102). These include doctors' offices, funeral homes, movie theaters, bus stations, amusement parks, museums, restaurants, and just about any other place where the public goes to eat, bank, shop, or engage in commerce or transact business (28 CFR 36 §104).

Although physical barriers often prevent access, some of the most significant barriers that adults with developmental disabilities face do not involve physical access. Rather, attitudinal barriers often prevent access and inclusion for those with developmental disabilities and their families. Whereas most look at Title III as a building code, in recognition of these nonphysical barriers, Title III also prevents the type of discrimination caused by attitudinal barriers that often result from fear, ignorance, stereotypes, and misconceptions about individuals with disabilities.

Before Congress made the ADA the law of the land, business owners could treat adults with developmental disabilities differently from other adults without disabilities. For example, a movie theater could require a wheelchair user to transfer into a regular theater seat to watch a movie or not allow wheelchairs in the theater at all. Congress intended the ADA to rid society of these kinds of barriers.

In addition to a plethora of architectural barrier–removal mandates, the ADA includes certain rules that theaters, malls, doctors' offices, and other places of public accommodation must follow to make it easier for individuals with disabilities, including developmental disabilities, to include themselves and participate in normal life activities. For example, suppose an adult with a developmental disability finds himself or herself unable to read information on a menu at a restaurant. The ADA requires that the restaurant provide a reasonable accommodation to enable access to the menu which, in this case, might include the server reading the menu to the customer (29 CFR §36.303).

Other ADA rules prevent places of public accommodation from segregating individuals with disabilities in the provision of goods and services (29 CFR §36.202). For example, a theater cannot require someone in a wheelchair to sit in the front of the theater just because he or she has a developmental disability and uses a wheelchair. As an accommodation, the theater must remove some of the seats to allow room for people using wheelchairs.

Under the ADA, places of public accommodation cannot treat people differently (e.g., charge them more money or not allow them in at all) just because they have a developmental disability (29 CFR §36.301). Just because a family member is in a wheelchair does not mean that management can force him or her to pay more money to sit in the handicapped section in the end zone at the football stadium. A restaurant manger cannot tell a family member who drools that he or she cannot eat in the restaurant, just because he or she drools.

The ADA also prevents people from treating family members differently. A restaurant manager cannot refuse to allow individuals to eat in a restaurant because their family member has a head injury. The concert stadium cannot make family members bring their own chairs to set next to their family members' wheelchairs at a rock concert. If everyone else is given a chair, they have to give family members or other attendants a chair, too.

The ADA's rules also make it easier for family members and others to care for adults with developmental disabilities (29 CFR §36.205). If family members travel and stop at a rest area on the interstate, they usually have two choices: a men's or women's restroom. What happens if a woman needs to help an adult son with a developmental disability into the bathroom? She must ask a worker at the rest stop to help clear people out or close the restroom. He or she will have to stand outside the bathroom and guard the door so the woman can help her son in either the men's or women's restroom. This is another type of reasonable accommodation that places of public accommodation must make (29 CFR §36.302). Newer facilities include unisex bathrooms.

There are many different types of accommodations, depending on the type of barrier one encounters and the type and extent of limitations found in the individual with a developmental disability.

Many places of public accommodation do not know about the ADA. They do not know about the rules they are supposed to follow. Sometimes, even if they know about these rules, they do not know anything about developmental disabilities, so they do not know what accommodations to make or how to make them.

As with the employment provisions of the ADA, to obtain reasonable accommodations under Title III's access provisions, one must request them. Occupational therapy clinicians can assist adults with developmental disabilities and their family members in identifying needed accommodations that enable inclusion in everyday life.

Some accommodations may be very difficult to make. For example, it may not be possible to install a wheelchair ramp to the door of a doctor's office in an old house. The ramp may cost too much money, or it may make it dangerous for other people to walk in the area. The doctor probably would not have to make this accommodation, because it is not a reasonable accommodation. The law only requires that places of public accommodation make reasonable accommodations.

Even though the law says places of public accommodation must make reasonable accommodations, many do not comply with the law, either out of ignorance or by intent. Occupational therapy clinicians may find their efforts to integrate adults with developmental disabilities into the community impaired by the physical and attitudinal barriers their clients face.

Clinicians must be aware of current laws that govern structural barriers and accessibility to community resources, which may include state and local ordinances as well as the ADA. Occupational therapists, as advocates, can increase the successful integration of individuals with developmental disabilities into their communities. Some physical barriers often encountered include unreachable store merchandise, inaccessible post offices, and inadequate or nonexistent access signs to buildings within the community. The following three provisions within the ADA address these problem areas:

1. The law requires that merchants not display their products too high (more than 54") or too low (less than 9").
2. The law considers post offices with only exterior and interior steps, high counters, and untrained personnel inaccessible under the ADA.
3. The ADA requires display of an international symbol indicating accessible entrances.

Ironically, Congress did not apply the ADA to itself until 1995. Senator Max Cleland (D-GA), an individual with a physical disability, encountered severe obstacles to serving in the Senate. According to the *New York Times* (November 8, 1996), he found bathrooms inaccessible, floors of the Senate chamber tiered, and no ramps in most hearing rooms. People with developmental disabilities with physical limitations also would find the House inaccessible.

Clinicians should serve as active advocates regarding these issues. This advocacy includes, among other things, bringing access issues to the attention of team members, agency officials, and community officials. Occupational therapy clinicians should make all efforts to encourage the removal of structural barriers that inhibit integration into the community (Parry, 1990).

Without ADA police to enforce this law, the ADA becomes a complaint-driven law. When a barrier is found in a place of public accommodation that the owner will not eliminate once notified, there are several methods for seeking a remedy. The U.S. Department of Justice maintains a complaint line to call to register a complaint: (202) 514-0301 (voice), (202) 514-0381 (TDD). Another alternative is to contact an attorney experienced with ADA litigation.

Human Rights of Individuals With Developmental Disabilities

The U.S. Constitution specifically guarantees fundamental rights, and *human rights* refers to the basic respect and dignity that should be afforded each individual. Congress can expand constitutional rights by passing federal laws. The ADA is an example of a federal law that expanded the rights of citizens.

In 1948, the General Assembly of the United Nations adopted the Universal Declaration of Human Rights. The Universal Declaration establishes uniform standards for the treatment of all people. In 1971, the United Nations adopted the Declaration of Rights of Mentally Retarded Persons (Association for Retarded Citizens, 1992).

Individuals with developmental disabilities, like all other citizens, have a vast array of protections under the law inclusive of the Universal Declaration of Human Rights that proclaims that all human beings are entitled to, among other rights, freedom of thought, conscience, and religion; freedom of opinion and expression; the right to work and choose one's work freely; the right to receive equal pay for equal work; and the right to an adequate standard of living.

Service providers, families, and advocates must be especially vigilant of their autonomy and right to equal protection under the law. Because of the long history of oppression, devaluation, and callous disregard for the rights of individuals with developmental disabilities, advocates must carefully monitor issues, such as the right to refuse and/or receive medical treatment or programming, to remain free from harm, and to marry and make informed decisions regarding sexuality and parenthood. Therefore, professionals and advocates involved in the provision of support services must maintain awareness of the ongoing risks and dangers that these individuals face on a daily basis.

Guardianship/Conservatorship

The law provides protection for individuals whom it considers unable to care for their own affairs or property or unable to meet some of their own essential health and safety needs. Although specific grounds and definitions vary from state to state, there are several commonalities. States appoint guardians or conservators to make financial and personal decisions for adults with developmental disabilities whom courts adjudge in need of this assistance.

When a client has a guardian or conservator, this individual makes decisions with regard to where the client will reside and what program the client will attend. In many of these situations, the clinician must look to the guardian or conservator for informed consent before initiating occupational therapy treatment given that, once adjudicated incompetent, the client lacks the legal capacity to give consent and sign documents on his or her own. Occupational therapy clinicians may find themselves facing ethical dilemmas in which the guardian or conservator refuses to consent to treatment that the ward desires or needs.

The Occupational Therapist as Advocate

As the team member professionally devoted to promoting independence in daily living, occupational therapy clinicians often will find barriers to this goal. Agencies, individuals, and institutions, among others, may cause these barriers by failing to comply with laws designed to guarantee certain rights. Failure to comply may result from intentional conduct as well as ignorance. Faced with barriers to achieving goals, occupational therapy clinicians may find that the most effective means of promoting their client's independence is to act as advocates. To effectively advocate for clients, occupational therapy clinicians should follow the Eight Rules of Advocacy.

Eight Rules of Advocacy

1. Know the laws.

Occupational therapists can familiarize themselves with laws that give rights to adults with developmental disabilities without the necessity of a law degree. Many laws provide rights for adults with developmental disabilities. Appellate courts reviewing ADA cases have restricted the ADA's employment provisions so that the ADA today does not cover situations that were originally covered. For example, when it originally became law, the ADA covered employment with state entities. In *University of Alabama v. Garrett* (2001), the Supreme Court ruled that the employment provisions of the ADA did not apply to employment with state agencies. Knowledge of these laws and the changes to them affects the goals therapists set with their clients, as shown in the example of Peter's employment. Occupational therapy practitioners should ensure that they prepare their clients to protect themselves and ask for their rights under the law. In many cases, this may require that clinicians take on the role of educator to teach clients their rights and how to assert themselves appropriately. Clinicians will find role playing very useful.

Knowledge of the pertinent laws also provides the basis for acting as an advocate for clients with developmental disabilities. One cannot take on an advocate role without having at least a rudimentary grounding in the rights for which one advocates. Without this basic foundation, the therapist runs the risk of looking foolish, and the client loses.

Occupational therapists advocating for clients with developmental disabilities cannot do their clients justice without an understanding of the Developmental Disabilities Act (42 U.S.C. §6000 *et seq.*) and the protections it affords. Congress passed the Developmental Disabilities Act (DD Act) to ensure that individuals with developmental disabilities and their families could participate in appropriate programs, services, and opportunities that would promote independence, productivity, and integration and inclusion into the community (42 U.S.C. §6000 {b}). The DD Act provides federal funding to support programs that work toward these goals. For states to receive this federal funding, each state participating in the program must create a protection and advocacy system empowered to do the following:

- "Pursue legal, administrative, and other appropriate remedies or approaches to ensure the protection of, and advocacy for" people within the programs
- "Provide information on and referral to programs" addressing the needs of people with developmental disabilities
- "Investigate incidents of abuse and neglect of [people with developmental disabilities] if the incidents are reported to the [protection and advocacy system] or if there is probable cause to believe that the incidents occurred" (42 U.S.C. §6042{a}{2}).

The DD Act also requires that the protection and advocacy system annually provide the public with an opportunity to comment on the priorities it establishes as well as its activities (42 U.S.C. §6042{C}). Further, the protection and advocacy system must establish a grievance procedure for clients or prospective clients of the system, to ensure that people with developmental disabilities have full access to the system's services (42 U.S.C. §6042{D}). The law requires the advocacy and protection agency to exist independently of agencies that provide treatment, services, and habilitation under the DD Act. The advocacy and protection agency must have reasonable access to individuals with developmental disabilities in facilities that provide services under the DD Act as well as access to their records (42 U.S.C. §6042{H}).

Occupational therapy practitioners may contact many sources to obtain additional information about relevant laws. They may contact directly the government agency charged with enforcing a particular law. For example, if there is a concern about a fair housing issue, they can call the Department of Housing and Urban Development. For an ADA issue concerning employment, they can contact the Equal Employment Opportunity Commission for additional information. The Department of Justice has a Web site that provides literature about the ADA, Fair Housing Act, and several other laws that protect clients' rights. The Advocacy Centers serve as excellent sources of information and good places to refer clients for attorneys and other professional advocates who are up to date on the laws for adults with developmental disabilities.

2. Read the regulations.

Whenever Congress passes a law, it assigns the responsibility for administrating that law to a federal agency. The federal agency's responsibilities include promulgating regulations. Regulations are the rules that give meaning to the law and its means of enforcement. For the most part, clinicians will find regulations involving laws protecting individuals with developmental disabilities written in relatively plain and understandable English. As an added bonus, many of these regulations are readily available on the Internet (through the Justice Department bulletin board) and sometimes in libraries. Clinicians need not fear reading the Fair Housing regulations to find out additional information about a client's housing situation or the ADA regulations to look into a client's discrimination situation. Reading the regulations can make the clinician more knowledgeable and facilitate advocacy.

3. Believe your client/patient has a right.
Before clinicians take on an issue, they should believe in the right they seek for their clients. Without this belief, clinicians will not make effective advocates.

4. Organize yourself; document your efforts and get everything in writing.
Most people associate the phrase "get it in writing" with attorneys. Only written documents provide the key evidence should the situation rise to a formal complaint or lawsuit. The prohibition against hearsay testimony—a popular objection on any television courtroom drama—prevents arguing over who said what in court. On the other hand, written documents hold the promise of credibility before an administrative investigator, judge, or jury.

Because many of our clients lack adequate skills for expressing themselves in writing, practitioners can help advocate for clients by helping them write letters. They may also write their own letters to engage the services of the protection and advocacy agency that must investigate the situations adverse to clients.

Advocates will find keeping a diary an invaluable tool for future reference in advocacy matters. Dates, places, and events, recorded in the diary, fill in the blanks for the advocate when memory leaves too many gaps down the road.

5. Start with the source of the problem.
Often advocates can solve problems by going to the source to complain. Ignorance of the law is often the reason behind many problems faced by adults with developmental disabilities, especially in the discrimination arena. Often the person at the "front desk" lacks proper training in the rules of the ADA or Fair Housing Act. Notifying the source and giving that person or company an opportunity to do "the right thing" can often solve discrimination problems and avoid future incidents.

6. Be specific; tell them exactly what you want.
When writing a letter or speaking to someone to advocate for a client, clinicians should be very specific about what is required to resolve the matter. Advocates should spell out specific steps they want taken before taking action.

7. File a complaint.
A good advocate need not "make a federal case" out of everything. Most of the laws discussed in this chapter provide administrative procedures for

remedying protected wrongs. In passing these laws, Congress charged various administrative agencies with the responsibility to promulgate regulations to enforce the law. The regulations include an outline of procedures one may take to resolve a complaint to enforce the law's protection using investigators employed by the government agency. These procedures allow the individual with a developmental disability to protect his or her rights without going to court.

8. Follow through.

Finally, advocates should not give up but must follow up and through on their complaints. Investigations under these laws often take a long time. However, frequent phone calls can accelerate investigations and make things happen.

Ethical Considerations in Advocacy

Occupational therapy clinicians acting as advocates will face many ethical dilemmas. Occupational therapy advocates may take positions that risk their jobs or risk funding. Accepting an advocacy role requires balancing interest in one's job with interest in the client's rights. At all costs, however, occupational therapy clinicians must not try to separate the human side from the clinical side. Therapists who find themselves embroiled in hot ethical issues may consult their institution's ethics committee.

Conclusion

There remain critical issues facing individuals with developmental disabilities. The uncertainty of health care reform, limited funding, and cuts in disability benefits will ultimately affect their quality of life. Clinicians committed to the provision of quality services should keep abreast of the laws that affect the lives of people with developmental disabilities. Informed clinicians make the best advocates.

References

Alliance for the Mentally Ill et al. v. City of Naperville, 8 NDRL ¶28 (N.D. Ill. 1996).
Americans With Disabilities Act, Pub. L. No. 101-336 (July 26, 1990).
Americans With Disabilities Act, Title III Regulations, 28 CFR §36.101 *et seq.*
Association for Retarded Citizens. (1992). *Human rights for people with mental retardation* [Position statement]. Arlington, TX: Author.
Bangertner v. Orem City Corp., 46 F.3d 1491 (10th Cir. 1995).
City of Cleburne, TX v. Cleburne Living Center, 473 U.S. 432 (1985).
City of Edmonds v. Oxford House, Inc., 114 S. Ct. 1776 (1995).
Developmental Disabilities Act, 42 U.S.C. §6000 *et seq.* (Supp. 1989).
Fair Housing Amendments Act of 1988, 42 U.S.C. §2601 *et seq.*
Fair Labor Standards Act of 1938 as amended, 29 U.S.C. §201 *et seq.*
Hasazi, S. B., Collins, M., & Cobb, R. B. (1988). *Implementing transition programs for productive employment.* Baltimore: Paul H. Brookes.

H.R. Rep. No. 711, 100th Cong., 2nd Sess., at 18 (1985).

Mangan, T., Blake, E. M., Prouty, R. W., & Lakin, K. C. (1993). *Residential services for persons with mental retardation and related conditions: Status and trends through 1991.* Minneapolis: University of Minnesota, Center for Residential Services and Community Living/Institute on Community Integration.

Nelson Souder et al. v. Secretary of Labor, 367 F. Supp. 808 (1973).

Oxford House, Inc., v. Township of Cherry Hill, 799 F. Supp. 450, 462, n. 25 (D. N.J. 1992).

Parry, J. (1990). The Americans with Disabilities Act (ADA). *Mental and Physical Disability Law Reporter, 14,* 292–294.

Potomac Group Homes Corp. v. Montgomery County, 823 F. Supp. 1285 (D. Md. 1983).

Rehabilitation Act of 1973, 29 U.S.C. 791 (1973).

Scheffer, A. (1994, Nov.–Dec.). People with disabilities move into their own homes, little NIMBY opposition reported. *The NIMBY Report (11).*

Shea, A., & Forrest, C. B. (1993). *Patterns of supported living: A resource catalog.* Napa: California Department of Developmental Services.

University of Alabama v. Garrett, 531 U.S. 356 (2001).

CHAPTER 2

Quality of Life: A Guiding Framework for Practice With Adults With Developmental Disabilities

Rebecca Renwick, PhD, COTA, OTR

Introduction

This chapter examines the growing concern with quality of life in contemporary practice with adults with developmental disabilities. Attention to this issue is reflected in the current emphasis on developing outcome measures of quality of life and on using these to demonstrate the effectiveness and accountability of interventions. This chapter also offers a definition of quality of life and examines the connections between engagement in occupations and quality of life. It summarizes some of the major advantages, disadvantages, and risks of focusing on quality of life, especially within the field of practice with people with developmental disabilities. It examines the value of applying quality of life as a guiding framework for occupational therapy practice with adults with developmental disabilities.

A brief review of the key themes of recent, major conceptual frameworks of quality of life provides a context for the introduction of the Centre for Health Promotion (CHP) approach to quality of life. The background and essential features of the CHP conceptual model are described. The importance of having a conceptual framework—particularly one that focuses on quality of life—that can be used to organize and guide assessment, intervention, and program planning with this population also is discussed. Examples of the application of the CHP model to those aspects of occupational therapy practice are presented. The chapter concludes with a discussion of other potential applications of the model (e.g., research, policy development, and advocacy) and implications for occupational therapists.

Increasing Emphasis on Quality of Life

Since the 1970s, but particularly during the past 15 years, there has been an increasing interest in understanding quality-of-life issues and planning human services that enhance quality of life for people who receive such services. Several influences have contributed to this growing interest. Fiscal constraints—and the associated trend toward cost containment in health and social services—and managed care have exerted pressure to systematically measure, evaluate, and maximize the outcomes of intervention. In essence, the drive toward "getting better results with fewer resources" (Brown, Renwick, & Nagler, 1996, p. 3) has been a powerful influence. However, contemporary trends in policy and legislation that emphasize equality, human rights, and independent community living for people with disabilities also have been important (Brown et al., 1996). Such policies and legislation have arisen during a period of activism promoting empowerment and inclusion in society for people with disabilities (Renwick & Friefeld, 1996). Although activism often focuses on specific issues (e.g., new definitions of disability, environmental factors in disability, societal attitudes, and empowerment), its overarching goals include fostering and enhancing quality of life. More detailed discussions of the forces that contribute to this burgeoning interest in quality of life are contained in works by Brown et al. (1996) and Renwick and Friefeld (1996).

It is no surprise that professionals and researchers from a variety of disciplines have begun to develop approaches and programs that will contribute to and support quality of life for people who have disabilities (Keith & Schalock, 2000; Renwick, Brown, & Nagler, 1996). Despite the current climate of fiscal restraint and diminishing government support, it is essential that members of vulnerable populations enjoy a good quality of life. In fact, it is a matter of concern—both from the perspective of social justice and for occupational justice—that must be addressed. These principles are discussed by Jongbloed and Chrichton (1990), Townsend (1993), Townsend and Wilcock (2004), and Wilcock (1998).

Those who work in the field of developmental disabilities have taken the lead in the development of such approaches and programs (Goode, 1994; Keith & Schalock, 2000; Schalock, 1990, 1996, 1997b). Several authors have identified important issues and articulated the need to apply specific quality-of-life principles in the planning and evaluation of services for people with developmental disabilities (Dennis, Williams, Giangreco, & Cloninger, 1993; Goode, 1990; Landesman, 1986; Renwick, Brown, & Raphael, 2000), and several approaches to conceptualizing quality of life have been developed (Brown, Brown, & Bayer, 1994; Felce & Perry, 1996; Renwick & Brown, 1996; Schalock, 1997b).

Several attempts to apply quality-of-life principles have been reported in the literature (R. Brown et al., 1994; Renwick, Brown, & Raphael, 1994; Schalock, 1997a; Schalock, Keith, Hoffman, & Karan, 1989), and the area continues to develop. Much work is still needed to clarify the application of theory to assessment and intervention and to translate concepts into practical terms that facilitate their use by practitioners. Translation of knowledge is particularly important for occupational therapists who work with people with developmental disabilities, as the discipline's professional literature does not yet provide much guidance concerning conceptual approaches to quality of life or their practical application. This chapter is intended to help link a potentially useful theoretical framework to practice with adults who have developmental disabilities.

The Meaning of Quality of Life

Although there have been many attempts to explain and quantify quality of life (Bowling, 1991, 1995), the concept is too frequently used without clear definition or thorough discussion of what the concept means (Renwick & Brown, 1996). *Quality of life* is such a deceptively simple concept. Although at first glance it seems like a straightforward idea, more thorough examination reveals greater complexity. Considerable philosophical and conceptual material can be drawn into a discussion about the meaning of quality of life, but for this chapter, a summary of some important ideas is a more useful and concise approach.

Quality of life embodies those characteristics we consider shared and expressed in some way by all human beings (Brown & Renwick, 1996). Specifically, everyone has a physical body and thoughts, feelings, beliefs, and values. Each of us seeks shelter and a safe place to call home. We need and seek the comfort, companionship, and support that relationships with others can provide. We want to be connected with others who share some of our values. We need access to services and resources in the community where we live. We also seek meaningful activities and occupations in several realms, including caring for ourselves and others, involvement in paid and unpaid work, participation in leisure pursuits, and engagement in occupations that promote our growth as individuals. All of those characteristics are readily understood because they are common to human beings.

When we speak of a good quality of life, we imply an excellent life, a life full of experiences that are thoroughly felt and enjoyed, a life full of meaning. Most people want quality in their lives and strive to attain it. But a good quality of life is the ideal and, for most people, life is not ideal. There are some aspects of life that we could improve and other aspects we would like to minimize (or eliminate) to have good quality of life (Brown & Renwick, 1996).

Thus, when we use the term *quality of life,* we are referring to both ideas: first, those characteristics that are common to all people and second, the degree to which life is excellent or approaches this ideal. Quality of life is the degree of excellence of the characteristics of human life. Thus, in asking about quality of life, we are really asking, *Considering the qualities of human life, how good is your life for you?* (Brown & Renwick, 1996). The question is relevant to all people, whether or not they have developmental disabilities.

Engagement in Occupation and Quality of Life

The rationale for using quality of life as a framework for occupational therapy practice is rooted in the powerful connections between engagement in occupations and the human experiences of well-being and our perceptions of enjoying a good life. Specifically, meaningful occupational engagement has been found to be positively associated with quality of life (Christiansen, Backman, Little, & Nguyen, 1999; Christiansen & Townsend, 2004).

Occupational engagement can lead to empowerment and contribute to the maintenance of identity, even to the extent of transforming the individual's sense of self (Christiansen, 1999). When people are prevented or constrained from participating in the necessary or chosen occupations that give meaning to their lives—especially for prolonged periods and by circumstances they cannot control—they can experience occupational deprivation (Wilcock, 1998). The consequences seem inconsistent with a good life: There can be a "sense of isolation, powerlessness, frustration, loss of control, and estrangement from society or self" (Wilcock, 1998, p. 257). Lack of engagement in meaningful occupations also results in many fewer opportunities for achieving competence or occupational mastery, and it can prevent people from exploring and fulfilling their occupational potential (Wicks, 2001). Thus, either satisfying engagement in meaningful occupations or a lack of such engagement can profoundly affect anyone, regardless of ability. In fact, it can be argued that occupational justice necessitates the right of every citizen to engage in meaningful and necessary occupations (Townsend & Wilcock, 2004) and that doing so is an important prerequisite for a good quality of life.

Historically, many people with developmental disabilities, particularly those in institutional or other segregated settings and those negatively affected by social stigma, have had a restricted spectrum of occupations from which to choose. Their occupational awareness, exposure, and participation have been limited. Consequently, many have been at risk of occupational deprivation, of having a decreased sense of competence and occupational mastery, and of experiencing a lack of fulfillment of their occupational potential. For too many adults with developmental disabilities, all or some of these issues are still problematic. Given the connections of quality of life with engagement in meaningful occupations outlined here, quality-of-life models that address related occupational issues are particularly relevant for informing and guiding practice with adults with developmental disabilities.

Quality of Life as a Framework for Practice

Integrating and Organizing Practice

Quality of life can be seen as an organizing framework to guide practice with adults with developmental disabilities. The material discussed in previous sections of this chapter and elsewhere (Brown et al., 1996; Renwick & Brown, 1996; Renwick, Brown, Rootman, & Nagler, 1996; Renwick et al., 1994, 2000; Schalock, 1997a) provides a rationale for adopting this approach. That is, quality of life can be the core, integrating concept for all aspects of practice—assessment, intervention, program planning, evaluation, and research—as well as for advocacy efforts targeted at funding and policy development. *Fostering, enhancing, maintaining, and restoring quality of life* is often stated as the overriding, ultimate goal of occupational therapy, and the links between participation in occupations and quality of life have been well documented (Christiansen et al., 1999).

Of course, a clearly articulated, coherent, detailed theoretical formulation is a prerequisite for using quality of life as a guiding and integrating concept for practice. Several potentially appropriate frameworks are noted, and one specific approach is discussed later in this chapter.

Advantages

There are several advantages of using a quality-of-life framework to guide, integrate, and evaluate practice. It can improve accountability to clients and their families, to the broader community, to specific funders of programs for people with developmental disabilities, and to the occupational therapy profession. It also can add coherence to and provide a solid foundation for practice. That is, it can provide a theory-based explanation for practice and a coherent set of guidelines for assessment, intervention, evaluation, and other aspects of practice. Such a theoretical foundation is consistent with the goals and the client-centered nature of occupational therapy practice. Adopting a quality-of-life framework for practice can enhance the credibility of the profession as a whole.

Cautions and Potential Limitations

The emphasis on developing outcome measures to evaluate the efficacy and cost-effectiveness of health and social interventions as a way to demonstrate accountability has been discussed elsewhere, for example, by the Canadian Association of Occupational Therapists (1997). It seems obvious, and even a

matter of common sense, that such measurement and evaluation are beneficial. However, there are issues that should be considered if quality of life is
chosen as a practice framework (e.g., if it is used to guide evaluation of interventions and the outcome measures selected).

There are cases in which it could be neither feasible nor desirable to try
to continuously improve quality of life in several or all areas of life, and doing
so is not always an appropriate or realistic goal of intervention. For example,
maintaining or preventing deterioration of quality in some areas of life that a
client already perceives as satisfactory could be an appropriate goal for that
person. In such situations, care must be taken to clearly specify quality-of-life
goals and to understand what they mean to that person, so that a lack of
improvement is not interpreted as a "failure" of the intervention, or the
client, or the therapist, or any combination of these. When a particular intervention, such as moving to a more community-based setting or starting a new
program or job, is stressful and disruptive to a client's daily routines, it can
be expected that quality of life will decrease in some areas until the client
begins to adapt to the changes. On the other hand, once quality of life has
improved in a given area of life, the person's expectations about the desired
degree of quality in that area are likely to shift upward, too.

The foregoing considerations highlight the need to assess changes in
quality of life regularly and carefully over long periods. Such continuous
assessment is appropriate with a population for whom change is often a slow
process. Furthermore, reliable and valid standardized outcome measures
often are desirable for formal program evaluations, although care must be
taken that such instruments are rigorously validated, found psychometrically
sound when tested with adults with developmental disabilities, and appropriately matched to the goals of the intervention. Qualitative information
that is consistent with the guiding conceptual framework also can be collected to provide a meaningful context in which to interpret the quantitative outcomes (i.e., information collected with standardized instruments). If a less
formal approach to evaluation is used, therapists can gather qualitative or
quantitative information, or both, through the regular process of assessment.
However, many of the same cautions noted above—concerning appropriate
quality-of-life goals that are personally meaningful to clients and concerning
the potential limits of improvement in quality of life—are relevant to such an
evaluation.

Recent Conceptual Approaches

The field of practice with people with developmental disabilities has been a
rich source of conceptual approaches to quality of life, such as those
advanced by Felce and Perry (1996), Goode (1994), and Schalock (1990,
1996). Collectively, those approaches have suggested some essential themes

that, taken together, form the foundation of a useful conceptual framework of quality of life (Schalock, 1996).

One important theme is the need to accord the greatest importance to the perceptions of people with developmental disabilities concerning their own quality of life (Brown, Bayer, & McFarlane, 1989; Brown et al., 1994; Goode, 1990; Schalock et al., 1989). That emphasis often is reflected in the concept of satisfaction as experienced by the individual. A second important theme is found in the concept of individual well-being, frequently expressed in terms of material and psychological resources and physical health. Renwick, Brown, et al. (1996) described approaches that emphasize this theme. Other themes include personal growth of and mastery by the individual (Brown et al., 1994; Felce & Perry, 1996) as important aspects of quality of life. Finally, the notion of connections between the individual and important others is a common theme (Felce & Perry, 1996; Halpern, Nave, Close, & Wilson, 1986).

The CHP approach to quality of life encompasses those themes, although it does so by considering broad areas of life that are essential to all people. The CHP approach interweaves those themes with other, new concepts (Renwick et al., 2000) to offer the unique conceptualization of quality of life (Renwick & Brown, 1996) that is the subject of the rest of this chapter.

CHP Quality-of-Life Framework

Development and Assumptions

The CHP approach was developed by a small, multidisciplinary group of researchers at the Quality of Life Research Unit of the Centre for Health Promotion at the University of Toronto (Renwick & Brown, 1996). The conceptual framework was developed by means of three concurrent processes: (a) a thorough review of the literature, (b) consultation with other researchers and experts working in the areas of disability and quality of life, and (c) consultations with individuals and groups with and without disabilities. We consider the last of these three items to have been the most important. The consultation was done through focus groups and in-depth interviews about what makes life "good" and "not so good" for the individuals participating (Renwick & Brown, 1996).

Although development of the conceptual framework was intended to guide research concerning quality of life as experienced by people with developmental disabilities, the researchers soon realized that this emerging model had broader relevance. That is, it applied to any adult, regardless of ability. Thus, during its formulation, the model was tested by means of case studies of the lives of real people, with and without disabilities.

Several broad assumptions guided the development of the CHP model.

See Woodill, Renwick, Brown, and Raphael (1994) for a more detailed discussion. However, some of the assumptions are useful to consider here:

- Individuals are best understood holistically, as is consistent with contemporary, client-centered approaches to occupational therapy that emphasize collaboration and partnership between client and therapist (Canadian Association of Occupational Therapists, 1997).
- Quality of life emerges from the continuous, dynamic relationship between the person and the environment and thus can change over time.
- Because quality of life has several aspects, its various dimensions can change at different rates and in different ways—positively or negatively—although some dimensions might not change much over the course of one's life.
- The basic dimensions or aspects of quality life are the same for everyone, regardless of ability.
- The basic dimensions of quality of life are consistent with broad, contemporary perspectives on health, health promotion (World Health Organization, 1986), and occupational well-being (Christiansen et al., 1999). Those perspectives include the view that social factors, such as poverty and unemployment, can significantly affect a person's health (Evans & Stoddart, 1990) and can lead to occupational deprivation (Wilcock, 1998).

Essential Concepts and Features of the Framework

Defining Quality of Life

The CHP conceptual framework is based on a specific definition of *quality of life*: "the degree to which a person enjoys the important possibilities of his or her life" (Renwick & Brown, 1996, p. 80). Those possibilities consist of the balance between opportunities and constraints in the various areas of a person's life, described in the next section. Of course, people encounter many possibilities in life, but it is the possibilities that have particular importance to the person and his or her way of life that have significant implications for quality of life. For instance, exercise is part of many people's lives, but for some, it takes on special significance. Exercise could be an important aspect of life for people who

- want to reach or maintain a healthy weight,
- want to improve cardiac fitness,
- need to walk their dogs several times each day,
- like to play sports or run with their friends,
- are in training for the Special Olympics, or
- are parents of lively young children.

Possibilities depend on the dynamic interplay of people and their environments. Some possibilities are influenced or controlled to varying degrees by choices and decisions, such as what to do for fun and with whom, where to work, and how to spend time and money. Other possibilities are difficult to influence or cannot be controlled or changed: the era and place of one's birth, the presence of serious disabilities from birth, and ethnicity. The enjoyment part of the definition of quality of life refers to the satisfaction people experience in the balance between their constraints and their opportunities, that is, in the possibilities in their lives.

Quality-of-Life Domains

Quality of life has dimensions that correspond to broad, fundamental areas of people's lives. The CHP model focuses on the possibilities that arise in three areas of life—*Being, Belonging,* and *Becoming* (Figure 2.1). Each domain encompasses three subdomains for which nine aspects of quality of life are represented in Figure 2.2. The quality-of-life dimensions are congruent with the domains of concern for occupational therapists and with contemporary occupational therapy principles—particularly the use of a holistic, client-centered approach that is guided by the social justice perspective (Townsend, 1993; Wilcock, 1998).

Being includes three dimensions of life that are concerned with who the individual is as a person. *Physical being* focuses on the body and on physical aspects of health. Included here are exercise and fitness, mobility and agility, nutrition, grooming, hygiene, and physical appearance. *Psychological being* refers to a person's thoughts, feelings, and mental health. This dimension encompasses self-esteem, self-concept, and self-control; the ability to cope

Figure 2.1. Three domains of quality of life.

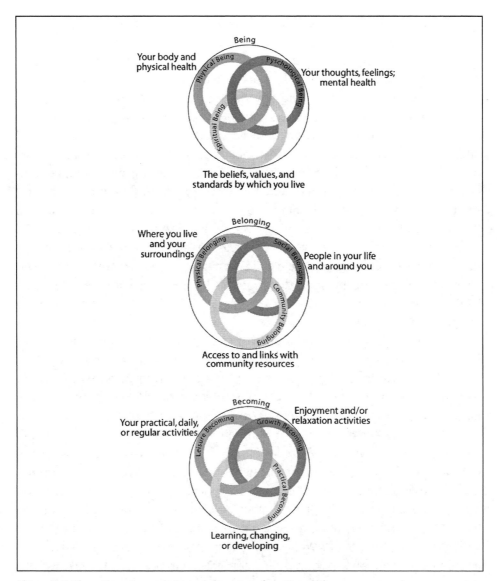

Figure 2.2. Three domains and nine subdomains of quality of life.

with anxiety; and the ability to initiate positive, independent activity. *Spiritual being* centers on the beliefs, values, and standards by which someone lives. Embodied here are an understanding of right and wrong, attaching meaning to life, feeling at peace within oneself, and celebrating special events in life (e.g., birthdays, holidays, and family events). It also includes the ability to help others and involvement in transcendent experiences, either religious or secular (e.g., engagement in activities and occupations associated with music, poetry, nature, organized religion, and meditation). Renwick et al. (2000) offered a more detailed discussion of spiritual being.

Belonging is the degree of congruence between a person and the environment. *Physical belonging* is concerned with physical aspects of a person's home; work, school, or program setting; neighborhood; and community. The major issues here are privacy, security, having personal possessions and a place to use or display them, and a feeling of being "at home" in one's physical surroundings. *Social belonging* refers to bonds and connections with significant people in one's life and with others with whom one has regular social interactions. This dimension includes meaningful relationships with a partner or special person, friends, and family members. Relationships with acquaintances; coworkers; neighbors; and members of cultural, faith, or interest groups are also encompassed here. *Community belonging* is concerned with the connections someone has with community resources. Having access to events, places, facilities, and services typically available in one's community is the major issue here. Among the usual community resources are employment, a source of money or income, education, health and social services, shopping facilities, and public events. Renwick et al. (2000) discussed community belonging in more detail.

Becoming is what a person does to fulfill hopes, goals, and aspirations. *Practical becoming* subsumes the practical activities—those someone wants or needs to accomplish regularly. Examples are involvement in work; volunteer activities; household chores; self-care; care of children, other family members, or pets; and attendance at school or other programs. It also includes making and attending appointments with providers of health, social, and educational services. *Leisure becoming* centers on what people do for fun or relaxation, including involvement in solitary, group, organized, or spontaneous activities that could be related to sports, hobbies, games, entertainment, or social interaction. This dimension also includes taking brief breaks from routine activities (e.g., a weekend away, a night out during the week) and taking vacations. *Growth becoming* emphasizes activities associated with learning, change, and personal development. Growth might involve the acquisition of new skills or the improvement of existing skills in formal ways (e.g., through courses or programs) or informal ways (e.g., learning from friends, social groups, or "how-to" books). The skills learned or further developed can be physical, interpersonal, or related to independent living. Growth becoming also includes seeking new challenges and adapting to changes in life.

Basic Quality of Life

Quality of life within each of the nine dimensions consists of both the degree of *satisfaction* and the degree of *importance* someone associates with the possibilities that arise in the continuing relationship with one's environment. Those determinants of basic quality of life are summarized in Figure 2.3.

Figure 2.3. Factors that determine and influence quality of life.

Personal Control

Personal control consists of two moderating factors that can either contribute to or detract from the degree of basic quality of life experienced by the individual in each of the nine areas of life. One factor consists of the *decisions* and choices a person makes. The other factor consists of the range of *opportunities* available as those decisions are made. Together, the two influencing factors constitute *personal control* (see Figure 2.3).

Applying the CHP Framework

The CHP model has several potential applications in occupational therapy practice with adults with developmental disabilities. The major applications examined here pertain to direct service and include assessment, intervention, program planning, and program evaluation. Additional applications are noted briefly in another section.

The CHP framework can be applied to identify those aspects of a person's life that add to or detract from quality of life. The application can serve to identify priority areas for goal setting, program planning, and intervention. It also can provide a way to determine a baseline for comparison of subsequent changes in a person's quality of life.

It is essential to note that, wherever possible, the perceptions of the person with developmental disabilities concerning quality of life should serve as the occupational therapist's major source of information. The client should have as active a role as possible in assessment, program planning, and intervention. As much as possible, evaluation of program effectiveness for a client or group of clients should draw most heavily on each person's experiences. According to the CHP approach, at every stage of occupational therapy involvement, the client should be as active a participant as possible (Renwick et al., 1994).

Other people who know the person well, such as family members, people who provide informal supports, and service providers, can be sources of additional or supplementary information. That source of information becomes much more important when clear communication between client and therapist is difficult or when the probability of misinterpretation of the client's perceptions is great, as, for example, when the client has a low level of cognitive functioning or a limited ability to express thoughts and feelings. In that case, information should be sought from at least two people who know the client well. Having adequate material from the appropriate sources is particularly critical in the assessment process.

Assessment

Assessment guided by the CHP framework can be quantitative; that is, instruments based on the framework can be used to determine quality of life for an individual in each area of life. The availability of such instruments is noted at the end of this chapter. Assessment also can occur more informally, through the systematic application of the CHP framework to interviewing the client and others as appropriate. Quantitative and qualitative assessment methods also can be combined. Whatever the approach, careful and thorough assessment greatly enhances the potential for planning meaningful interventions and achieving positive outcomes.

Because a qualitative interview is more likely to be used by therapists who provide direct service, this application of the framework to client assessment is examined further here. All nine areas of life can be assessed in terms of basic quality, and specifically, a determination can be made of how much importance and enjoyment or satisfaction the client attaches to the items included in each area of life. The items in each area also can be assessed with respect to personal control. Specifically, an assessment can focus on the extent to which clients perceive that they make choices and decisions and on the range of opportunities available to the client from which to make such choices and decisions. In assessing personal control, it is essential for the therapist to explore how much control the client is comfortable with or can deal with and wants to have in each area of life. For example, a client could be quite comfortable with making more decisions and choices related to physical being, such as

- when to wash his or her hair,
- choosing to have a bath instead of a shower,
- what to eat for breakfast, or
- deciding to get some exercise by going for a swim.

The client might also want to have more variety in the opportunities available to select from when making those choices and decisions. On the other hand, he or she might feel comfortable with the amount of personal control already exercised in other areas, such as leisure, illustrated by

- being able to watch favorite television programs each week,
- going bowling one night a week with fellow group home residents, or
- being able to make arrangements to stay at a family member's apartment for a weekend each month.

However, in other areas of life, the client could feel overwhelmed by the number and variety of choices and decisions he or she feels pressure to make. For instance, if growth becoming presents such a problem, the client could find it difficult to decide what social or independent-living skills to improve. More structure, assistance, or guidance might be required to facilitate decision making.

One important aspect of assessment is the exploration of the range of opportunities available to the client in the areas of life in which quality most needs to be enhanced. This process requires thorough consideration of the options—that is, of the constraints relative to the opportunities present in each area of life. In essence, alternative resources—people, groups, settings, programs, and activities—as well as strategies or courses of action the person can draw on to enhance quality in a particular area of life must be balanced against factors that would make improvement difficult or impossible. Some resources could be too costly, require too much travel, or require too lengthy a waiting period for the client to obtain access. Some strategies could be inappropriate to a client's current skills. In such situations, the therapist can discuss with the client what alternative resources and strategies would be acceptable and of interest.

Another crucial aspect of assessment is careful attention to how much the client's environment promotes, could promote, or detracts from quality in each area of life. The environment in which the client lives, works, goes to school, participates in programs, and engages in leisure occupations should be included in the assessment. Consideration should be given to the nature of the client's environment, including its physical, social, cultural, legal, and political aspects.

Two levels at which the environment can contribute to quality of life also should be explored. First, quality-promoting environments are those that meet the client's basic requirements for food, shelter, safety, and social contact. Second, such environments also offer the client a range of choices and opportunities from which to make decisions that are congruent with the client's capacity and comfort level and that can result in supporting or enhancing enjoyment or satisfaction in several of the nine areas. Assessment of the client's environment using the CHP framework can help the therapist identify those areas of life in which the client's environment for living, working, engaging in leisure pursuits, and so on is likely to promote quality as well as those areas in which it is not likely to do so.

Program Planning and Intervention

The assessment will enable the therapist, with as much participation as possible by the client, to identify which areas of life most require quality enhancement, particularly those areas that are very important but not currently satisfying to the client. Those priority areas become the focus for goal setting, program planning, intervention, and implementation of the plan as a way to reach the planned goals. The interdependent processes focus on strategies that are targeted to increasing the client's enjoyment or satisfaction in the most important areas and to decreasing dissatisfaction with activities that are not as enjoyable. Other essential strategies would be used to increase the amount of personal control in the areas of life in which the client wants to exert more influence.

At the same time, the amount of control experienced by the client can be decreased in those areas in which the demands to exert more personal control produce more pressure and anxiety. Increases or decreases in personal control can be achieved by expanding or narrowing the range of opportunities for choice and decision making and by increasing or decreasing the environmental demands on the client to exercise personal control.

If the environmental assessment indicates that the client's living or work environment, or both, do not promote quality—or in fact that they undermine it—some environmental modification strategies might need to be planned and built into the intervention. Strategies could include identifying and cultivating opportunities for the client to meet new people, to try new leisure activities, or to explore new settings or programs.

Evaluation

Application of the CHP framework to evaluation of how well the intervention addressed program goals can be done with individual clients or with groups of clients, such as those who share common program goals, have similar needs, or live in the same home. As with the initial assessment to establish baselines for the client, evaluation might consist of a formal, quantitative approach; of a less formal, qualitative approach; or of a combination of quantitative and qualitative methods.

Regular follow-up assessments (quantitative, qualitative, or combined) can determine whether the client's quality of life is improving, deteriorating, or static. The object is to determine whether satisfaction has increased in more important areas and dissatisfaction has decreased in less important areas. Attention also should be given to determining whether control has increased or decreased, as appropriate, to a desired or manageable level for the client. Finally, the therapist should ascertain whether a range of opportunities has been made available to the client that the client can access with or without facilitation from the therapist. If the client's goals are not being reached, the results of reassessment can guide the therapist in working with the client to make adjustments to the goals or to the overall program plan and intervention strategies, as appropriate.

Other Potential Applications

The CHP framework has been used to guide a large-scale, longitudinal study of quality of life for adults with developmental disabilities who live in Ontario, Canada (Renwick et al., 2000). The provincial government's Ministry of Community and Social Services at the time of the study was actively implementing policy to move those adults from institutions to more community-based settings for living, working, and participating in educational and other programs. The study was done by researchers at the University of Toronto's Quality of Life Research Unit, in part to assess the consequences of these public policy decisions for quality of life for adults who had moved to new places of residence or who had begun to participate in work or in programs in community settings. The research included the use of quality-of-life measures in the form of a psychometrically sound instrument package that was based on the elements of the CHP model. Future research could be designed such that the instruments would serve as outcome measures to test the relative efficacy of different interventions with adults who have developmental disabilities.

The CHP framework also can be used to guide the analysis and evaluation of existing policy, without necessarily requiring a specific research study of the kind noted above. It could be used, for instance, in a qualitative examination of specific policies and for summarizing and interpreting existing statistical reports relevant to them, to determine whether current policies adequately address the important aspects of quality of life for adults with developmental disabilities. Those applications of the CHP model could identify the aspects of quality of life that are inadequately addressed by a particular policy and indicate, in general terms, how gaps might be filled. The framework could be useful in guiding development of new health and social policy designed to target or include people with developmental disabilities.

Finally, the CHP approach can provide a platform for advocacy. That is, it can help to highlight issues for use as focal points of advocacy efforts. The framework also can be used to provide shape and direction for efforts aimed at changing policy, securing funding, and establishing or enhancing programs that support good quality of life for adults with developmental disabilities.

Conclusion

This chapter describes the CHP conceptual framework of quality of life and discusses its usefulness as a coherent, systematic guiding framework for occupational therapy practice with adults with developmental disabilities. Several aspects of the model make it appropriate for application by occupational therapists who work with that population:

- It is consistent with the holistic view and the client-centered approach that are hallmarks of the occupational therapy profession.
- It is relevant to important occupational issues that are common, and often problematic, for adults with developmental disabilities, including fulfillment of occupational potential, occupational exposure and engagement, and the risk of occupational deprivation.
- It focuses clearly and in detail on the nature of quality of life and how it might be promoted, fostered, enhanced, supported, or restored. This focus is highly congruent with the overarching goal of occupational therapy.
- It is grounded in the real-life perceptions of real people, with and without disabilities. Thus, the concepts associated with the framework are readily applied to all major aspects of occupational therapy practice, including assessment, intervention, and evaluation.
- It has been used successfully, over time, in a large-scale research study on the quality of life of people with developmental disabilities (Renwick et al., 2000).

Acknowledgments

The development of the CHP framework, the associated instrumentation, and the conduct of the study discussed in this chapter (Renwick et al., 1994, 2000; Renwick & Brown, 1996) constituted a program of research, the Quality of Life Project, which was funded by the Ontario Ministry of Community and Social Services. However, the views expressed here do not necessarily represent the views of the ministry nor of the government of Ontario.

The author gratefully acknowledges the assistance of Ted Myerscough, Quality of Life Project research unit manager, who designed the figures for this chapter. More information on the assessment instruments is available from the Quality of Life Research Unit, http://www.utoronto.ca/qol, or by writing to quality.oflife@utoronto.ca.

References

Bowling, A. (1991). *Measuring health*. Milton Keynes, UK: Open University Press.
Bowling, A. (1995). *Measuring disease*. Buckingham, UK: Open University Press.
Brown, I., & Renwick, R. (1996). *Improving quality of life*. Toronto: Quality of Life Research Unit, Centre for Health Promotion, University of Toronto.
Brown, I., Renwick, R., & Nagler, M. (1996). The centrality of quality of life in health promotion and rehabilitation. In R. Renwick, I. Brown, & M. Nagler (Eds.), *Quality of life in health promotion and rehabilitation: Conceptual approaches, issues, and applications* (pp. 3–13). Thousand Oaks, CA: Sage.
Brown, R. I., Bayer, M. B., & McFarlane, C. (Eds.). (1989). *Rehabilitation programmes: Performance and quality of life of adults with developmental handicaps*. Toronto: Lugus.

Brown, R. I., Brown, P. M., & Bayer, M. B. (1994). A quality of life model: New challenges arising from a six-year study. In D. A. Goode (Ed.), *Quality of life for persons with disabilities: International perspectives and issues* (pp. 39–56). Cambridge, MA: Brookline.

Canadian Association of Occupational Therapists. (1997). *Enabling occupation: An occupational therapy perspective.* Toronto: Author.

Christiansen, C. (1999). Defining lives: Occupation as identity. An essay on competence, coherence, and the creation of meaning. *American Journal of Occupational Therapy, 53,* 547–558.

Christiansen, C., Backman, C., Little, B. R., & Nguyen, A. (1999). Occupations and subjective well-being: A study of personal projects. *American Journal of Occupational Therapy, 53,* 91–100.

Christiansen, C., & Townsend, E. (2004). An introduction to occupation. In C. Christiansen & E. Townsend (Eds.), *Introduction to occupation: The art and science of living* (pp. 1–27). Upper Saddle River, NJ: Prentice Hall.

Dennis, R. E., Williams, W., Giangreco, M. F., & Cloninger, C. J. (1993). Quality of life as a context for planning and evaluation of services for people with disabilities. *Exceptional Children, 59,* 499–512.

Evans, R. G., & Stoddart, G. L. (1990). Producing health, consuming health care. *Social Science and Medicine, 31,* 1347–1363.

Felce, D., & Perry, J. (1996). Exploring current conceptions of quality of life: A model for people with and without disabilities. In R. Renwick, I. Brown, & M. Nagler (Eds.), *Quality of life in health promotion and rehabilitation: Conceptual approaches, issues, and applications* (pp. 51–62). Thousand Oaks, CA: Sage.

Goode, D. A. (1990). Thinking about and discussing quality of life. In R. L. Schalock (Ed.), *Quality of life: Perspectives and issues* (pp. 41–57). Washington, DC: American Association on Mental Retardation.

Goode, D. A. (1994). (Ed.). *Quality of life for persons with disabilities: International perspectives and issues.* Cambridge, MA: Brookline.

Halpern, A. S., Nave, G., Close, D. W., & Wilson, D. (1986). An empirical analysis of the dimensions of community adjustment for adults with mental retardation in semi-independent living programs. *Australia and New Zealand Journal of Developmental Disabilities, 12,* 147–157.

Jongbloed, L., & Chrichton, A. (1990). A new definition of disability: Implications for rehabilitation practice and policy. *Canadian Journal of Occupational Therapy, 57,* 32–38.

Keith, K. D., & Schalock, R. L. (2000). *Cross-cultural perspectives on quality of life.* Washington, DC: American Association on Mental Retardation.

Landesman, S. (1986). Quality of life and personal satisfaction: Definition and measurement issues. *Mental Retardation, 24,* 141–143.

Renwick, R., & Brown, I. (1996). The Centre for Health Promotion's approach to quality of life: Being, belonging, and becoming. In R. Renwick, I. Brown, & M. Nagler (Eds.), *Quality of life in health promotion and rehabilitation: Conceptual approaches, issues, and applications* (pp. 75–86). Thousand Oaks, CA: Sage.

Renwick, R., Brown, I., & Nagler, M. (Eds.). (1996). *Quality of life in health promotion and rehabilitation: Conceptual approaches, issues, and applications.* Thousand Oaks, CA: Sage.

Renwick, R., Brown, I., & Raphael, D. (1994). Quality of life: Linking a conceptual approach to service provision. *Journal on Developmental Disabilities, 3,* 32–44.

Renwick, R., Brown, I., & Raphael, D. (2000). Person-centred quality of life: Contributions from Canada to an international understanding. In K. D. Keith & R. L. Schalock (Eds.), *Cross-cultural perspectives on quality of life* (pp. 5–21). Washington, DC: American Association on Mental Retardation.

Renwick, R., Brown, I., Rootman, I., & Nagler, M. (1996). Conceptualization, research, and application: Future directions. In R. Renwick, I. Brown, & M. Nagler (Eds.), *Quality of life in health promotion and rehabilitation: Conceptual approaches, issues, and applications* (pp. 357–367). Thousand Oaks, CA: Sage.

Renwick, R., & Friefeld, S. (1996). Quality of life and rehabilitation. In R. Renwick, I. Brown, & M. Nagler (Eds.), *Quality of life in health promotion and rehabilitation: Conceptual approaches, issues, and applications* (pp. 26–36). Thousand Oaks, CA: Sage.

Schalock, R. L. (1990). *Quality of life: Perspectives and issues.* Washington, DC: American Association on Mental Retardation.

Schalock, R. L. (1996). Reconsidering the conceptualization and measurement of quality of life. In R. L. Schalock (Ed.), *Quality of life: Vol. I. Conceptualization and measurement* (pp. 123–139). Washington, DC: American Association on Mental Retardation.

Schalock, R. L. (1997a). Can the concept of quality of life make a difference? In R. L. Schalock (Ed.), *Quality of life: Vol. II. Applications to persons with disabilities* (pp. 245–267). Washington, DC: American Association on Mental Retardation.

Schalock, R. L. (Ed.). (1997b). *Quality of life: Vol. II. Applications to persons with disabilities.* Washington, DC: American Association on Mental Retardation.

Schalock, R. L., Keith, K., Hoffman, K., & Karan, O. (1989). Quality of life: Its measurement and use. *Mental Retardation, 27,* 25–31.

Townsend, E. (1993). Occupational therapy's social vision. *Canadian Journal of Occupational Therapy, 60,* 174–184.

Townsend, E., & Wilcock, A. (2004). Occupational justice. In C. Christiansen & E. Townsend (Eds.), *Introduction to occupation: The art and science of living* (pp. 243–273). Upper Saddle River, NJ: Prentice Hall.

Wicks, A. (2001). Occupational potential: A topic worthy of exploration. *Journal of Occupational Science, 8*(3), 32–35.

Wilcock, A. (1998). *An occupational perspective of health.* Thorofare, NJ: Slack.

Woodill, G., Renwick, R., Brown, I., & Raphael, D. (1994). Being, belonging, and becoming: An approach to quality of life of persons with developmental disabilities. In D. A. Goode (Ed.), *Quality of life for persons with disabilities: International perspectives and issues* (pp. 57–74). Cambridge, MA: Brookline.

World Health Organization. (1986). *Ottawa charter for health promotion.* Ottawa, ON: Canadian Public Health Association.

PART 2

Profile
of Needs

CHAPTER 3

Clinical Issues
Characterizing Adults With
Developmental Disabilities

Hollis A. Kellogg, OTR/L

Introduction

Paula is a 23-year-old who spends her day in a wheelchair. She keeps her hands and arms in a flexed position. She does not use her hands to reach, grasp, or hold any objects, including food. She is nonverbal and does not utilize any gestural or pictographic communication. When upset, she yells. She is thought to be cortically blind. She is totally dependent in all aspects of self-care, and records indicate she has been so since birth. Such an individual, and others not nearly so dependent, are the subjects of this chapter.

Individuals who have mental retardation make up 2.5%–3% of the population. Of this, 13% have IQs under 50 and serious limitations that require institutionalization or special care (Association for Retarded Citizens [ARC], 1982). Within this 13%, there is a still smaller percentage of individuals such as Paula. When compared to the entire mentally retarded/developmentally disabled (MR/DD) population, this is a small number of people. Many programs do not adequately serve their needs, and clinicians are not routinely taught about this population in baccalaureate-level programs. As states began to downsize large, overpopulated, and substandard institutions in the 1970s, the most dependent residents were often the last to be relocated. These people were described as a very difficult-to-serve population averaging 1,000 per state. Techniques for training them to leave the facilities had not been adequately developed (Stark, Baker, Menousek, & McGee, 1982), so the highest functioning residents were deinstitutionalized first.

In New York, this trend was seen in the state institutions. In 1977, 46% of the institutionalized residents were considered profoundly handicapped,

86% were toilet-trained, and 25% had behavioral disorders. By 1987, 62% were seen as profoundly impaired, and those with behavioral disorders and toilet dependency increased by 20% (Lakin, Hill, & Haydn, 1989). This was due primarily to the placement of the higher functioning residents into small group homes and day programs. To complete the closing down of the state facilities, some day programs had higher functioning consumers discharged from their facilities to make room for the most dependent consumers still awaiting placement. At present, New York has mostly completed this first phase, and some day programs have at present a large census of those considered the most dependent. The next trend might be the phasing out of day programs, causing elimination of or changes in clinical services to the participants.

As these cost-cutting trends swing in various directions, clinicians working with those who present the greatest challenges will need frames of reference, methods, and information resources.

It is difficult to take people with developmental disabilities as a whole and then to clearly separate those with the most-challenging deficits from the rest. Generally, these are people who are defined as profoundly retarded, with an IQ of 20 or less as determined by standard psychological tests such as the Vineland or Stanford Binet scales. Terms such as *profound, severe, moderate,* and *mild* are still used to describe degrees of retardation, just as the old terms *cretin, idiot, moron,* and *imbecile* were used until they became anathematized. Another classification system contains the terms *educable, trainable,* and *subtrainable.* The terms *educable* and *trainable* were adapted by the White House Conference on Children and Youth in 1930. The term *trainable* was a catch-all for the most dependent, and what then may have been known as *subtrainable* individuals were included. Programs for this group were almost nonexistent then (Dussault, 1989).

The American Association on Mental Retardation also no longer wishes to use the *mild* to *profound* labels, instead emphasizing strengths and weaknesses across four dimensions:

1. Intellectual/adaptive skills
2. Psychological/emotional considerations
3. Physical/health/etiological considerations
4. Environmental considerations.

These areas are assessed after administering a formal intelligence test. Then, levels of support are assigned four levels of intensity:

1. Intermittent
2. Limited
3. Extensive
4. Pervasive (ARC, 1996).

The subjects of this chapter could be described as those who generally require extensive to pervasive support across all four dimensions.

Etiology

The group of individuals marked by extreme dependency have etiologies similar to the general MR/DD population, such as Down syndrome, Fragile X syndrome, fetal alcohol syndrome, and low birthweight. However, these and other etiologies do not indicate accurately the degree of handicap an individual will demonstrate in later life. For example, a study showed that only 20% of very low-birthweight babies had significant handicaps, with the rest described as intellectually competitive (Stahlman et al., 1988). Children with retardation may be developmentally delayed at birth by genetic abnormalities or prenatal damage from alcohol or drugs. A child who is normal at birth may suffer postnatal neurological insult from ingesting toxins such as lead paint or suffer from head trauma, hydrocephalus, and various diseases that destroy or damage parts of the brain. Those born normally who experience significant central nervous system damage before age 21 may be classified as retarded. Those who suffer such damage after 21 are considered brain injured and generally will not be placed into the MR/DD system.

Other factors weigh significantly in degree of dependency. Some have dual diagnoses: developmental delay plus mental illness. Affective disorders are reported to occur in 3%–6% of the general MR/DD population, but rates are much higher for adults than for children younger than age 10 (Reiss, 1996). Adults with dual diagnoses who test in the severe or moderate range can exhibit behaviors that inhibit independent functioning, and this may subsequently place them in a profound level of function. Cerebral palsy, in its most severe quadriplegic forms, and other diseases that significantly affect motor function may seriously decrease the functional capacity of individuals and place them in the most dependent status. Because adults with mental retardation have been living longer, the incidence of age-related dementias and Alzheimer's disease has become more prevalent in this population. For example, virtually 100% of those with Down syndrome older than age 40 have significant Alzheimer's neuropathology (Haxby & Shapiro, 1992). Another secondary diagnosis is familial or environmental deprivation. When a child with retardation is raised in a dysfunctional family or in a barren environment within an institution, the initial handicaps that result may be amplified or compounded by adulthood.

Characteristics and Capabilities

In this population, deficits may be seen in all or nearly all areas but are *very* varied. Sensory functions may be intact, absent, or impaired or may indicate sensory integration problems. Motor function may or may not be impaired. Some may be fully ambulatory and even show good fine-motor skills. Others may ambulate with a stable if primitive gait, whereas others require assistance or a wheelchair. Fine-motor skills can range from being able to tie shoelaces, to gross grasping, to not using one's hands in any functional manner, even for feeding. Self-stimulatory and/or self-abusive behavior may be seen. Self-stimulation often is in the form of

- rocking, twirling, or head rolling (vestibular);
- string fixation or finger weaving (visual/tactile);
- sexual self-stimulation; or
- auditory self-stimulation in the form of vocalizations.

Self-abuse may be seen in the form of hitting the head with hands or on surfaces, grinding teeth (bruxism), picking skin, and biting hands or other body parts.

The individual may exhibit obsessive, sometimes sensory-related problems, such as disrobing; fecal smearing; tearing clothes; licking the floor and objects; flinging objects; eating paper, dirt, or other nonedibles; and many other, even more bizarre, behaviors that are difficult to analyze.

Communication is limited, with expressive capacity usually lagging far behind receptive ability. Some may be minimally verbal, use a few signs, or point to pictures or objects they want, whereas others will show preference only when food or stimuli are offered to them, and they accept or they refuse in the form of pushing away or becoming agitated.

History: The Effect of Long-Term Institutionalization

At the present time, many adults with severe developmental disabilities attend day programs and live in state-run or proprietary residences. Some of these adults still live with their families. Many day program attendees may have a long-term state institutional background.

Large-scale, long-term institutionalization of people with retardation has a troubled past. Through the first half of the 20th century, it was a common belief that people with retardation were hereditary aberrants and the defective results of "bad stock." In the manner of criminals, it was felt appropriate that they should be separated from society. This belief was particularly easy to maintain with the most dependent, such as someone who could not engage in basic self-care or effectively communicate, as opposed to an adult considered "feeble minded" (that is, someone who could perhaps help out in the grocery store on the corner). At that time, institutionalization was heavily used by poor families who had no resources to support their children with disabilities at home. In many states, large numbers of these individuals, born during the 1930s up to the beginning of the 1970s, were placed in state facilities that eventually housed several thousand. Some spent their childhood and much of their adulthood in such settings.

In New York, these settings deteriorated severely due to the withdrawal of funds during the 1960s, and it took a class-action lawsuit to begin reform. Willowbrook (the Staten Island Developmental Center, New York) was so bad that some residents who were relocated from it were placed under a "Willowbrook decree" and assigned public advocates. At one time in this facility, many residents huddled unclean, half-clothed or naked, in bare, filthy rooms and got the barest minimum of custodial care, with one staff member to 30 or 40 residents (Kihss, 1977). The Faribault state institution in Minnesota in the late 1960s was equally horrible. Other states had similar situations, and at one time an estimated 92,000 adults with retardation were living in comparable substandard conditions in the United States (Thompson, 1971).

The legacy of this kind of long-term neglect is that day programs at present have hundreds, perhaps thousands, of residents who were formerly in state institutions. Even though the number of survivors diminishes with each day, these people continued to be a presence through the year 2000. Of this population, those residents with severe and profound handicaps appear to have suffered the most. With impaired mobility or confinement to a wheelchair, with sensory impairments, with little or no capacity or opportunity to make needs and wants known, and with little more than a shoelace or scrap of paper to play with for year after year in a bleak ward, these individuals show the effects of neglect. I have observed that individuals with profound disabilities who lived for many years in underfunded institutions tend to show more deficits than similar individuals raised in home environments.

In 1954, a child named Eric was 2 1/2 years old. He was born with Down syndrome and showed profound developmental delay, and on the advice of a doctor his family placed him in a large state institution at that time. No early intervention services were easily available, whether through state, federal, or private sources. For 32 years, he lived in a limited, highly segregated environment in which funds for adequate supplies and staffing were gradually withdrawn. In 1986, the state instituted reforms, and he was moved to a small group home. In 1988, he was enrolled in a day program, and I met him for the first time. I found a 44-year-old man, ambulatory but with a minimal interest in his environment. His only interest was string, which he would dangle in front of his face and make "suckling" motions while he fondled it. Was this type of limited, repetitive, self-stimulatory behavior caused by a sensory-deprived childhood? What would have happened to Eric if, in his infancy, he was placed in a well-run, early intervention program? Answers to these questions are subject to discussion, but I suspect that Eric and others like him were affected in a very negative way by institutionalization and with better care would have matured with a significantly higher skill level.

Justification of Service and the Professional's Challenge

Why serve those who show a minimal level of independent purposeful function? I once met a professional who felt that individuals who function at the very lowest levels should simply be euthanized. For the slightly higher functioning, he felt most therapy was a waste of time. A therapist, however, is a practitioner of health who is concerned with maximizing and maintaining function. Regardless of whom a therapist is asked to treat, the therapist should have a commitment to maximizing each consumer's potential: assessing, finding a problem, and redressing the problem.

The problems related to deficits in self-care, work, and leisure areas are so numerous that a beginning therapist may be overwhelmed and not know where to begin. These problems are further magnified by public underfunding and apathy. The adult with developmental delay who cannot work even in a sheltered workshop, and who needs a great deal of support and supervision, is seen by the general public as a burden on society like other chronically disabled people. Most facilities for adults with retardation are remnants of old, underfunded state-run programs or Medicaid-supported county not-for-profit institutions or proprietary programs run on shoestring budgets. There are exceptions, in the form of well-financed private programs, but these are usually inaccessible to those of low income and are few in number. The therapist choosing to work with this population will more often than not find an underfunded program with underdiagnosed and underserved consumers, just as one would expect to find in agencies serving those with a chronic mental illness and impoverished. These facts alone justify intervention with this population, in which well-trained and dedicated professionals probably always will be in very short supply.

In the facility where I work, I am required to cover the needs of over 200 adults in three different day programs. This type of caseload forces ethical decisions on the therapist. An adult who is able to speak in simple sentences, work independently on simple tasks, and make simple decisions is a far better candidate for a variety of therapy interventions than a nonverbal adult who shows poor adaptive skills and limited receptivity to verbal and physical prompts. In making such a choice, a therapist has to weigh different factors and develop a priority system. The main questions will be, What resources do I have and, given these resources, with whom can I accomplish the most?

Resource Questions

1. *Equipment:* Do I have what I need? If I want vestibular stimulation, do I have a swing, rocking chair, or similar device?
2. *Environment:* Is the consumer's present environment conducive to my therapy goals? Do I need space, quiet, and accessibility?

3. *Time:* Can I accomplish my goals in a reasonable amount of time? Will a specialized sensory program, designed to change a consumer's behavior, produce results that will be worth the time invested?

4. *Assistance:* If I am an OTR, do I have a COTA or therapy aide capable of understanding and carrying out my therapeutic ideas? If I am a COTA, does my supervising OTR support my ideas and give me a caseload I can realistically handle? Do other clinicians (physical therapist, speech therapist, registered nurse, psychologist) support or agree with my therapy ideas?

5. *Carryover of therapy by nonprofessionals:* How much of what I hope to accomplish is dependent on nonclinical staff?

The last question is of particular concern. An OTR's interventions with this population often depend on staff showing understanding and following recommendations. Most adult day programs have a job description for direct-care staff, and one of the basic job duties is to "follow clinical staff's recommendations." As many clinicians who have worked in this field will report, compliance can be far below average. Many direct-care staff I have encountered have no college or specialized education related to MR/DD and leave the field in a year or less. Some agencies experience a turnover rate of 50%–100% within a year (Gardner & Chapman, 1985). Some direct-care staff members have attitudes detrimental to any kind of therapeutic relationship: "He doesn't need therapy—he is just lazy," "clinicians make big bucks—we don't need them," or "clinical recommendations are unimportant and a nuisance—we won't bother to follow them." I have encountered direct-care staff and even program administrators with these kinds of attitudes, and getting therapy carried over with such people in charge is nearly impossible. However, most agencies may have as many people who support the clinician's ideas and therapy programs. The therapist must not give up hope.

In summary, the therapist serving the needs of those with profound disabilities will need to

- Obtain a physician's referral
- Establish the consumer's functional needs
- Prioritize who will be treated
- Identify resources available such as equipment, professional assistance, environment, staff support, and time.

Functional Category Guidelines for Treatment Intervention

To assist the therapist in developing appropriate programs and expectations, some classification of those with profound disabilities is useful. Some have argued against this, stating that

advocates for persons with profound retardation are often caught in the classic bind of simultaneously articulating the deficits or differences that characterize this particular group of individuals. . . . [T]he standards, expectations, and criteria that have emerged in the field for persons who are "moderately" and "severely" handicapped apply perhaps equally to those who are the most profoundly disabled. (Evans & Scotti, 1989, p. 84).

This reasoning is laudable on the point of preventing overly negative expectations, but if different criteria are used for different categories in a careful and methodical manner with full consideration that one may move from one category to another, then this labeling will be helpful rather than harmful.

Knowledgeable and informed professionals will be aware of normalization needs and will not segregate or neglect people just because they fall into a category. The following is a simple protocol that will help to organize the deficits and develop appropriate methods of intervention.

Categorization Guidelines for the Most Dependent

Category I

1. The consumer is nonverbal and does not use signs or point to picture symbols.
2. All movements of the body are limited. The individual usually is severely physically handicapped but, if not, will only show limited movement.
3. Little or no interest in or interaction with the surrounding environment is shown. The individual will not reach, grasp, hold, or manipulate most objects. They may insert their hand in their mouth, chew on clothing, or make other repetitive or stereotypic movements but generally will not respond to external stimuli. If responses are made, they are "short chain" in nature, such as a startle reflex or withdrawal response, and do not lead to learning or adaptive patterns.
4. The individual may show little or no visual regarding. Looking at faces or objects may be very transitory if seen at all. Those who do show some ocular motor function or sustained gaze will not use this function to obtain objects.
5. The individual usually will not feed himself or herself.
6. The individual usually will be incontinent of bowel and bladder.

These individuals usually have significant differences from the profoundly handicapped population as a whole, but they are often grouped with others without regard for their special status. Some of the words used to describe states of awareness after a head injury form an interesting description with which Category I individuals correlate. For example, *stupor* indicates spontaneous movement and groaning in response to various stimuli. This term is not used with the MR/DD population but may depict the functional level often seen in Category I. Category I individuals make up a very small number of those with developmental disabilities. In a day program setting where I have worked, five people qualified out of a census of 80. In another setting I counted approximately 10 out of a population of 130. Different states and different institutions will vary in the number of these individuals placed in one setting.

Category II

Individuals in Category II show some awareness of and interaction with the environment. They may look at faces or objects and reach for them. They may hold objects and manipulate them. They may have some primitive but consistent means of communication. They will show some connection with the world around them, unlike the client in Category I, who appears to be interested only in his or her own body. Even if their interactions with the environment are primitive and repetitive, there are observable connections that are not seen with the Category I client. These individuals may have their cognitive deficit compounded by problems in one or more of the following areas: mobility, perception, and behavior. Because of their great diversity, the client in Category II is hard to separate from others of higher function. Some may have splinter skills, such as self-feeding and toileting, but may be extremely dependent in nearly all other areas. Two elements stand out to distinguish them from others less dependent:

1. An apparent lack of or use of long-term memory
2. Initiation of purposeful activities.

The majority of those who attend day programs often present the characteristics of Category II.

A point of reference: Category I individuals correspond to the lowest segment of the profoundly retarded population, with IQs of 10 or much less. Those in Category II may also be classified as profound (with IQs of 20 or less) but may also test within the severe range (20–35). Those who test in the upper severe and moderate ranges (approximately 30–36) and who are functioning within average expectations for this range are not seen as qualifying as subjects of this chapter.

Category III

Category III people have mobility and communication impairments that are so severe that they are totally dependent in nearly all domains. However, they have cognitive capacities that are significantly higher than their physical capacities. If they did not have these physical restrictions, they might conceivably be working in a sheltered workshop and showing independence in activities of daily living (ADL) routines.

An example is Ronald, a 43-year-old man who tests in the severe IQ range and might score in the moderate range if his motor abilities were not so impaired. He has spastic quadriplegic cerebral palsy and is confined to a wheelchair that he cannot self-propel. His only intact functional movement is in his head, face, and left hand. He is able to feed himself with a universal cuff and other adaptations. He is nonverbal but can draw attention by yelling and is able to point to a wide variety of pictures with good accuracy. His memory for people and day-to-day events is good. His attention span is also good in comparison to his peers, and he is cooperative and friendly. Such a person is a good candidate for occupational therapy but also can present great challenges. In my experience, this type of day program attendee is rare. In 8 years, I have encountered only 3 or 4 people who fit this description.

In some facilities, such people may be grouped together so a teacher or therapist can maximize their potentials with assistive technology, such as computers and environmental control devices. Unfortunately, many day programs or group homes do not have the budgets to provide such expensive items or to hire clinicians skilled in their use. There also may be little incentive to spend a lot of scarce funds on just one or two individuals. Some individuals are given expensive and sophisticated communication and mobility equipment in their school-age years, which may not be used later on when they enter a day program. If the equipment needs repair, modification, or replacement, funding that was available when they were of school age may be unavailable now that they are adults. Often this equipment requires assistance and encouragement from others for the consumer to use. Some direct-care staff may be unfamiliar with the function or importance of the device and will not use it, causing it to be virtually abandoned. Assistive technology does not always guarantee a consumer significantly more function. Without these devices, extra staff support, and specially adapted activities, a Category III individual may be grouped with the most dependent, just because he or she cannot physically work on the tasks that others in higher functioning groups can.

A person can drift between Category I and Category II status, and conceivably a Category III person may decline in function and qualify as being in Category II or I. If a person considered Category I shows a Category II action, then that action should be encouraged and promoted. The purpose of the categories is simple: to have a frame of reference from which to build interventions. Not everyone who is classified as being in one of the above categories will necessarily stay there for the duration of his or her life, but the characteristics of one category will often predominate.

Assessment and Choosing Areas of Intervention

Assessment of adults with severe and profound handicapping conditions is difficult. Traditional means of evaluation are often inappropriate. The primary focus when working with people with profound disabilities is, *What does the individual initiate?* Those in Category I may initiate only a limited repertoire of movements. Those in Category II may initiate little more than feeding and stereotypic behaviors. This means that the therapist must have excellent observational skills and an open mind with which to interpret what seem to be meaningless and aimless behaviors. Some common characteristics to watch for are

- A receptive capacity or an ability to follow simple directions that is far greater than expressive capacity
- Odd behaviors that may be related to sensory-processing abnormalities
- Significant challenges associated with the initiation of purposeful or adaptive actions.

In behavioral terms, the last characteristic mentioned above would indicate a lack of operant behavior in the environment.

Each individual, even someone who is extremely dependent, tends to show some kind of distinctive pattern of response and arousal to stimuli. These patterns should be considered when making assessments of ability to perform a purposeful action. Although it seems the functional capacity of these individuals can be determined relatively quickly, the therapist must be wary of making judgments based on too few observations made in only one or two environments. The consumer may not exhibit specific abilities to some examiners or will show certain actions or behaviors only in certain environments. I recall a case of an adult care worker who tried unsuccessfully for several years to get one of the adults in her care to write his name. He would make a few letters only poorly. Then one day, when he did not know she was looking, he wrote his full name legibly. Another man presented himself to me as nonverbal and would not utter a sound in all of our interactions. However, with others, he would speak in sentences. These types of circumstances may often be seen with individuals with autism, who may demonstrate a splinter skill in an unpredictable manner. Another typical situation often encountered is when the parent or house caregiver states, after hearing about how the individual behaves in a day program, "Bobby never shows that behavior with us." In view of this, the therapist must interview different staff and observe the individual in as many different environments as possible to get the most accurate information.

Establishing Priorities in Providing Therapeutic Interventions in a Day Program

The following is an example of a typical day program classroom.

The classroom is a 25' × 12' room with one entrance; a wall with some windows; and a few old battered metal cabinets, tables, and chairs. Two training specialists are assigned to a group of six consumers. The two staff members have little with which to work. Their cabinets are mostly filled with bibs, diapers, and economy foodstuffs. They have an odd mixture of program materials: children's toys, a Mr. Potato Head™, preschool puzzles with missing pieces, pegboards, and many homemade items. There is a dirty cardboard box with empty bent-up soda cans, parts of broken toys brought in from home, shoe boxes of clothespins, straws, beads and Popsicle™ sticks, old clothing, stuffed toys, plastic Easter eggs, and piles of ragged women's magazines. The training specialists are young with little knowledge of developmental or physical disabilities. They also have limited knowledge of the needs or past histories of their clients. They are given a brief introduction to the people to whom they are assigned and then are expected to supervise and provide a goal-based program for nearly 4 or 5 hours, 5 days a week. In classrooms for the most dependent, a great deal of time is spent toileting. Because toileting and changing some individuals may take over 20 minutes, often six or more clients are supervised by only one training specialist. Because the program budget will not allow the hiring of enough direct-care staff and because of high staff turnover and absentee rates, clinicians and program administrators frequently need to spend time in the classroom to provide coverage.

This particular classroom contains six individuals, all conforming to Category I–III criteria. The characteristics of all these individuals are closely based on real people with whom I have worked.

- *Ray,* a 42-year-old man with tubular sclerosis, is hyperactive. He runs about the room, grabbing any object he sees, and quickly flings it when it no longer interests him. The staff have resorted to hiding most all materials to prevent them from being flung, broken, or accidentally striking another person.

- *Nate* is a 38-year-old man who has severe spastic quadriplegia. He is positioned in a wheelchair that he does not self-propel, is nonverbal, and has severe visual impairments. When taken out of his chair, he assumes a fetal position. He has contractures in various joints and does not use his arms to reach for any nonedible objects placed within his reach. He is often constipated and may "dig" himself, necessitating a major cleanup operation.

- *Mildred* is 56 years old and blind. She will not work on any table-top activities but sits rocking, singing to herself, and chewing on her shirt. Occasionally, after she is tired of sitting, she will stand and fling over her chair.

- *Richard* is a 42-year-old man with right hemiparesis. He is fully ambulatory and has good use of his left arm and hand. He has lived at home all of his life and has been fed, dressed, and toileted by his mother. He will not eat in the day program and will not use the toilet, having adjusted himself to only doing those things at home. He does not engage in any purposeful task in the day program, preferring to wander, to sit in a rocking chair, and occasionally to have a tantrum when he is bothered by certain noises or redirected.

- *Margret* is a 34-year-old with a severe self-abusive problem. On a daily basis, she will strike her head with her hands or bang it on hard surfaces, sometimes causing bleeding. It may take two or more staff to stop her from self-abusing. At other times she will be calm and may fall asleep.
- *Joseph* is a 41-year-old man with spastic quadriplegia and is positioned in a wheelchair that he cannot self-propel, like Nate. Unlike Nate, he shows good awareness of people and objects. He is non-verbal but can gesture and point to some picture symbols with accuracy. He is very mobility impaired and feeds himself with difficulty, using adapted devices. He is friendly and recognizes favorite staff, greeting them with a yell.

The six disparate people making up this classroom present a therapist with multiple problems:

- Which of the six should be treated with a formal therapy program?
- Who should be treated first?
- What types of therapeutic interventions should be used?

The occupational therapist with a background in holistic thinking should have many questions with which to deal.

To begin, I gathered all the known information I could on each individual: the past history, past therapies if any, diagnoses and, as available, descriptions of the family or institutional environments in which he or she had lived since birth. My clinical decisions were as follows.

Ray

Ray was treated first. His grabbing and flinging behavior was disrupting the entire classroom, making it very difficult for staff to use materials or give any attention to others in the room. First, I observed Ray in the day program environment. I considered him a Category II. He would not sit for much more than a few seconds, despite concerted efforts to train him. He would run about the room, grabbing all manner of objects, observe them, shake them briefly, and then fling them. Often he would return to the flung object and pick it up, only to quickly fling it again. He would be extremely restless and forage about obsessively, damaging property and sometimes knocking people over to get something. I provided the classroom with a large, brightly colored box in which I put a number of interesting objects and worked one-on-one with Ray for several weeks. He was allowed to choose whatever he wanted out of the box, but if he flung it, he had to pick it up and put it back in the box. This was partially successful. Then, I observed that some objects seemed to interest him longer than others. A large rubber spider was particularly interesting to him, giving him visual stimulation to which he did not quickly habituate. Eventually I made him a spiderlike object: a sturdy plastic ring with short lengths of rope attached. This became his object and held his attention

through most of a program day. His foraging and destructive behavior greatly decreased. I also felt it was important for a hyperactive and restless person
like Ray to get outside his room, so I took him outside and around the building for walks. This provided him with significant amounts of proprioceptive,
visual, auditory, and other stimulation, and he did not need his object when
on the walks. The fact that he did not need this "stimulator" on these walks
indicated that the classroom space provided inadequate movement and stimulation. The walking activity also provided me with opportunities to work with
him on simple ADL routines, like putting on and taking off his coat.

Nate

Nate was not as high a priority as Ray. He did, however, require some intervention. He was seen as possibly falling into a Category I status, largely
because of his severe limits in mobility. His marginal self-feeding needed some
monitoring of his adaptive equipment, which consisted of a high side dish and
a spoon in a universal cuff. He needed sensory stimulation because he could
not explore or reach for objects. A range-of-motion maintenance program was
developed by the occupational and physical therapy departments. His staff
was instructed in techniques for (a) providing guided movement (described
later), (b) maintaining his self-feeding, and (c) providing adequate sensory
stimulation. His digging problem—not uncommon with those who are constipated and incontinent of bowel and bladder—was monitored by staff and
addressed by providing movement and keeping a regular changing schedule.

Mildred

Mildred required intervention to address her chair-flinging behavior, which
had a high potential for injuring others. A chair with a heavy base fixed to
the legs was fabricated by a COTA, and use of this prevented her from toss-
ing it. By why did she do this? Perhaps she needed to walk. Perhaps she felt
unable to walk by herself because of blindness. She did not show the requi-
site skills to learn cane use or blind mobility techniques like trailing. In her
attempts to walk she would often get up and bump into something before
staff members could get to her. Staff members were often unable to leave the
room to walk with her, because they had to supervise the others. Intervention
in a case like this might involve putting her into a sensory environment
designed so she could not hurt herself but in which she could explore freely.
If this were not possible, arrangements could be made to give her walks and
multisensory experiences suited to her needs.

Richard

Richard was seen as having a number of problems, including sensory integration deficits. He showed hypersensitivity to noise. He was dependent in

basic self-care skills. He was self-abusive and aggressive toward others at times. He was nonproductive, even though he showed some potential for following simple instructions. A program to get him to feed and toilet himself was very difficult, because his mother was unable to relinquish her role as a mother of a dependent son, whom she continued to spoon-feed. In her 80s and partially deaf, she was difficult to counsel on Richard's need to be more independent. She also would not cooperate in administering behavior medication to him, and he would not easily take medication from anyone except her. It naturally fell to the occupational therapy department to intervene. In this case, an intuitive COTA who had known and worked with him for years was the impetus for positive changes. She went to a conference given by Patricia Wilbarger on sensory defensive behavior and how it can be treated with a tactile stimulation program. This program involved vigorous brushing with a soft plastic brush over arms, legs, and back. Richard tolerated this program well and appeared to show some improvement in behavior. This treatment alone was not sufficient; he needed to be trained in purposeful activities. It was known that he immensely enjoyed walking despite a hemiparetic leg. In the past, staff would let him wander about the building. This was structured into something more purposeful. He would stay in a classroom part of the day, and the COTA would come to get him and set him up with some simple tasks like carrying bags of clothes to other classrooms and helping to push wheelchair-bound consumers around the day program. Gradually, his self-abusive and aggressive behavior decreased.

Margret

Margret showed a severe self-abusive problem. In her case, it appeared that the primary reason for her behavior was a craving for specific stimuli. After consulting with a therapist who had worked with her in the past, it was found she craved vestibular stimulation in the form of spinning. A large, pediatric floor saucer was found, and fortunately this woman was small and could fit into it. All self-abusive behavior ceased immediately when she experienced gentle spinning, and the effect would sometimes last for hours after a session.

Joseph

Joseph fit into Category III. He had certain capacities but was so physically impaired that he could do very little. His mother and brother felt that he could "do nothing" for himself. After evaluation, it was found that he was able to do certain things with adaptive devices. He could feed himself with adaptive equipment. He could press switches to turn on a radio, fan, or battery-operated toy. He remembered people and objects, could follow simple instructions, and could point to pictures. With these capacities, the therapist could facilitate some independence.

Summary

The six individuals just described illustrate the three categories of those with profound challenges and suggest certain methods of intervention. Also, the need to prioritize problems is demonstrated. These individuals were co-existing together in a confining space, and the actions of one individual could affect all the others. For example, treating Ray first was important, because his behavior would have undermined interventions that the therapist would attempt to do with others.

Key Treatment Considerations

Positioning

Positioning problems are most frequently seen with Category I and Category III consumers. Kyphosis and scoliosis of the spine may keep them in a poor posture. Hemiplegia may cause lateral leaning and other problems. Those who sit for long periods and who are unable to shift weight are at risk for decubitus ulcers. When intervening with such problems, the therapist should know as much as possible about the individual's specific orthopedic pathology. Often the individual has already been placed in some kind of customized wheelchair or seating arrangement. Over time, this seating system may need modification. The therapist needs to get a full workup of the diagnosis and any past interventions that have already been done or attempted. Then the therapist must examine the individual in his or her environment. Is the positioning problem affecting eating, working on tasks, or mobility? For example, one very dependent consumer who needed to be spoon-fed had a tendency to extend his head while eating. This head position created a higher risk for aspiration, so a head rest was installed. Another consumer was partially ambulatory and used a regular armchair to sit in, but he tended to lean significantly to one side. A small, firm, rectangular cushion was custom-made to support him in a more upright posture on that side.

A very common problem is table height and dangling feet. Many clients are of short stature (some under 5 ft. tall), and standard tables and chairs are not appropriate. Firm cushions can raise individuals up in their seat. Getting their elbows to rest on the table in 90 degrees of flexion is ideal but may be unrealistic, and another position that increases function is often acceptable. Feet should be supported. A foot box can be made to the correct height so feet can rest comfortably. Some may wish to attach the footrest to the chair so its use will be guaranteed, but if the individual transfers independently, he or she must be able to do so without tripping on the rest.

Some consumers (mostly Category I status) may have what is known as a "tilt-in-space" wheelchair. This is a large, complex chair that enables the entire seating component of the chair to tilt back within the frame; it differs from a reclining back wheelchair, where only the back of the chair tilts. The tilt-in-space chair is used for people with severe mobility impairment who need to be in an upright posture but also need pressure taken off of the coccyx and ischial areas. Pressure relief is gained by placing them in at least 45 degrees of tilt for part of the day.

Positioning those with severe orthopedic problems is a science in itself. Unless a therapist is particularly knowledgeable, he or she could do more harm than good when attempting significant interventions. It is best to consult with experts. If a whole new seating system is being planned, then the therapist needs to work with the physical therapist, orthopedist, wheelchair vendor, and other significant professionals. In this team approach, the OTR may need to speak up on certain issues related to occupational therapy practice. For example, a physical therapist may recommend that a consumer be placed in a fully reclining position due to hip contractures. The OTR, in turn, might indicate the significant perceptual problems such an individual might experience when placed in that position.

Positioning adults who have been accustomed to abnormal postures most of their lives is difficult. They may have developed habits of walking, sitting, or lying that are comfortable or acceptable to them, and interventions at this stage may be uncomfortable or unacceptable because they are simply different. One man with whom I worked had a leg-length discrepancy and hip and back deformities. He could work on simple tabletop tasks, but he preferred to stand and lean on a table to work. I experimented with cushions that put him in a very functional seated position. Because he was verbal, I asked him if he was comfortable, and he said he was. However, he removed all of the cushions after I left and went back to his old pattern of standing and leaning. The therapist must be aware of the pitfalls of intervening in such positioning problems and proceed carefully before spending lots of money or time.

To summarize, the therapist working with positioning must
1. Have a good knowledge of the consumer's positioning history, diagnosis, and any pertinent pathologies
2. Assess needs as related to respiration, eating, swallowing, task function, stress on joints, functional vision, and safety
3. Consult as needed with others
4. Experiment before ordering or making expensive alterations
5. Be sensitive of how the positioning device will fit into the consumer's lifestyle and be accepted or tolerated by him or her.

Suggested Treatment Interventions to Teach to Staff and Use as Formal Therapy

Guided Movement

Guided movement as described here is not a special technique and may resemble other methods with the same or with more complex names. It is simply a means to give movement to the consumer who initiates minimal movement. Most importantly, it is meant as a technique that the therapist can teach to direct-care staff. The Category I consumer is most frequently suited to this type of intervention, but some Category II consumers may benefit also. The consumer would usually be in a wheelchair. He or she would tend to keep the limbs in one position, often making some limited, repetitive, self-stimulatory movements. He or she may or may not have contractures.

To guide movement, the staff members would first let the person know that they are going to move his or her arms or legs. This is especially important if the person startles easily and should be done regardless of whether the consumer understands what is being said. The staff may say, "I am going to move your arm up so your hand can touch your head." Staff then gently guide the person's arm in that direction. If the person begins to pull away, the staff member goes with the consumer's movement. The staff should not try to move the limbs in directions in which the consumer resists moving, or cannot move, due to range-of-motion limits. Instead, the staff should attempt to guide the limbs to move in ways they might move if the consumer showed more cortical control and motivation to do so.

Some Category I consumers will favor a fetal-like position with flexed arms. Gradually, they may develop contractures and lose range, first in shoulder flexion and then elbow and wrist extension. Although it may slow this loss, guided movement is not passive range of motion (PROM). If PROM is recommended by the occupational or physical therapist, the therapist treats the consumer. Guiding or encouraging movement, however, is not the specific stretching of soft tissues with outside forces. It can be done by nonclinical staff. Some therapists may feel it is risky to train nonprofessionals to do this. However, direct-care staff members make the consumers go through such movements anyway (when they dress, toilet, and transfer them). Some staff also need this training to feel less inhibited about touching the people to whom they are assigned. Furthermore, one therapist cannot go about a program with 100 consumers and do all the therapeutic handling that is required.

The seven basic tenets of guided movements are as follows:

1. They are not performed to passively stretch joints to maintain ROM but to give proprioceptive and tactile stimulation, as well as to maintain a consumer's sense of his or her own body.

2. They can be taught to direct-care staff. The therapist makes the judgment as to the capability of the staff members to learn the technique with a specific consumer and then trains them with the consumer.

3. The staff goes with the self-initiated movements of the consumer and gently guides the movements and expands on them. For example, a consumer fixates on twirling the hair on the left side of her

head. The staff encourages and guides the consumer's hand to her ear or other body parts.

4. All movements are slow and gentle. If the consumer pulls in a direction opposite to the staff, the staff goes in that direction. The staff stops the procedure if the consumer becomes agitated or too resistive.

5. Guided movement should be a part of the Category I consumer's daily multisensory experiences.

6. Staff performing this procedure are regularly monitored by a clinician.

7. They are often used with Category I consumers and sometimes with Category II consumers who show limited volitional movement.

Assisted Function

Unlike Category I consumers, many Category II consumers are reaching, grasping, and moving their limbs in purposeful ways. However, many have difficulty completing most actions successfully. For example, they may grasp a spoon but are unable to use it to feed themselves. When someone uses a hand to guide/prompt a consumer's movement during eating or other functional tasks, the desired movement is being *assisted*. This method can be used for all activities involving reaching, grasping, holding, and placing. If consumers show some improvement in completing an action by themselves, then the hand-over-hand assistance can be phased out. This should proceed from distal to proximal, first to hand, then to wrist, and finally to forearm. This basic method has been used for a long time with children and adults and has been detailed by Whitman (Whitman, Scibak, & Reid, 1983) and others, but it is amazing how few staff who work with this population apply it.

Category II consumers are usually able to understand some verbal instruction. Verbal prompts alone should be used first before immediately providing assisted function, to check if the consumer needs the physical help. To encourage independence, it is good practice for all staff at home as well as at day programs to use assisted function techniques on a regular basis. Assisted function should not be confused with facilitated communication. The latter was a controversial technique used to assist nonverbal people in communication by providing support to the dominant hand/wrist/arm so that letters could be typed in sequence and, in turn, words could be spelled.

Assisted Function Is Not Used If the Consumer Consistently
Does Not Maintain Grasp on Varied Objects

Consider the following example: A client uses his hands to grasp string to self-stimulate and uses his hands to scratch himself or to suck on fingers. He will consistently not grasp any object, even if it is placed in his hands. However, staff members attempt to hold his hand around a pencil or paintbrush so as to artificially make lines or patterns that he is exerting no effort himself to make. In addition, he shows no awareness of the action or inaction of his limbs in this or other tasks. After evaluation and careful review of the client's history, a determination can be made that it serves no purpose to use assisted function. Such an individual is in a Category I status and should receive guided movement as opposed to assisted function.

Basic Tenets of Assisted Function Techniques

1. They are used with clients who will consistently grasp and hold a variety of objects and who show some awareness of and appropriate response to the external environment.
2. Hand-over-hand assistance should be phased out proximal to distal.
3. They can be used at times with Category I clients as an experiment, but therapists should counsel staff if they feel guided movement is more appropriate.
4. Verbal prompts should be used first. If there is no or inadequate response, the same verbal prompts should be used with the assisted function.

Other Activities

Dressing, grooming, toileting, eating, and other ADLs seem to be the first areas to address in this population. The therapist, however, should expect to see little significant progress in the development of new skills. Often the individual has had a lot of self-care training in childhood and, if not, there may be important behavioral/cognitive reasons.

Nonetheless, an assessment of the client's present skills and a concerted effort to preserve these skills should be made. For example, direct-care staff often need frequent reminders not to give full assistance. A 45-year-old man may not be able to signal his need to go to the bathroom and may wear an adult protective garment. With prompts, he will undress and assist in changing himself. A 32-year-old woman will bring a spoonful of food to her mouth but does not scoop the food herself. In both cases, the therapist should make sure the staff is letting the client do as much of the task as possible. Sometimes an assistive device will help. Assistive devices for eating, such as high-sided dishes; covered, spouted cups; and built-up utensil handles are often helpful in reducing spillage. Assistive dressing devices, such as long-handled shoehorns, sock aides, and dressing sticks are much more difficult to use with this population. Simpler dressing adaptations that require little or no training are more appropriate. A roller brush that will brush one's hair no matter how the handle is held is much better than a comb or a one-sided brush. Velcro®-tie shoes or elastic shoelaces that transform a tie shoe into a slip-on shoe are preferable as long as they provide support. I have seen many individuals who would have been independent in donning shoes if staff had used a substitute for laces.

Use of Toys and Switches

Toys

The use of toys with this population is controversial because of the need to provide age-appropriate activities. Although a therapist would be unlikely to give a client an item that is obviously a child's toy, such items often find their way into day programs. Some clients also may be oriented to certain items that would be considered toys. Often the item may not function as a true toy to a client but rather as something that provides sensory stimulation. For example, a client may hold a doll and pick at the hair or buttons on it, getting tactile stimulation or visual stimulation while shaking it. The direct-care staff is not always aware of the relationship an individual has with an object. Because the clients appear childlike to them, it may seem natural to give them children's toys. The staff may be unaware that the individual does not have representational thought: an ability to engage in make-believe that is usually seen emerging in normal children at about age 4 years. The sensory value of an object should be considered. A ball and a stuffed animal both provide sensory stimulation, but the ball will move more freely when pushed. Different objects need to be introduced to someone so he or she has a choice. Some adults may seek out a doll or stuffed toy over a more age-appropriate item, but they should not then be given only those items. Battery-operated toys such as cars or animal figures could be used, but only if the consumer shows some sustained eye contact or response. Ideally, such toys should be hooked up to a switch so that the individual can operate them independently. It is often a judgment call as to whether a toy is appropriate for an adult. Obvious infant items such as rattles and teething rings should be avoided.

Some items can be adapted. In the aforementioned case of Ray, a ring with strings attached was a less childlike object than a toy spider. Another caveat is to prevent toys from becoming a fixation, like a security blanket, from which a person cannot separate. Also, there is a choking risk with small items when used with clients who mouth items, as well as hygienic concerns.

Switches

Therapists and staff often get excited over the possibilities of switches but may be unaware of their limitations. It is easy to buy or make battery interrupter switches that will activate things when touched. The first problem that arises is, Will the client use it? The Category I client probably will not. He or she does not show a sense of cause and effect and usually is unaware of how his or her actions change the environment. A motion switch, however, may be useful to break stereotypic behavior in a Category I individual. For example, a man always inserts his hand in his mouth. A motion switch is attached to his wrist, and when he lifts his hand to his mouth, it activates a diversionary stimulus such as a vibrator. This may not always work, because the person can habituate quickly to the diversionary stimulus.

Switches may be useful with the Category II individual, but results also will vary considerably. The variance of the stimulus may be important. Such people may "outwit" the purpose of the switch. One Category II individual simply laid an object on a switch so it would continue to activate a music-producing computer while he walked away from it. This is good problem-solving training, but the therapist will need to make such a system more sophisticated and adaptable if he or she wants further purposeful interaction.

With Category III individuals, switches are often the most useful. These people are aware of their actions on the environment and desperately need some method to gain whatever independent control can be given to them. The therapist will need to find the right activity, then adapt and position it so it can be used independently.

What can a switch activate? Some suggestions and problems:

- A battery-operated toy can easily be hooked up to a switch. The result is usually only a limited amount of repetitive visual and auditory stimulation. These items are often fragile and break easily.
- Radios and tape players make a good choice if the consumer responds to music and voices, and these can be varied. The consumer will probably need to tolerate headphones, if he or she is in a classroom, so that others will not be disturbed.
- Lights are a limited stimulus but may be set up in such a way so that they can be varied.
- Fans, again, are a limited stimulus and somewhat difficult to find in a battery-operated form that is safe, but this has possibilities for some individuals.
- Computers can also be operated by simple switches and may be a valuable communication device. They are expensive, and the therapist needs access to and knowledge of software and keyboard adaptations.

Self-Abuse and Self-Stimulation: Treatment Considerations

It is hypothesized that adults with severe and profound retardation who engage in self-injurious behavior (SIB) and stereotypic self-stimulation do so because they lack stimulation from their environment. If the appropriate amount of stimulation is provided, including positive social interaction, then the SIB is expected to decrease or stop. In more sensory-integrative–based theories, the person's internal thresholds for experiencing stimuli may be abnormally high or low. Then, the problem is seen as more neurological, but the result may be the same: The individual engages in SIB or self-stimulation to compensate. Both of these perspectives must be put into the context of the specific individual and not vice versa. There is no simple formula for dealing with such behavior. For intervention, each person will need a custom-tailored program.

This subject covers a large area and is presented here in an introductory manner. Readers are urged to research the literature and consult with psychologists and behavioral specialists. Nonetheless, it is important to note the distinctions between SIB and self-stimulatory or stereotyped behavior.

SIB

SIB is an action that is self-inflicted and causes physical harm. It may be done as a form of temper tantrum, a response to redirection, or an act of frustration. It also may be done in response to internal pain or an outside stimulus such as noise. SIB also may be done as a means to provide neurological stimulation (Belfore & Dattilio, 1990).

SIB causes some kind of lasting damage such as a bruise, laceration, or other more serious injury. A common form is head banging: The person strikes his or her head against a hard surface or slaps or strikes it with hands or fists. People with chronic problems like this are often seen wearing helmets and receiving contingency/reinforcement programs set up by a psychologist. Hand or arm biting may also be seen. Sometimes the skin is broken and blood is drawn; sometimes only calluses are produced. Skin picking, usually on arms, hands, or face, may be seen. This can produce a small, mildly callused or reddened area, or a large area of scar tissue. Hair or fingernails may be pulled out.

Finding a specific etiology for SIB is difficult. Although aspects of this behavior demonstrate that it is very likely the result of learning processes, biological causes are implicated as well (Cataldo, 1988). In regard to psychiatric causes, a study of SIB in 251 severely and profoundly retarded individuals found no specific psychiatric disease associated with the behaviors (King, 1995).

Chronic SIB, especially in its more serious forms, attracts attention. If manifested in childhood, there usually has been some attempt to treat it. The therapist makes note of this, and it is significant if the behavior is of more recent origin. More commonly, the person is profoundly disabled, noncommunicative, and has a history of SIB, usually of a specific nature. In an attempt to analyze a person's SIB, one must look first to an internal pain, such as a toothache, headache, or ear problem (e.g., otis media). If pain is ruled out, then one must look to environmental causes. Is the person bothered by stimuli in the environment? Does the person engage in SIB only when certain stimuli are present? For example, one nonverbal man would bite his hand only when objects dropped on the floor or when someone turned on a faucet. SIB also is often a form of tantrum exhibited only when the person is redirected or frustrated.

SIB is sometimes the individual's only means of communication. Some have learned to use SIB as a means of communicating that they want attention or to gain something. One woman learned that by pulling off hangnails and causing bleeding, she could get to go to the nurse's office and get a Band-Aid™, on which she fixated. These reasons for SIB are usually easy to identify when consistently seen and may be remediated with behavioral approaches, environmental changes, and/or sensory methods.

Self-Stimulatory Behavior

Self-stimulatory or stereotypic behavior differs from SIB in that it does not usually cause damage to the person. One of the most common examples is rocking while seated or standing. People may also engage in twirling or spinning around. They may make repetitive arm or hand movements, such as shaking or flapping a hand in front of their face. They may make repetitive vocalizations or noises. Objects may be used. One favorite object used in self-stimulation is a string; individuals fondle or dangle a string, shoelace, or similar object in front of their face.

There may be a blending of self-abusive and stereotypic behaviors. Sometimes a stereotypic behavior such as finger sucking can produce damage by breaking down the skin. Excessive rubbing of one area of skin can also produce damage. Bruxism (teeth grinding) can damage teeth. Some repetitive behaviors can cause injury by accident. For example, someone who frequently swings his head around may inadvertently strike it on an object. In such cases, the therapist might intervene to provide some environmental adaptation to protect the person. In the case of self-stimulatory yelling, something should be done to protect others in the same room from auditory abuse. The therapist or another staff person should be able to take the loud consumer out of the room to give the other consumers and staff a respite. Repetitive self-stimulatory behavior that does not injure the consumer or bother others is usually not seen as needing intervention, although such behaviors may upset parents and caregivers who are attempting to get the individual to behave as normally as possible. The therapist should offer the team members suggestions for activities or methods but should remind them that some behaviors may arise from sensory needs and may be a chronic and "necessary" action for the consumer.

Interventions for SIB

Sensory Substitution

One simple method to deal with sensory behaviors is sensory substitution, or finding an alternative way to provide a stimulus the person seems to crave. The substitute stimulation is safe, whereas the original stimulation causes harm. For example, a woman picks the skin on her arms and produces numerous small lesions. She is given a soft plastic brush to rub briskly on her arms, producing a similar sensation without causing harm. In another case, a man strikes his chin, impacting his inner lip on his teeth and causing a lesion. He is offered a vibrator and encouraged to try it on his chin. In both examples a substitute stimulus is used to replace the original, harmful one.

Alternative Activity

When using alternative activities, one is basically using the old behavioral methods of differential reinforcement of incompatible behavior or differential reinforcement of other behavior. In one example, a woman picks at her hand until it bleeds. She is given a computer game to play that occupies both hands. In all cases, the individual is not forced in any way to comply but is shown the activities and encouraged to engage in them. As with all such interventions, the activities are offered *noncontingently*—that is, they are not offered only when the person self-abuses. If they receive the activity or are given attention only when SIB is shown, the risk is present that the SIB will be reinforced.

Somatosensory and Sensory-Integrative Approaches

Somatosensory refers to bodily sensations as distinguished from visceral or cortical influences. Noncontingent sensory stimulation has been suggested as a method to reduce SIB based on the presumption that certain levels of somatosensory stimulation are necessary or desirable for human beings. If such stimulation procedures are successful, direct-care staff could use them to reduce SIB in the severely and profoundly retarded nonambulatory population (Hiramu, 1989). In 1989, Hiramu completed a study in which SIB was reduced in eight teenage subjects by the use of noncontingent tactile stimulation. The stimulation was in the form of stroking, squeezing, and pressing specific areas of the body.

Sensory defensiveness, most commonly seen in the form of tactile defensiveness, can produce symptoms of SIB or antisocial behavior. Here the person's nervous system is overreacting to familiar stimuli, and negative behaviors may result. One somatosensory approach to address this problem in children ages 2–12 was to brush specific areas of the body vigorously with a soft plastic surgical brush. A treatment session was believed to produce effects that would last about 2 hours (Wilbarger & Wilbarger, 1991).

Both of the above techniques emphasize the use of *deep* pressure as opposed to light touch, which has a different neural pathway and affects different behavioral outcomes.

Vestibular stimulation has been frequently used with children with developmental delays and is a valuable technique with some adults as well. In the above-mentioned case of Margret, vestibular stimulation in the form of gentle swinging in a swing or spinning on a large floor saucer would immediately calm her down, and she often would remain calm for hours afterward.

To organize one's thinking about sensory-related behavior, the following steps and questions should be kept in mind:

1. Is there any evidence that an acute pain is the cause of behavior? For example, a client striking her face is found to have a bad tooth.
2. Does the behavior warrant intervention? Is it harmful to the individual or to others?
3. Is the behavior best remediated with a behavioral/contingency program? If so, the psychologist/behavioral specialist should intervene.
4. If the behavior is sensory in origin, does it seem to be manifested primarily because of outside stimuli, internal processing problems, or lack of stimuli?
5. Should the approach be in the form of a sensory substitute, environmental adaptation, alternative activity, or sensory stimulation program?
6. Can direct-care staff safely and effectively administer the program?

If treatment is decided on, the following should be done:

1. Consult with the team regarding the why, the how, and the where of therapy.
2. Secure a physician's order. A specific form should be used with a description of the SIB, prior diagnosis, current medications, and description of treatments to be used. The form should indicate that certain reasons for the SIB have been ruled out, such as a medical condition or means to communicate anger or frustration or to seek attention. It is important to justify the intervention of an OTR rather than a nurse or psychologist.
3. Make an accurate method of documenting the incidence of the target behavior before, during, and after treatment.

Environments: Safe, Suitable, and Sensory Enriched

Typical day programs and home residences for adults with profound disabilities may often be structured and furnished in ways that are unsuitable for the needs of the consumers. Often a day program may be in an older building designed for a completely different purpose. The building may have been formerly an old factory, department store, or religious seminary. Sometimes the building is fairly new but, due to severe budget restraints, may be greatly lacking in important features. Residential homes can also vary widely in suitability. They may be new modern structures designed to serve mobile, independent people, but instead, over time, the beds are given to people with more severe disabilities. They may be large estates "converted" into group homes. Sometimes they are dilapidated structures that pose a variety of hazards and limitations to the residents.

The following are important environmental elements for which a clinician should advocate.

1. Handicapped Accessibility and Safety

It seems incredible that people with wheelchairs and physical disabilities can be placed in homes and day programs lacking basic wheelchair accessibility, but this happens all too frequently. Ramps built to the code of 1 foot of ramp to 1 inch of elevation should be in place where needed. Sinks and tables should not have obstructions that prevent consumers in wheelchairs from using them. Individuals of very short stature should have the choice of using small chairs that allow them to sit and have both feet resting on the floor, if they will not or cannot use a foot box. Double railings and grab bars should be provided where required; sharp edges of furniture and other potential hazards should be padded or modified as needed.

2. Adequate Space

Category I individuals have limited or no mobility and may not need a large space. Category II individuals are more mobile and need to have the opportunity to explore the environment. Sometimes these mobile individuals are confined to absurdly small spaces and drab classrooms. Sensory materials and supplies can be brought into these spaces, but the space itself often needs to be changed to deliver the most effective interventions. If mobile clients have behaviors such as food stealing or tendencies to wander or are at risk of falling, there is often an attempt to keep them in an enclosed classroom that may be very small and confining. Those are unacceptable reasons to limit their freedom. A large recreational space should be available, where they can move about freely and safely for at least part of every day. An outside area, fenced in and with an area protected from the sun, is essential.

3. Bathrooms and Sinks

Every room should have a sink or be in close proximity to one. Hands and supplies frequently need to be washed for hygienic reasons. As many consumers have toileting accidents, the room they are in should have a bathroom within or in close proximity, equipped with changing tables, lifters, and all needed supplies. This is important not only for client-training purposes but also to expedite the whole routine. Otherwise, some clients end up spending a large part of the day in a toilet routine.

4. Sensory Room

The so-called classroom equipped with tables and chairs is often unsuitable for the clients who are the subjects of this chapter. They need a place to sit, but they are not usually people who work at tables. The rooms in which they are placed should offer them sensory interest. It may be suitable to have mats on the floor and large balls and bolsters about the room. There should be boards with different textures for tactile experiences. Objects such as mobiles and balloons should be suspended from the ceiling to provide visual stimulation. If possible, a special room may be set aside for such an environment where clients may be brought for part of a day. At the Young Adult Institute in Tarrytown, New York, for example, a sensory "obstacle course" was built in one room. This 20' × 19' structure was the product of a multidisciplinary core team, composed of an occupational therapist, physical therapist, and special education teacher. It was carpeted and designed to encourage a consumer to engage in a variety of experiences that stimulate gross motor and sensory functions. This structure contains mats, tunnels, and hanging bolsters, as well as textured walkways, mirrors, lights, music, and a "smell station." Several features of this environment were activated by the individual by means of switches. If such an environment as this could be made in units that could be adapted and modified as needed, it would truly be an asset to any house or day program seeking to provide a sensory-enriched environment.

The Therapist as Educator

The treatment team may consist of direct-care staff (training specialists), clinicians (occupational, physical, speech, nursing, psychology), a physician, supervisors at the day program, house managers, social workers, parents, consumer advocates, and/or significant others. Each plays a role as part of a team that ideally works together for the consumer's benefit. The occupational therapist communicates with all needed team members. In my experience, I have found that the occupational therapy perspective is very important with this population, and occupational therapy staff often need to bring specific issues to the attention of the team. Providing in-services to training specialists and others is also very important.

Sometimes staff, even clinicians, harbor certain attitudes that one may find necessary to address. Staff may need to have neurological and sensory impairments explained to them, as well as why it is wrong to always assume that the client is being lazy or engaging in a manipulative behavior when he or she does not meet expectations. Sometimes, a client will have a disease, physical/sensory impairment, or drug-induced syndrome and, additionally, exhibit behaviors that confuse staff. One individual I worked with developed a Parkinsonian movement disorder and had a long history of being given neuroleptic drugs. At times he would be able to move very fast, and at other times he would become very stiff with "cogwheel rigidity" and would tend to fall. Because of these inconsistencies of movement and because he would smile or show a flat affect to pain and falls, many staff felt he was exhibiting only attention-seeking behaviors. Because of this attitude, these staff members did not respect his disabilities. The therapist needs to intervene in such cases, sharing his or her professional judgment and providing education.

Conclusion

Working with this population delivers job satisfaction for those who have patience, persistence, and motivation to meet therapeutic challenges. Key elements needed to achieve meaningful outcomes include

- Making effective, appropriate assessments
- Prioritizing treatment issues and empowering direct-care staff for nonskilled issues
- Being willing to take calculated risks and try varied approaches
- Using resources effectively
- Reviewing progress regularly and monitoring for necessary changes.

It is quite possible that, with advances in genetics, biomechanics, and early intervention access, the members of this population may decrease in number in the future. They may also be served in programs and with methods that are simpler, more streamlined, and more effective than ones that now exist across the country. The drive to cut costs will continue to harm progress in this area. The essential element to improving quality of care, however, will be a better understanding on the part of the public of the nature of people with these disabilities and their needs.

References

Association for Retarded Citizens. (1982). *The prevalence of mental retardation.* Silver Spring, MD: Author.

Association for Retarded Citizens. (1997a, September). *Introduction to mental retardation: How is mental retardation diagnosed? Questions and answers.* Retrieved January 13, 2004, from http:// www.thearc.org.

Association for Retarded Citizens. (1997b, September). *Introduction to mental retardation: How many people are affected by mental retardation? Questions and answers.* Retrieved January 13, 2004, from http://www.thearc.org.

Belfore, P. J., & Dattilo, F. (1990). The behavior of self-injury: A brief review and analysis. *Journal of Behavioral Disorders, 16*(1).

Brown, F., & Lehr, D. H. (1989). *Persons with profound disabilities: Issues and practices.* Baltimore: Brookes.

Burkhart, L. (1982). *Homemade battery-powered toys and educational devices for severely handicapped children* (2nd ed.). Baltimore: Burkhardt.

Cataldo, M. (1988). Analysis and modification of disruptive behavior. In J. Kavanagh (Ed.), *Understanding mental retardation: Research accomplishments and new frontiers* (p. 272). Baltimore: Brookes.

Durand, M., & Kishi, G. (1987). Reducing severe behavior problems among persons with dual sensory impairments: An evaluation of a technical assistance model. *Journal of the Association for Persons With Severe Handicaps, 12*(1), 2–10.

Dussault, W. (1989). Is policy of exclusion based upon severity of disability legally defensible? In F. Brown & D. Lehr (Eds.), *Persons with profound disabilities* (p. 45). Baltimore: Brookes.

Evans, I., & Scotti, J. (1989). Defining meaningful outcomes for persons with profound disabilities. In F. Brown & D. Lehr (Eds.), *Persons with profound disabilities* (p. 84). Baltimore: Brookes.

Gardner, J. F., & Chapman, M. S. (1985). *Staff development in mental retardation services.* Baltimore: Brookes.

Haxby, J. V., & Shapiro, M. B. (1992). Longitudinal study of neuropsychological function in older adults with Down syndrome. In L. Nadel & C. J. Epstein (Eds.), *Down syndrome and Alzheimer's disease* (pp. 35–50). New York: Wiley-Liss.

Heller, L., & Lockwood, J. (1991). *Designing a sensory motor environment.* Presentation at NYS/ADTP Statewide Meeting, Young Adult Institute, Tarrytown Day Treatment Program, New York.

Hiramu, H. (1989). *Self-abusive behavior: A somatosensory approach.* Bethesda, MD: Chess.

Iwasaki, K., & Holm, M. B. (1990). Sensory treatment for the reduction of stereotype behaviors in persons with severe multiple disabilities. *Occupational Therapy Journal of Research, 9,* 170–183.

Janicki, M. P., Heller, T., Seltzer, G., & Hogg, J. (1995). *Practice guidelines for the clinical assessment and care management of Alzheimer's and other dementias among adults with mental retardation.* Washington, DC: American Association on Mental Retardation.

Kihss, P. (1977, February 26). Court-ordered winds of change touch Willowbrook. *New York Times,* pp. 21, 41.

King, B. (1995). *Self-injurious behavior (SIB) in individuals with mental retardation.* Retrieved from http://www.mrrc.npi.ucla.edu/mrrc95/research/clinres/bking.htm.

Lakin, K. C., Hill, B., & Haydn, M. (1989). *Directory of residential centers for adults with developmental disabilities.* Phoenix, AZ: Oryx Press.

Luiselli, J. K. (1995). Reinforcement methods and variations in the clinical treatment of challenging behaviors. *Habilitative Mental Healthcare Newsletter, 14,* 2.

Lynch, K., Kiernan, W., & Stark, J. (1982). *Prevocational education for special needs youth.* Baltimore: Brookes.

Parrete, H., Strother, P. O., & Hourcade, J. J. (1986, Fall). Microswitches and adaptive equipment for severely impaired students. *Teaching Exceptional Children.*

Peck, C., & Hong, C. (1989). *Living skills for mentally handicapped people.* London: Croon & Helm.

Reisman, J., & Hanschu, B. (1990). *Sensory integration inventory for adults with developmental disabilities: User's guide.* Minneapolis, MN: PDP Press.

Reiss, S. (1996, August). *Mental illness in people with mental retardation.* Retrieved January 13, 2004, from http://www.thearc.org.

Stahlman, M. T., Grogaard, J., et al. (1988). Neonatal intensive care and developmental outcome. In J. Kavanagh (Ed.), *Understanding mental retardation.* Baltimore: Brookes.

Stark, J., Baker, D., Menousek, P., & McGee, J. (1982). Behavioral programming for severely mentally retarded/behaviorally impaired youth. In K. P. Lynch, W. E. Kiernan, & J. A. Stark (Eds.), *Prevocational and vocational education for special needs youth: A blueprint for the 1980s* (p. 215). Baltimore: Brookes.

Thompson, T. (1971). Preface to the first edition. In T. Thompson & J. Grabowski (Eds.), *Behavior modification of the mentally retarded* (2nd ed.). New York: Oxford University Press.

Whitman, T., Scibak, J., & Reid, D. (1983). *Behavior modification with the severely and profoundly retarded.* New York: Academic Press.

Wilbarger, P., & Wilbarger, J. (1991). *Sensory defensiveness in children aged 2–12: An intervention guide for parents and other caretakers.* Santa Barbara, CA: Avanti Educational Programs.

CHAPTER 4

Using a Sensory Approach for Adults With Developmental Disabilities

Bonnie Hanschu, OTR

Introduction

This chapter describes how we came to understand the significance of a frame of reference and how a sensory-oriented frame of reference made the significant difference for adults served by occupational therapy in an institutional environment. The term *frame of reference* refers to a particular clinical perspective that has guiding principles to govern the treatment and evaluation of people who have severe disabilities. A frame of reference provides a consistent set of assumptions to direct, control, or judge one's clinical approach. It guides clinical activities, but it does not provide a recipe or formula for action (Mosey, 1981; Reed, 1984). Service providers maintain a responsibility to accurately identify needs and then to adjust what they do according to the effectiveness of programs designed to meet those needs.

Consider several individuals for whom a sensory orientation made a big difference. In each case, viewing the person's responses through sensory-oriented eyes helped us to understand that self-stimulatory or maladaptive behavior could reflect a sensory need. If that was appropriate, we were curious to find out what would happen if we were to respond by providing a strong, pleasurable sensation. To guide our choice of sensation, we observed what each person sought through his or her own behavior, and we incorporated the results of offering each a variety of sensations to identify those that elicited approach versus avoidance responses. We kept in mind a priority concern that we avoid any sensation a person seemed to not like or to find unpleasant.

Case 1

Before

A 41-year-old woman had a well-established history of picking at herself. The picking resulted in broken skin and oozing sores that required medical treatment. This behavior and its progression were documented all the way back to early childhood and remained her priority problem despite attempts to intervene with medications and a variety of intense behavioral strategies. Behavioral attempts included differential reinforcement of alternative or incompatible behaviors and the use of aversives and restraints. Nothing had altered the frequency or intensity of the picking, and this behavior alone was the barrier preventing this woman from moving to a less restrictive setting.

After We Started Using a Sensory Approach

A program was started in which the woman was given doses of proprioception and pressure touch for about 10 minutes every hour, on the hour, during her waking hours. Following the dose of sensation, a helper invited her to participate in an activity she was expected to enjoy. Within 6 months, her rates of picking dropped from an average of approximately one pick per minute during her awake hours to only a few picks per several hours. Her team had a goal of finding her a community-based placement within 4 years before she began the sensory treatment. Because of the success of the program, she was successfully placed within 7 months in a homelike foster care environment with a couple, their dog, carpeted floors, and live plants. The couple continued the program of sensory doses throughout the woman's transition to her new home, fading the frequency of the doses to only occasional use of the technique in preparation for events that were expected to be more stressful. At the end of the 6-month post-discharge period, the placement was still rated a success by everyone involved, and the picking behavior had not returned (Reisman, 1993).

Case 2

Before

A 24-year-old woman had an established history of recurring episodes during which she became totally out of control. When she was doing well, she had many abilities and was relatively adaptive. She dressed and fed herself. She was continent and took care of her toileting activities with only occasional prompts to flush, use soap, or turn off the faucet. She was good humored and complied with requests. She smiled and showed evidence of pride when helping household staff with routine domestic chores, such as carrying dirty dishes to the sink, wiping the table, or putting chairs in place. Unfortunately, after just a few days like this, her adaptive behavior would disintegrate, and she would rapidly escalate to being out of control.

During these times she was incontinent of bladder and bowel. She would not eat and would take only occasional sips of liquid. She whined or screeched almost continuously as if she were in severe distress. She was intolerant of clothing and stripped or ripped her shirts as fast as they were put on her. She ran from one place in the room to another and abruptly flung herself into solid brick walls. Her cheeks were a ruddy bright red from slapping herself. She would throw her mattress and any piece of heavy furniture she could get to, posing a threat to anyone who happened to be in the path. It was impossible for anyone to console or calm her. Month after month she would have 20 or more days like this, spending most of that time being held in a prone position on a thick floor mat to protect her and those around her. The only interventions that helped get her through these episodes were physical containment and heavy sedation.

After We Started Using a Sensory Approach

She was started on an intensive program of sensation that involved being bounced gently on a trampoline, being held tightly from behind and swayed gently from side to side, being gently stretched in a supine position, and being swung slowly and rhythmically in one direction at a time in either a swing or a hammock. In a matter of several months, she had improved to the point of being able to leave the campus to perform work in the community. She dressed appropriately and made the trips successfully with just her job coach. She ate in public eating establishments; used public restrooms without incident; and carried out a job at a local church, vacuuming the carpets and polishing the pews. She was a changed person.

Case 3

Before

A 36-year-old woman, totally blind since birth, had a terrible time tolerating touch from others. Her physical problems were substantial; her hips disarticulated in a wind-swept deformity. She could not sit without total support, and her wheelchair was adapted with cumbersome modifications to ensure her comfort as well as her safety. She required total care and had to be handled multiple times a day to meet her most basic needs. Whenever she was transferred, fed, dressed, cleaned up after an accident, or repositioned, she screamed and cried as if someone were tearing her limbs from her body. When she was left alone, she would gently rub a spot on the side of her head, smiling and occasionally making playful sounds. These were the only times she did not seem to be in acute distress.

After We Started Using a Sensory Approach

She was started on a program that involved transferring her as quietly as possible to a hammock swing and then gently swinging her for several minutes.

This was accomplished by using a specially designed transfer pad that enabled care providers to move her without touching her. She got the swinging at least three times a day and at least twice in the evenings. After the swinging, she was provided with several minutes of pressure touch to her legs and arms, and soft objects were pressed gently into her lap. After the sensory services were started, one of her more consistent direct care providers had an idea. She made the woman a weighted poncho that had a snug-fitting hood for her head and heavy fabric that covered most of her body. The woman would smile and relax immediately after the poncho was put on her. The sensory strategies seem to make her much more comfortable, and her team credited them for enabling her to get through morning and evening cares without becoming upset.

Case 4

Before
A 32-year-old man, blind from birth, displayed no sense of balance when walking and would fall over unless he could hang onto someone's arm or a handrail. He did not tolerate shirts and stripped them off and flung them away as fast as someone tried to put one on him. He was typically found sitting on the floor, tailor fashion. He would rapidly scoot away in the opposite direction when anyone approached. He would not sit in chairs unless someone insisted by pressing him into it and holding him down at the shoulders. When left alone, he made almost continuous clicking noises and displayed almost continuous hands-in-the-pants behaviors.

After We Started Using a Sensory Approach
He received increasingly intensive sensory services over the course of 3 years. At the end of the 3 years, he was walking on his own with a reciprocal gait rather than a side-to-side sway. He sat in chairs routinely, and he even liked to get into suspended equipment to swing, something he had refused to do through almost 3 years of encouragement to try. Videotaped "before" and "after" films at 1-year intervals revealed significant progressive structural change, as well as dramatic changes in his behavior and interaction. Initially his legs were severely bowed. By the end of 3 years, his legs had actually straightened. In the third tape, there was a complete absence of clicking noises. He approached care providers on his own and would sit in a chair and interact with someone who talked to him. He accepted help from someone who stood behind him, reaching around to guide his hands through a task. This was a kind of close contact he would have no part of before. Throughout his sensory service, his medications were steadily reduced until psychotropic medication was eliminated entirely. This man ultimately moved to a community-based group home with three other individuals. He did work-

for-pay in a structured day program to which he rode the bus without difficulty. None of this had ever been considered for his plan because goals of this nature were considered to be an unrealistic expectation for him. The time coinciding with the introduction of sensory-based service for him was the first time in the course of his 20-plus years of institutionalization that he showed any progress, let alone the steady trend of progress in all of his active treatment goals.

Figuring Out a Better Approach

These were four people whose lives were stuck in time until they were provided with a treatment approach that met their needs. They are similar to adults with developmental disabilities being served in long-term-care settings all over the United States. What we learned about what made the difference for them is the subject of this chapter. The chapter describes the setting where their stories took place and how a conflict arose concerning the prevailing frame of reference. The chapter goes on to detail the search for a more fitting frame of reference and emphasizes that finding a better approach sometimes requires figuring out a better approach. The chapter closes with a discussion of the new frame of reference, now being called the "Ready Approach," and what we learned from developing and implementing an untested sensory approach.

Perhaps the most important lesson we learned from the experience described in this chapter was that, when people are not improving, it may be because we have not yet come up with the right approach to help them. The 1990s have been called the "Decade of the Brain," and neurologists have discovered that even damaged brains can be remarkably resilient. When they are given even a little bit of help, the results can be stunning.

Background

The Setting

Our facility was a placement of last resort for adults with severe developmental disabilities. Some were physically able but severely behaviorally challenged. Others had physical disabilities and problematic behaviors. Still others were totally physically dependent, and occasionally also medically fragile. Even some of the medically fragile individuals had challenging behaviors. Every person had complex and profound functional and performance deficits and serious combinations of interdependent problems. Almost all had grossly impaired or absent communication.

Aggression, defensiveness, and self-stimulation were the order of the day. In some households and in many day programs, staff struggled to get through each shift with no one getting hurt. Unless someone was working with them directly, those who were physically able spent their time stripping, engaging in hands-in-the-pants behaviors, mouthing, eating inedibles, and making nerve-racking sounds. Programming was almost at a standstill, and lack of active treatment was a source of recurring multiple citations during licensing surveys.

Most of the people we served had been challenged by brain damage since birth. The rest incurred severe brain damage during their formative years. The damage was usually associated with biological factors such as genetic faults, chromosomal abnormalities, metabolic disturbances, infections, or anoxia; other causes included traumatic injury, disease, and damage from chemical or toxic agents. Regardless of the cause, each person ended up with devastating brain damage. The vast majority had lived in an institutional environment since infancy or childhood. As a result, they had developed additional secondary problems associated with sensory deprivation, lack of opportunity, and all the other depersonalizing factors that are so hard to eliminate in large institutions.

No matter what teams identified as priority needs, the ever-present stereotypic, self-stimulatory, and self-injurious behaviors continued to demand attention. Staff made concerted efforts every day to focus on "positive programming," in which the goal was to develop new skills or abilities. However, those attempts were derailed every day by the need to control, or at least manage, problem behaviors. It eventually occurred to us that those behaviors reflected the significance of unmet sensory needs, but it was hard to think "sensory" when we were so focused on behavior.

The Prevailing Approach

Behaviorism was well established as the predominant frame of reference at our institution. There were at least two good reasons for that. First, it was well known that people who have mental retardation sometimes learn new skills best when they are trained with highly structured, consistent reinforcement of positive responses. Second, many people served in our institution faced significant obstacles to community-based opportunities and less restrictive placement because of maladaptive behavior. Therefore, behavior modification was a top priority.

It was appropriate for a treatment facility like ours to have a wide range of behavioral expertise available, and it did. In addition to a well-staffed behavioral psychology department, every team had its own behavior analyst. The roots of behavioral thinking went even deeper, because people with behavioral expertise were also the team leaders, the supervisors, the managers and, in general, the people most influential in all programmatic and organizational decisions.

No one questioned whether behaviorism had an important place in the treatment of people with developmental disabilities. An approach does not become the predominant view, recommended by experts around the world as the premier choice, unless there is good evidence it has merit. Behaviorism has a long, well-documented history of producing results with hundreds of thousands of people who have severe disabilities.

Because behaviorism was *the* frame of reference in our organization, other alternatives were not considered. Yet social changes were leading to legislative initiatives, such as the required downsizing of our institution's population from 2,000 to a few hundred. When we got to 400 clients it was clear that behaviors were the greatest barrier to community integration. As we approached 200 residents, it had become urgent for staff to figure out more effective ways to deal with challenging client behaviors so people remaining in the institution could be served more safely and transitioned into community settings with more success.

We began to see that there were several indications that a behavioral frame of reference was not the best alternative for the remaining group we were trying to serve. Yet, behaviorism had been the predominant approach in settings like ours for so many years. It was hard to break away from behavioral thinking.

Conflict for Occupational Therapists

Occupational therapists, as well as other therapists in our organization, frequently experienced conflicts in such a behaviorally oriented setting. Everything about the people we served needed to be described in behavioral terms so that its frequency, intensity, or duration could be observed or tested using objective means. Therapists were even cautioned about how to discuss muscle tone or other sensorimotor issues in their reports and admonished to focus on observable behaviors that could be improved, for example,

- How far a person could reach,
- How many seconds a position could be held, and
- How many objects a person could move to a specified location.

Therapists understood the need to operationalize desired outcomes by describing them as something that could be observed or measured. How else could we obtain objective and reliable data on which to make decisions? However, describing behaviors is different from applying a behavioral frame of reference, and that difference was not always understood. Many therapists consequently felt pressured to abandon their sensorimotor orientation in favor of a behavioral perspective, an outcome that severely compromised the value of having therapists on interdisciplinary teams in the first place.

It was their sensorimotor frame of reference that helped therapists recognize the inappropriateness of people with significant postural and motor control problems being conditioned with edibles or other reinforcers to improve their task performance. Such training often took place at mealtime for people

- Who could not sit in chairs,
- Who had no stable base of proximal support,
- Who had insufficient motor control to grade muscle actions, and/or
- Whose inadequate integration of primitive reflex patterns made it difficult for them to control extraneous movements.

In rare instances, aversive behavioral procedures were used to get people to open their mouths to receive food, completely missing how much difficulty they had coordinating their suck–swallow–breathe patterns. Everyone knows better now, but these examples show that, when we do not understand the nature of a need, we can make well-intended, but potentially harmful, decisions.

Therapists also questioned another implication of behavioral approaches—the tendency to view everything a person does as adaptive or maladaptive behavior. Human nervous systems are truly remarkable in their capacity to protect us from what we cannot manage. From a sensory perspective, it is possible to argue that some maladaptive behavior might actually be a clever compensation on the part of a nervous system struggling to keep a person safe, comfortable, or free from demands that are beyond the person's ability. In such instances, behavior labeled "maladaptive" might actually be quite adaptive (Reisman & Hanschu, 1992).

We see lots of behaviors in an institutional setting that, from a behavioral perspective, need to be modified. From a sensory perspective, those same behaviors provide evidence of just how much pressure we are putting on someone's nervous system. Misinterpreting such behavior could result in adding to, rather than decreasing, the amount of stress on someone's nervous system. That could explain why there was mounting evidence provided by ongoing programmatic data that our people were not improving, and their behavior seemed to be getting worse in some cases.

Behavioral training did not seem to be working. In fact, medical and program records of the people remaining in our care indicated that, if behavioral interventions had ever worked, there was only a temporary gain, and there was evidence a person could actually regress after intensive behavioral intervention. This observation in our setting was consistent with the results of multiple studies reported in the psychological literature that short-term success in eliminating or decreasing maladaptive behaviors may be achieved, but targeted behavior sometimes returns with a vengeance, or new, more troublesome behaviors emerge in its place.

Unfortunately, when there is little or no improvement, especially with adults, care providers, including therapists, sometimes attribute lack of progress to limited potential for change, citing limitations associated with age, severity of disabilities, or disabilities being well established over so many years. They may emphasize the need to maintain abilities the person already has, believing it is unrealistic to expect improvement. We now have reasons to view that line of thinking as erroneous for many individuals (Bidabe, 1991). It is also easy to blame lack of progress on administrative issues such as staffing or funding, especially when there is frequent organizational upheaval associated with downsizing. With so many possible explanations for lack of progress, there is little reason to suspect that it might be most directly related to the program's prevailing frame of reference.

Power of Management

We might have continued on the same course indefinitely, if not for a licensing survey that prompted a change in our top management. Along with the new leadership came a mandate to provide effective service or prepare for the consequence, which was assumed to be closure. This executive agenda cut through months (potentially) of discussion and created a more united effort to solve overall programmatic problems.

In occupational therapy we saw the management change as a significant opportunity to help make a difference. We were guardedly optimistic that program philosophies more compatible with our view might be considered. We had been using the Model of Human Occupation, a frame of reference that helps occupational therapy practitioners use a uniform approach and terminology to identify functional abilities and life tasks that need attention. This model helped us isolate functional and performance deficits, but we were still left with basic questions. What were the underlying causes of the person's functional deficit? How much improvement in function could we expect? What needed to change for the function to improve? We had to apply more specific clinical frames of reference for answers to those questions.

In addition to behaviorism, neurodevelopment and sensory integration are frames of reference commonly applied by occupational therapists in the field of developmental disabilities. These last two seemed to be particularly important for therapists who serve adults with multiple handicapping conditions and severe sensorimotor problems. As therapists, we had tried applying them separately, and then we tried mixing and melding ideas from each. No matter what we tried, we kept coming to the same conclusion. Each alternative explained many things we observed, and each offered methods and techniques that helped in some situations, but none quite matched our clinical experience. They were useful, but we still did not have a clinical perspective that was consistent with our experience.

Meanwhile, the situation for people being served remained intolerable. We finally concluded that we would not be able to rely on an existing frame of reference and that we would instead have to figure out, at the very least, a variation of an existing approach. We needed a way to describe our people that would enable us to make a greater—and more predictable—therapeutic impact. In view of the pressure from licensing, finding that way became our Number 1 challenge.

Search for a Better Way

Despite our efforts, we could find no one approach that provided the answer for our situation. We had to figure out how to do things better, but we were not even sure what "better" involved. Our only remaining option was to review our clinical reasoning and to evaluate our own clinical observations and experiences.

We knew that the major problem for all people in our care was brain damage, and as occupational therapists we believed that was significant. Therefore, we reasoned that we should know more about the relationship between brain damage and the performance problems displayed by the people we served. Because behavior was so frequently the focus of a person's program, we felt it was especially important for us to look at challenging or excessive behaviors as a possible reflection of what goes on in the brain. These lines of reasoning took us directly to a sensory perspective.

We decided to see what would happen if we were to interpret the challenging behaviors as evidence of a priority sensory need (Reisman & Hanschu, 1992). Relying on sensory integration and neurodevelopmental principles to guide us, we proceeded to introduce individual programs with strong sensory elements. We started to emphasize the importance of heavy work and taught staff how to safely give therapeutic "doses" of sensation, including direct compression or stretching at joints and pressure touch to backs, arms, and legs to provide stronger body sensation. We got equipment into household and day program areas so that people could swing before challenging events or major transitions. We even organized therapy staff to provide direct service in the work areas, scheduling extended blocks of time according to the number of people with sensory needs in the area. We also figured out how to incorporate strong sensation at strategic times in the daily routine, namely, during transitions, mealtimes, morning care, and medical appointments.

Benefits became evident almost immediately, but we still were not sure how to explain or predict what was happening. We believed the improvement had something to do with increased opportunity to get strong sensation because nothing else had changed. Enhanced sensation was simply structured into the person's experience. As clients began to look more comfortable and more settled, they became more initiating, indicating what sensory activity they wanted and when. Rather than frantically going for vigorous sensation or engaging in insistent self-stimulation, they looked like they were comparing choices and selecting what they preferred. Although we often controlled their choices, being able to choose from alternatives made it more possible for them to lead us rather than our controlling the interaction. This was quite a new development for many of them.

We were encouraged by results associated with sensory techniques, but we did not yet have a frame of reference, consisting of logically connected ideas, that we could support with scientific evidence. Sensory integration theory, which in many ways was so helpful at getting us closer to the nature of the need, actually held us back a bit. It did not easily or fully explain what we were doing or seeing. We spent a lot of time and effort trying to reconcile our experience with the theory before we began to realize that a different theory might be more applicable. Explanations that fit our population did not start to emerge until we got beyond sensory integration to the more generic concept of sensory processing and until we started to delve into what scientists were discovering about the neurobiology of behavior. Until then, we were trying to get a theory about sensorimotor function to explain behavior, as if sensorimotor function and behavior were one and the same. The limitations were not in sensory integration theory; they were in how we were trying to use it. Nevertheless, sensory integration theory got us started in the right direction: thinking sensory.

Thinking sensory was one thing; trying to reconcile a sensory perspective with the prevailing behavioral view was another. We immediately encountered conflicts and inconsistencies that made it difficult to use the two approaches together. For example, the behavioral approach for designing individual programs took no account of neurology, that is, the brain damage experienced by the people we served (Crick, 1994; Edelman, 1992). In contrast, sensory approaches were dependent on an understanding of neurohabilitative considerations. Another conflict was that behavioral approaches relied heavily on learning theory, whereas sensory theory suggested the possibility that learning might be blocked.

The discrepancies between the two approaches magnified our concern that behavioral thinking might actually result in significant misunderstanding or misinterpretation of behaviors displayed by many of the people we served. This concern had been raised by prominent behavioral psychologists who were starting to acknowledge sensory explanations for some behaviors (Durand & Crimmins, 1988; Lovaas, Newsom, & Hickman, 1987). We envisioned a future in which teams might need to choose one approach over another, but we realized their task would be formidable unless we could offer clearer explanations of the sensory issues and defend what we said. That got us searching the neuroscience literature, particularly what it had to say about the neurobiology of behavior.

Closing in on Priority Issues

Many authorities on the nervous system describe how behavior is dependent on sensation coming into the brain and being processed. Different authors offer different perspectives of the processing involved, such as anatomical (Brodal, 1992) and biochemical (Rahmann & Rahmann, 1992; Shepherd, 1988). Although there are still many questions about how the brain processes sensation, scientists believe they are getting much closer to the answers. What is known provides us with possible, if not probable, explanations for how the brain registers and integrates sensation and how sensation influences emotion, awareness, cognition, and behavior (Chopra, 1989; Churchland, 1993; Gazzaniga, 1988, 1992, 1995; Goleman, 1995; Kandel & Schwartz, 1991, 1995; Kotulak, 1996; LeDoux, 1996; Masters & McGuire, 1994; Nuland, 1997; Pearsall, 1996; Ruden, 1997; West, 1991). In general, *processing sensation* enables the brain to do several things related to experience: make sense of it, organize responses to it, and form memories of it (Kandel & Schwartz, 1991, 1995; Kotulak, 1996; Ruden, 1997). This raises another question about behavioral approaches: If someone's brain is unable to comprehend the meaning of experience, how would reinforcing aspects of that experience promote learning? How can one learn something that makes no sense? Perhaps there was a neurobiological explanation for why the most carefully designed, consistently applied behavioral interventions might have no lasting effects, as was the case for the people in the remaining group at our institution, with whom such interventions had been tried over and over again for many years.

Neuroscientists also tell us that most of a person's sensory processing involves neural activity in lower centers, such as the brain stem, cerebellum, and limbic structures—centers that work well below the level of consciousness (Kotulak, 1996; Masters & McGuire, 1994). This processing enables humans to do all kinds of complex tasks automatically, without any thought, often without awareness of doing them. Those of us who have cars and routinely drive back and forth between two familiar locations, such as work and home, can probably relate to the experience of finding ourselves at one of the locations with no memory of having driven there. Our brains can do extremely sophisticated tasks for us, such as driving a large piece of expensive equipment through heavy traffic, calling for our attention only if something unusual occurs. Adequate sensory processing frees people to live full lives, to give their conscious attention to what most interests them. Some people actually make a nice living capitalizing on highly efficient sensory processing—for example, professional athletes.

There is obviously a wide range along the continuum between functional and dysfunctional sensory processing. That range made us all the more aware of the degree of disordered sensory processing in our clients who did little that was automatic, unless it also involved strong emotion. Then they could move in a flash. Otherwise their actions often seemed delayed and deliberate, as if they were paying attention to every detail. We also saw the problem of experience apparently not being stored in memory. Numerous direct-contact staff reported the observation that "If we've done it once, we've done it a million times, the same way, every time; yet, it's always like it's the first time." Neuroscientists tell us memory does not store confusion.

Given such observations and seeing how our clients responded in various situations, it seemed highly likely that their sensory processing was significantly disordered. Not only did their sensory processing seem insufficient to support the development of a repertoire of automatic responses, it was also too disordered for most clients to get enough meaning out of their experience to form adequate memory of that experience. We now know much more about memory mechanisms and how they influence behavior. Joseph LeDoux's work clearly differentiates emotional memory from something we could call "rational memory" (LeDoux, 1996). Emotional memory is thought to be fully functional at the time of birth, laying in memory circuits that can be, as Daniel Goleman (1995) described it, trip-wired to provide immediate, strong emotional reactions in the presence of just a few stimuli that trigger the memory. In contrast to emotional memory, rational memory is not fully functional until around age 2 years. Rational memory is provided by circuitry that enables the brain to interpret experience, to understand what is happening, and to provide a context for what one may be feeling. That we recognize a face is a product of rational memory; that we have feelings about the person with that face is a product of emotional memory.

The day-to-day reactions of our clients seem to perfectly illustrate emotional memory dominating responses without the benefit of rational memory's mediation. Other factors may have contributed, but we certainly could argue that disordered sensory processing probably made it difficult for our clients to form rational memories of their experience. How could anyone's brain interpret what it experienced and mediate that person's response to experience, if it could neither get the meaning nor store memories of the experience?

The more we came to understand how the chemistry and circuitry of the brain influence behavior, the more we had to rethink assumptions about several aspects of the people we served. However, our ability to rethink assumptions was still complicated. We had lots of new ideas and were excited about how perfectly they seemed to fit our clinical observations, yet we still lacked a cohesive set of consistent and compatible assumptions to guide our clinical reasoning. When we tried to use sensory integration theory to explain the needs of our group, we ran into limitations. For example, experts on the topic emphasize that sensory integration requires active participation to plan, organize, and generate adaptive responses (Ayres, 1972; Fisher, Murray, & Bundy, 1991). How could we justify, as a treatment technique, giving strong sensation to someone who remained essentially passive? This, according to the sensory integration experts, was nothing more than sensory stimulation (Fisher et al., 1991). Some sensory integration experts also stress that effectiveness of sensory integration is reflected by sensorimotor ability (Ayres, 1972; Fisher et al., 1991). Therefore, we had trouble explaining how some individuals could have so many functional, performance, and behavior problems, yet the quality of their sensorimotor ability could seem quite intact. How could they move with ease and finesse, when they wanted to do so, if disordered sensory integration was a fundamental problem?

We faced another conflict in our ability to rely on sensory integration theory when we got the Wilbarger explanation of *sensory defensiveness*. According to Patricia and Julia Wilbarger (1991), defensiveness can occur in anybody at anytime. If faced with circumstances that severely tax the protective mechanisms managed by the brain's limbic structures, any of us, even as adults, can develop sensory defensiveness. The idea that defensiveness can occur in anyone at any time is also consistent with Joseph LeDoux's (1996) explanation of fear responses in his book *The Emotional Brain*. Yet, according to experts on sensory integration theory, sensory integration dysfunction includes tactile defensiveness (Royeen & Lane, 1991) and results from damage to lower brain centers early in the life of the brain, usually before age 3 years (Fisher et al., 1991). This tactile problem seemed to be the same tactile defensiveness that the Wilbargers had described as the most common form of sensory defensiveness, with sensory defensiveness being a condition that can arise anytime in the life span.

It seemed we needed to figure out if sensory defensiveness might more appropriately be viewed as a separate and distinct problem. Our need to figure this out became even more compelling when we saw the degree to which the distinction influenced our diagnosing. Using the Wilbarger explanation, we saw defensiveness all around us in our adult population. If we viewed defensiveness as one aspect of sensory integration dysfunction and followed the criteria advocated by Fisher et al. (1991), the problem was less rife. However, we also found that the treatment protocol developed by the Wilbargers achieved more significant improvement, much faster, than any of the other sensory strategies we had tried. This presented still another conflict in trying to explain sensory defensiveness as an aspect of sensory integration dysfunction because, according to the Wilbargers, if necessary, you impose the treatment. Yet, imposing strong sensations is considered to be inappropriate from the perspective of sensory integration theory.

It was becoming increasingly obvious to us that we probably could not rely solely on sensory integration theory to explain the needs of, or plan an appropriate intervention for, our adult population. In addition, it looked like any frame of reference we developed would have to be able to explain sensory integration and sensory defensiveness as two distinct aspects of a more generic brain mechanism or activity. For adults served in an institutional environment, we decided the more generic activity, sensory processing, was the issue on which to focus our attention.

Sensory Processing and Neural Plasticity

Neural plasticity was another well-documented aspect of brain activity that captured our interest. *Neural plasticity* accounts for a person's ability to recover from a stroke as well as the ability to learn increasingly complex information and skills. *Plasticity* is the capacity of the human brain to improve its circuitry for better communication among various neural networks (Aoki & Siekevitz, 1988; Brodal, 1992; Churchland & Sejnowski, 1993; Kandel & Schwartz, 1991, 1995; Kotulak, 1996; Kuno, 1995). Plasticity even enables the brain to repair or modify circuitry that becomes damaged (Levitan & Kaczmarek, 1997; Nicholls, 1994; Rahmann & Rahmann, 1992; Shepherd, 1988). This highly dynamic, ongoing process helps the brain achieve and maintain maximal efficiency. It is known to be present in the human brain, even damaged brains, for the whole of the life span.

We were fascinated by the phenomenon of neural plasticity because of our observation about sustained improvement in the adults with whom we were using sensory techniques. There were indications in many of the individuals who improved that the improvements were stable. We observed this stability in more and more people the longer we continued to use sensory techniques. We found, for example, that with some people, there came a time when we could fade the frequency and intensity of service without seeing any regression. Now, after years of experience with this approach, we find this same "permanence" in the progress made by many children who are treated for sensory processing problems. We think the relatively permanent change results from improved circuitry that helps the brain become more efficient in its ability to adapt to varied situations. It seems to be a manifestation of neural plasticity in action. This is not to imply that there is never regression, but even in the adult setting, where some of our patients were in their 50s, those receiving sensory services could sometimes have three medication reductions before displaying any signs of regression. When regression did occur, it was relatively minor, and a short period of more intense sensory service would help the person recover a more adaptive level of performance. Our conclusion: Sensory strategies and enriched sensory experience appeared to be facilitating sensory processing and neural plasticity. This was very exciting indeed!

Brain Stem Sensations

Changes associated with plasticity are known to involve the brain's chemistry and circuitry. Both are influenced by experience, but both are influenced first and foremost by brain stem sensations. Brain stem sensations "wake up" the nervous system and help it become "ready" to support increased neural activity associated with our being alert and doing something. Brain stem sensations are important to maintain responses like

- Muscle tone,
- Equilibrium reactions,
- Physical sense of self,
- Modulated arousal, and
- Focused attention (Brodal, 1992; Kandel & Schwartz 1991, 1995).

Brain scientists tell us that about 80% of what we do is managed for us by lower brain centers, which process sensations and generate adaptive responses automatically, without our having to give a single conscious thought to what we are doing. That 80% relies directly on efficient processing of brain stem sensations. When sensory processing is disordered, one of the first things that gets compromised is the ability to do things automatically, to act adaptively without having to think about what we are doing. The 80% starts to become the 20%. That is what happens in people who have disordered sensory processing.

Of all the sensations coming into the brain, the brain stem relies most on three types of sensation to help it know when to activate and turn up the firing in multiple central nervous system mechanisms. They are

- Tactile or touch sensations,
- Proprioceptive or joint sensations, and
- Vestibular sensations from movement of the head and the pull of gravity.

Patricia Wilbarger calls these the *power sensations* because they have such an enormous influence on all aspects of brain activity. These are the same three sensations that occupational therapy practitioners have found to be so effective in their sensory techniques. For over 30 years, inspired by the likes of Margaret Rood, A. Jean Ayres, and Lorna Jean King, occupational therapists have been making it a specific point to incorporate these sensations into various treatment programs.

If you ask 100 people to name the basic senses, they will probably name touch, taste, smell, vision, and hearing. Many science textbooks do the same. Even therapists may forget to include proprioception (joint sensations) and vestibular sensations (detection of gravity and movement). Yet, we have experiences everyday that point out how important movement and joint sensations are. Think about lying back in a recliner to take a few moments to rest after a busy day. You are likely to find that you quickly become drowsy. The next thing you may notice is a voice in your head telling you it is important to get out of the chair before you fall asleep, but when you finally decide to get up you find it is impossible to move. Your brain decided that, because you were going to rest you would not need muscle tone. Consequently, it significantly reduced the messages to muscles that tell them to maintain a tonal-ready state. Why should the brain expend effort to provide something you do not need? When you decided to get up, you momentarily caught the brain off-guard. Muscle tone was needed and the brain was not prepared. Your alternative was to rely on *cortical mediation,* activity in the higher centers of the brain that involve awareness, thinking, and intention, so you could do something that would otherwise have been automatic, namely, moving. This may be akin to the experience our clients have when they have to use cortical mediation for responses that are normally automatic. It would explain their seriousness, the intensity of their concentration, their deliberateness, and their slowness to respond.

When you finally got out of the recliner, you probably discovered that, by the time you got to where you were going, you felt wide awake. In the process of moving, your brain got the strong brain stem sensation it needed to increase your alertness naturally—sensation from muscles and joints and from the vestibular apparatus in each ear. General alertness relies much more on brain stem sensations than on vision and hearing. Visual and auditory sensations are processed by higher brain centers that analyze and interpret the meaning of what you experience. To compare the difference between brain stem sensations and sensations that are processed primarily in higher brain centers, we can contrast the difference between being awake and alert versus knowing exactly where we are and what is happening once we are awake and alert. The knowing part of the equation comes from vision and hearing.

Experience has shown that sensory techniques using powerful brain stem sensation are extremely helpful with many individuals. Authors from many different fields attest to the benefits of strong brain stem sensation (Brocklehurst-Woods, 1990; Grandin, 1992; Iwasaki & Holm, 1989; McGimsey & Favell, 1988; Pearsall, 1996; Reisman, 1993; Rosenthal-Malek & Mitchell, 1997; Silver, 1993; Tomporowski & Ellis, 1985; Trott, 1993; Watters & Watters, 1980). Providing brain stem sensation takes advantage of how the human brain naturally uses sensation. Therefore, sensory techniques are relatively safe when used by someone who understands the principles of neurohabilitation. Occupational therapists have a natural treatment alternative with the potential to achieve impressive results without being intrusive or expensive. With so many benefits, one might expect a sensory approach to be embraced with open arms by service providers, especially in situations in which nothing else seems to be working. That such eagerness may not be present is an example of how lower brain centers can also influence the human response to any prospect of change.

The Challenge of Change

When occupational therapists in our institution started advocating a sensory perspective as an appropriate "primary" frame of reference for everyone, they had in mind the benefits of viewing clients first and foremost in terms of sensory needs. Knowing how effectiveness of sensory processing influences everything a person does, therapists reasoned that sensory needs could be a barrier to every person's ability to benefit from other services. Therefore, it made sense to therapists for teams to know when sensory needs were likely to be something to take into consideration.

Of course, that implied that everyone on the team accepted the legitimacy of a sensory perspective. As it turned out, this was not the case. We were advocating something many involved did not support or even understand. Therapists were not only asking strong, behaviorally oriented treatment teams to make a significant shift in their thinking, they were actually asking the whole institution to make a monumental change in how it operated. Taking sensory needs into account as a primary consideration meant that responses previously assumed to be learned behaviors might have to be interpreted in a different light. That created the possibility that intervention plans might need to be significantly modified, and that led to the strong possibility that team members might need to interact with clients in a new way. Allowing for primary sensory needs presented the possibility of major change for many levels: individual service providers, teams, design of individual programs, as well as probable overhaul of the whole organizational program. For such a major shift to occur, teams, supervisors, managers, and administrators had to make many tough, sometimes unpopular, decisions. The fact that it was a large organization, with a multidecade history of doing things one way, did not help. Even if it is not working, there can be something reassuring about doing what is most familiar.

We knew it would take time and careful planning to have minimal disruption of essential services. We knew our roles and responsibilities could change dramatically, and we were apprehensive about managing the increased demand on our time, attention, and expertise. We were also working in an organization that was dealing with recurring periods of downsizing. As the number of staff decreased, we had to keep collapsing and reconfiguring groups, which meant reorganizing staff and program locations. Downsizing also meant periodic closure of older buildings, so major relocations were needed more than once. It was a complicated and challenging work environment, not the best of circumstances for encouraging people to think about significant changes in program philosophy. Consequently, even though we understood and believed in the benefits of making the necessary changes, we, who were therapists, had our own trepidations to overcome.

Meanwhile, it was decided that the therapy department should proceed, person by person, to redesign individual program plans to take sensory needs into account. Fortunately, almost as fast as redesigned programs got started, positive results became evident. Seeing the benefits for clients so quickly certainly made it easier for people to consider a sensory frame of reference with a more open mind. The case examples at the beginning of this chapter illustrate why, despite the upheaval associated with all the changes, many people were quite positive about the new sensory perspective. Even the skeptics contributed to the effort by forcing us to answer questions and figure out solutions we otherwise might have overlooked.

Eventually, we had the opportunity to see the benefits of a fully integrated sensory model. With the change came tremendous improvement in clients, well beyond anything we would have predicted. The benefits of the change could be seen in other aspects of the institution's operation as well. For example, instead of getting citations on every standard in the licensing regulations as before, once the sensory orientation was fully in place, the program got no citations; it actually got commendations! The mask of sensory issues that made it so difficult to see the abilities and potential of the people we served had finally been removed, and people evaluating our services were as enthused and impressed by the change as we were.

The Ready Approach

In retrospect, it is evident that we were on our way to developing a new frame of reference. In the years to follow, the ideas that started to emerge from our experience in that adult program have become more crystallized. They are now assembled in a frame of reference called the *Ready Approach*. Advances in the brain sciences continue to refine our understanding of the neurobiology of behavior and how sensation can be used to influence that neurobiology. That information has helped us to further refine the theory that underlies the approach we developed for the institutionalized adults. We now know from firsthand experience that the Ready Approach can make a dramatic difference for adults and children, even those who have the most severe sensory processing problems. Even though the approach still needs to be formally tested, it has been introduced with positive results in programs for people of all ages, in all kinds of settings, all over the United States. Service providers are hungry for an approach that works, especially with adults who have severe behaviors. The Ready Approach appears to be a promising alternative that is worthy of consideration.

The frame of reference that made such a difference turned out to be a sensory perspective based on a set of assumptions rooted primarily in both

sensory integration theory and what neuroscientists tell us about the neurobiology of behavior, cognition, emotion, and consciousness. It provides an
organized approach that enables service providers to consistently and systematically

1. Determine priority needs,
2. Make appropriate recommendations to treatment teams,
3. Get visible or measurable improvement, and
4. Predict how soon and to what degree those changes are likely to
   appear.

It seems to be especially well suited for children or adults who have the most
challenging behaviors, but therapists are reporting that it enhances progress
in many other individuals as well. It is believed that the approach helps by
enhancing the ability of a person with disordered sensory processing to
respond more adaptively. It helps the disorganized or struggling nervous system to become *ready* to respond, *ready* to interact, and *ready* to catch on to
what is happening and what it means. Giving people time and sensation that
bridges the gap between being ready and just being expected to respond
seems to be a key difference. It is not unusual to see the benefits of the
approach in a single interaction, showing up as more adaptive behavior,
social interaction, or task performance.

Positive changes associated with the approach that are typically
observed or reported first include improvements in

• Alertness,
• Ability to regulate arousal,
• Interest and attention,
• Sleep-related behavior,
• Eating habits and mealtime behavior,
• Willingness and ability to dress or stay dressed, and
• Initiation of interaction with others.

Individuals served with this approach often start to look happier and
more comfortable. Over time, they are likely to spontaneously express new,
relatively complex skills that familiar care providers describe as "amazing"
and "something the person was never taught." We used the techniques associated with this approach with a man in his 30s who was blind and who
would never wear shirts. He became upset if attempts were made to put one
on him and would frantically strip as soon as someone succeeded in getting
one on him. One day, the certified occupational therapy assistant who
worked with him handed him a T-shirt and asked him to put it on. He took
it, faced it in the right direction, and put it on correctly with no assistance
whatsoever. A colleague reported her experience with a man in a different
institutional environment. He had frequent toileting accidents and never used
the toilet without maximal assistance and prompting. He had never removed

his pants or put them on by himself during toileting or any other time. One day, he just went to the bathroom without prompting, undressed to use the toilet, finished and redressed, flushed the toilet, and came out to wash his hands. All this with no assistance. The staff who worked with him could not believe the change in his degree of independence.

These are not unusual reports, nor are they isolated examples. Direct contact staff working with people getting this approach in our organization frequently reported new abilities in the daily log that they described as "incredible," something "never seen before." They described clients who for the first time approached them for positive interaction, brought them a piece of sensory equipment, like a brush, and indicated they wanted sensation. They described people who had always avoided peers who suddenly seemed to want to be with other people. Medical and dental personnel reported that clients tolerated an examination without medication and that they arrived for the appointment on their own with just one escort to assist. They found this change particularly remarkable in individuals who had been unable to tolerate examinations, who typically had needed several escorts, sometimes as many as six or seven, to get them to the appointment, at which time they would be medicated to relax or sedate them.

The ideas that now define the Ready Approach made a profound difference in our institutional setting. Many of the people we served made remarkable progress; their lives changed for the better in ways we would never have imagined possible. After years of no progress or regression, everyone started to improve. Our institution went from being threatened with decertification, which would have meant forced closure, to being identified as a model program. On every index, from personnel issues, such as sick leave use and workers' compensation claims, to measurements regarding the progression of medication reductions and the success of community-based placements, our numbers improved (Reisman & Hanschu, 1993).

Today, many organizations are still downsizing, creating recurring episodes of havoc for people who live or work in large institutions. In states across the country, political changes are altering the philosophies and financial priorities for public and private agencies, sometimes necessitating sweeping changes that drastically affect how adults are served. For years, many people have believed that it is not realistic to expect major progress in adults with severe, long-standing, well-established problems. It turns out that this kind of thinking may have a devastating consequence for the people we serve, limiting what we see as possible and, therefore, limiting what we are willing to try.

Ironically, studies reported in the *Autism Research Review International*, Volume 11, No. 1, suggest that movement out of institutions into community settings may not be the best alternative for everyone. Nevertheless, the days of large institutions seem to be coming to an end. For service providers and the people being served, these can be difficult times, when funding and politics can make our work a discouraging and frustrating experience. In the face of all that, the Ready Approach offers hope for people who have seemed unreachable. It is an alternative that can remind us all of the remarkable resilience of the human brain and its ability to recover from and rise above its experience, even when that experience is less than ideal. Occupational therapy practitioners who participate in the process are likely to find that working with adults who have the most challenging problems turns out to be an exciting, rewarding, and most enjoyable experience, regardless of the environment in which the adults are served. Our experience is also a reminder that, when we get it right, people can accomplish amazing progress. One of the great pleasures of being an occupational therapist is the opportunity to witness such improvement; but even better, we help make it happen.

A New Way to View Old Problems

The sensory processing perspective that underlies the Ready Approach is simply a frame of reference, an alternative way to view the needs of people with complex handicapping conditions associated with developmental disabilities. As a frame of reference, it influences what we see, how we describe it, what we identify as important issues, and what we consider to be an appropriate course of action. As is the case when we use any frame of reference, nothing about the person actually changes. All we are doing is looking at the same old problems in a new way. This section will describe the view from the perspective of the Ready Approach. In the Ready Approach, the concern is whether or not someone's sensory processing is effective enough to enable the person to respond adaptively. We could say the Ready Approach makes the difference between instinctive reactions and conscious responses. The crucial questions become, Is the person ready to respond, ready to interact, and ready to do something that has meaning to that person?

We have established how readiness is compromised by disordered sensory processing. But sensory processing is also compromised by lack of readiness. The brain takes in sensation. Everything enters the brain as sensation. Normally, various brain mechanisms then go to work to decode and translate the sensations into recognizable perceptions. The perceptions become information that enables the brain to catch on to what is happening, to get the meaning of what the person is experiencing. When the brain has trouble recognizing the relevance of specific sensations within the full range of sensations we experience, when certain sensations are given too much importance and other sensations are not given enough, then the brain computes a flawed set of perceptions. Meaning computed on the basis of faulty perceptions will invariably be flawed itself. This meaning, however flawed it may be, gets stored in memory for future reference. Then, when similar stimuli are present in the future, the brain decodes the sets and patterns of the stimuli from that flawed perspective, and the stage is set for a vicious cycle of disordered sensory processing.

Readiness Is the Ability to Respond

Responding occurs after the brain has analyzed the sensations coming in, computed the meaning of what we are experiencing, weighed options, considered consequences based on prior learning, and then figured out an organized response based on all it wants to accomplish through what we do. Responding is a form of replying to one's experience. It is hard to reply to something if the brain's attention is diverted to other matters. This is the problem for people who are not ready. Their brains miss important information to be gleaned from the present experience, because 80 percent of brain activity and attention is riveted to safety, survival, comfort, being free of pain or confusion, and feeling in control. Consequently, the brain disregards other information that would be relevant, and the person becomes increasingly stuck on safety and comfort needs.

Reacting is not as adaptive as responding in everyday circumstances. Reacting is important when we are in danger, so we do not waste time thinking and analyzing. Instead, our actions are triggered by the sensory stimuli in the situation. This gets us out of harm's way quickly, sometimes before we are even aware of being at risk (Goleman, 1995; LeDoux, 1996). Reactions are driven by the most primitive, pleasure-seeking, pain-avoiding brain centers. These centers do not think before they do; they do not weigh options and consider the consequences. They just fire off strong urges, moving us toward or away from specific stimuli. That is fine in emergencies, but in everyday, routine situations, reactions are clumsy and incomplete, like pieces of responses. The incompleteness makes them less than adaptive.

Because everything coming into the brain enters as sensation (Ruden, 1997), Ready proponents believe the key to facilitating more adaptive responses, to enhancing readiness, is to improve the effectiveness and efficiency of sensory processing by influencing the sensation a person takes in. This brings us to two basic goals for helping people who have disordered sensory processing. They amount to either taking something away or adding something in, to influence the sensory intake equation at any particular time.

Goal 1: Lower Demands on a Struggling Nervous System

This involves changing the environment. One option is to move someone to an environment that is already structured to lower sensory demands. Another option is to modify how people experience time, space, interactions, and activities in their present environments. Pressure on a struggling nervous system will be lowered if there are fewer distractions and interruptions, if there are more cues available to help the person predict what is going to happen next, and if there is plenty of time to settle and get reorganized before being asked to respond again. Implementing environmental changes that take sensory needs into account can sometimes make enough difference, all by itself, to bring about more adaptive behavior (Duker & Rasing, 1989; Merrill, 1990). We have observed this over and over again.

Goal 2: Provide Sensation to Enhance Brain Efficiency

People who have disordered sensory processing need increased opportunities to obtain direct, strong doses of helpful sensation. When it comes to the fundamentals of sensory processing, the most helpful sensations are brain stem sensations, like touch, proprioception, and vestibular sensation. These are the sensations that activate helpful brain chemistry, that nurture and nourish neural circuitry, that enhance the computation of meaning by giving context and perspective to the brain's interpretation of what it is experiencing.

Enhanced opportunities to get strong brain stem sensations can be provided to someone through three alternatives:

1. Hands-on techniques, such as pressure touch to body surfaces or compression or stretch to joints
2. Activities with natural opportunities to move, exert, or have physical contact, such as doing heavy work
3. Activities set up or structured to incorporate strong brain stem sensation, such as going through an obstacle course.

The most powerful results are achieved when therapists are skilled in (a) determining and treating the nature of someone's specific sensory needs and (b) designing enriched sensory diets. Ideally, services are designed to achieve both sensory goals, that is, decrease pressure on a struggling system and provide helpful sensations. Given that so much can safely be accomplished by providing an enriched sensory diet, we will consider that option first.

Enriched Sensory Diets

The term *sensory diet* refers to the kinds of sensory opportunities and experiences available to a person as part of that person's daily routine (Wilbarger & Wilbarger, 1991). Sensory diets can be influenced by modifying the environment to simultaneously add opportunities to get strong brain stem sensation while removing excessive pressure on a struggling system. People with sensory processing problems need enriched sensory diets, meaning that someone has taken special care to structure the natural day to maximize sensory benefits. Diets are especially likely to include opportunities to get large doses of helpful sensation at strategic times of the day. Some individuals get enough benefit if they just have periodic opportunities to do heavy work, that is, physical exertion using the large muscles of the body. For example, to provide heavy work opportunities at strategic times, one might structure an opportunity to stack furniture or carry books to a storage site shortly before going to the cafeteria for lunch. At the extreme of severity are people who are so overwhelmed that they have gone into a relatively permanent state of shutdown. They need sensory diets that start out being much more subdued. Until they can tolerate more sensation, such individuals may need to be served in quiet environments where the lights can be dimmed, where there are no distractions or interruptions, and where someone approaches them gently or not at all.

Enriched sensory diets almost always need to be planned on an individual basis, but many enriching opportunities can be shared by more than one person in a particular setting. It is important to remember that all human nervous systems benefit from opportunities to get strong brain stem sensation, so sensory opportunities structured to help one person often benefit everyone in a group.

Successful Treatment Depends on Effective Evaluation

Clinical reasoning is always required to match treatment choices correctly with treatment needs. In the Ready Approach, clinical reasoning begins with the ability to interpret behavioral indicators of the effectiveness of someone's sensory processing. Many therapists use the Sensory Integration Inventory for individuals who have developmental disabilities to get a profile of sensory indicators (Reisman & Hanschu, 1992). The inventory can usually be used with anyone older than age 2, but the therapist who interprets the results must be able to rule out indicators that can be explained by something else. Behaviors can look like sensory indicators but actually be symptoms of a motor control problem; an attempt to communicate; an attempt to achieve comfort from physical or emotional distress; a learned response; or a frank pathology, such as Down syndrome.

Even if someone does not have a fundamental sensory processing problem, the person may still benefit from sensory techniques based on the Ready Approach or sensory integration theory. It is important to not call something a sensory processing problem if there is another explanation that explains the symptoms nicely. It is also important to remember that, whenever we use any clinical frame of reference, whether it be behaviorism, neurodevelopment, or a sensory approach, our interpretations and conclusions can be no more than our best educated guess. The fact is, no one knows the full picture of what may be influencing someone's behavior at a particular time. We deal in possibilities and sometimes probabilities, but rarely in certainties.

It is good to know as much as possible about different clinical frames of reference, so we do not overlook the significance of a particular interpretation because of our own ignorance. Considering how often functional problems manifest as maladaptive, excessive, or challenging behaviors, it is wonderful that so many people are becoming more knowledgeable about how brain chemistry and circuitry influence behavior, especially because that influence typically affects behavior in ways that are well beyond the person's understanding or control. When we understand better, we automatically take a lot of pressure off their systems.

Recognizing Four Sensory Processing Problems

It is possible to differentiate four distinct sensory processing problems. Each relates to separate and discrete neural mechanisms involving how sensation is detected, filtered, interpreted, and incorporated into the brain's computation for readiness. Disorder in one mechanism can greatly influence or create disorder in other mechanisms. A person can have one or more of the four problems at the same time, but it seems that optimal results are usually obtained when problems are treated in this order:

1. Sensory defensiveness,
2. Disordered sensory modulation,
3. Inadequate sensory registration, and
4. Sensory integration dysfunction.

Sensory Defensiveness

There are two characteristics of someone's response that increase the probability that the person has sensory defensiveness. The first is an exaggerated avoidance of specific sensations that is out of proportion to the situation. The second is the element of surprise. Most defensive people have periodic episodes of unpredictable dramatic behavior. No one can provide an explanation for the reaction, including the person who reacted. The reaction seems so illogical that people who spend time with the defensive person may feel they need to be on their toes at all times to avoid anything that might "set the person off."

Most of what we know about defensiveness is based on the work of two occupational therapists, Patricia and Julia Wilbarger, a mother and daughter team who have collaborated in studying the issue of sensory defensiveness for many years. Patricia Wilbarger was a partner of Jean Ayres and, with Dr. Ayres, cofounded Sensory Integration International. Patricia is considered by most to be the premiere occupational therapy expert on the issue of defensiveness, having devoted the main part of her career to this single specific condition.

Joseph LeDoux's 1996 book, *The Emotional Brain,* provides an interesting take on defensiveness from the perspective of primitive memory mechanisms responsible for what he called "fear reactions." His insights, combined with those of the Wilbargers, are enabling therapists to understand, recognize, and treat defensiveness as never before, in people of all ages and functional abilities, around the world.

Defensiveness is a serious disorder that can affect anyone at anytime in his or her life span. It seems to be a crucial piece of the sensory puzzle, because it is both a common and a serious problem. In some environments, where people with severe sensory processing problems are served together in groups, the incidence of those displaying evidence of defensiveness can approach 75 percent or higher. Defensiveness to touch is by far the most common, present in about 80 percent of defensive individuals, according to Wilbarger and Wilbarger (1991). Their estimate is certainly consistent with our observations.

People can also be defensive to movement (vestibular sensations), oral sensations, and sounds and even to visual stimuli and odors. It is not unusual to work with people who are defensive to more than one type of sensation. As far back as the 1970s, Barbara Knickerbocker, the occupational therapist who gave us the term *sensory defensiveness,* was already reporting dyads and triads of sensation, especially the triad involving touch, sounds, and olfactory sensations (Knickerbocker, 1980). She had observed that, if the children she served displayed an aversion to one of the sensations in the triad, they were likely to display some degree of aversion to the other two. Many people with developmental disabilities find movement unpleasant or even frightening. Individuals who display defensiveness or an aversion to movement or postural changes, like those who are defensive to touch, tend to be hypervigilant or too preoccupied with the potential for the offending sensations to give adequate attention to other matters. Thus, defensiveness alone can create the appearance of significant sensory processing problems, which may disappear once the defensiveness has been treated.

It is not hard to see how defensiveness creates a major barrier to a person's ability to interact freely and benefit from other treatments. Occupational therapy practitioners should be familiar with the diagnosis and treatment of sensory defensiveness because this processing disorder is easy to miss, especially in its more subtle forms. Given what we know now, it is difficult to justify defensiveness remaining in someone's system when the Wilbarger protocol can be such an effective treatment.

Disordered Sensory Modulation

This is a significant problem affecting self-regulation of arousal. In some settings, it is likely to be as, or even more, common than defensiveness. Sensory modulation problems usually show up as overarousal (hyperactivity), attentional problems (distractibility), or shutdown—a paradoxical problem of looking underaroused when you are actually so overly aroused your brain dampens sensation to keep you more comfortable. Disordered modulation can also show up in the form of fluctuating arousal and underarousal, in which someone has difficulty maintaining sufficient alertness to even remain awake or aware of the environment. Overarousal and distractibility often go hand-in-hand. People with both are likely to engage in stereotypic behaviors, especially persistent self-stimulation. In general, self-stimulation can be evidence of other problems, but when it is present in people who also have difficulty with transitions, it is important to consider the probability that the person has disordered sensory modulation.

Inadequate Sensory Registration

This is a problem that can involve heightened as well as diminished detection of specific sensations, either having the potential to cause significant secondary problems. An example of overregistration would be the person who fixates on visual stimuli in the ambient field. When we focus attention on one type of stimuli, registration of other stimuli is dampened (Hobson, 1994). Hyperfocusing can lead to an imbalance in how stimuli in a particular sensory channel are registered. Registration problems, however, show up most commonly as underregistration of vestibular sensation (movement) that tends to make the person uninterested in moving. The subsequent lack of movement can lead to something akin to sensory deprivation, with secondary underregistration of proprioception (joint and muscle sensations) that, in turn, can lead to inadequate physical sense of self, directly compromising someone's ability to get the meaning of what they experience (Damasio, 1994; Greenspan, 1997). Impaired tactile discrimination, another form of inadequate registration, often improves on its own as registration of vestibular and proprioceptive sensation improves, again showing that problems registering sensations in one system can lead to impaired registration of other sensations. Adequate vestibular processing does seem to be a basic need. It is important for all movement—for bilateral abilities, perceptual abilities, and most task-related responses. We frequently see individuals whose inadequate vestibular registration severely compromises their overall functional skill and independence. Fortunately, this is a problem that seems quite amenable to treatment, and the main challenge for the therapist is to recognize when it is present.

Sensory Integration Dysfunction

Sensory integration involves the ability of the central nervous system to take in sensations from different sensory channels at the same time; to filter, organize, and sort the sensations, in order to discern their meaning; and then to use the sensation and its meaning to generate an adaptive response. The differentiating feature of sensory integration and sensory registration is the difference between processing multichannel sensations entering the nervous system at the same time (integration) and the ability to discriminate aspects of specific stimuli entering through one sensory channel (registration).

Sensory integration is the most sophisticated aspect of sensory processing, in that it requires effective communication between lower and higher brain centers to ensure that responses are well suited to the situation, well planned, and well executed. It is difficult for sensory integration to be adequate if one or more of the other sensory processing mechanisms is disordered or inefficient. Nevertheless, unless sensory integration is itself disordered, improvement in the other aspects of sensory processing almost always leads to direct improvement in sensory integration. Therefore, it is wise to withhold judgment about someone's sensory integration until all other sensory processing problems have been treated.

Therapists who specialize in the application of sensory integration theory have much to offer individuals whose sensorimotor difficulties are more subtle. For example, children with learning disabilities or attention deficit disorders often benefit greatly from sensory integration therapy designed to improve their gross and fine motor abilities. One of the most common referral requests for children with sensory integration dysfunction, for example, is the need for help to improve handwriting ability. The child's behavior and general responses may seem relatively appropriate, but motor tasks requiring rapid and precise adjustments may be difficult. Sensory integration dysfunction can be present in people whose behavior may seem adaptive. This can be contrasted with people who have defensiveness, sensory modulation, or sensory registration problems, in which evidence of a problem manifests as too much, too little, or inappropriate behavior.

Sensory integration has been regarded by many therapists as something of an umbrella ability, with modulation and registration considered to be aspects of sensory integration. Our severely challenged adults taught us that it is important to differentiate them as separate problems in order to treat them as separate problems. Treating the problems separately yields much faster and much bigger improvement, especially in people with severely disordered sensory processing.

This does not diminish the importance of diagnosing and treating sensory integration dysfunction. Sensory integration is likely to be a higher priority concern in people who have more adaptive behavior than in those who benefit most from the Ready Approach. If sensory integration is disordered and left untreated, it invariably leads to secondary social and psychological problems, even in people who appear to be quite capable. Nevertheless, in adults who have the most severe sensory processing problems, there are usually higher priority needs to address, related to defensiveness, and modulation or registration problems. Sensory integration is usually the least of our initial concerns.

Following Through Based on the Sensory Profile

Once there is evidence of priority sensory needs, the next step is to formulate a hypothesis about how much each of the four sensory processing problems is a factor for the person. Sorting out the nature and relative effectiveness of different sensory processing mechanisms is important, because it is easy to do too much too fast. Donna Williams is an incredibly articulate woman who struggles on a daily basis with severe sensory processing problems. In her remarkable 1996 book *Autism: An Inside-Out Approach,* she describes the kinds of sensory challenges faced by many people with autism and explains how using a sensory integration approach may be an example of trying to do too much, too soon. We have ample clinical evidence that doing too much, too fast overwhelms many struggling nervous systems, compromising the results we can achieve. People with the most complex and severe sensory processing problems find it much more helpful to take things in order, one step at a time. When this is done, the brain is much better able to keep up and benefit from the sensory opportunity, forming improved circuitry, including memory circuits, which make it easier for the brain to build on what it is learning. Rather than slowing down the rate of progress, taking things more slowly and in order helps the brain keep up and improve its efficiency faster which, of course, translates to faster improvement in adaptive behavior as well.

Transdisciplinary Teamwork

It is clear that the more fully a sensory perspective is integrated into a person's ongoing experience, the better and faster the results. There simply is no substitute for everyone being able to respond whenever sensory needs arise, and needs can arise anytime, anywhere. Therefore, when a sensory processing perspective, such as the Ready Approach, becomes the frame of reference for a treatment program, everyone involved needs to understand sensory processing disorders and how to help. The more they understand, the more likely they will automatically start working together more closely in a transdisciplinary team model. In such a model, specialists shift some of their focus from direct client service to educating and collaborating with coworkers. Such a shift can be hard for teams and parents to support (unless they have experienced its benefits), especially if their experience has been one of dwindling service associated with consultative models.

Transdisciplinary teamwork is not about consultation; it is about working side-by-side to get the job done. When therapists participate in a transdisciplinary model, they do not relinquish responsibility for sensory services. To the contrary, they maintain accountability even as they strive to share and exchange roles with team members to facilitate fuller integration of services.

People who have sensory processing problems and developmental disabilities have what the general systems theorist, Russell Ackoff, calls a *MESS* of problems: multiple, complex, and interdependent. People with messes of problems rely on us to provide services that fit their needs. That means our services are organized and delivered by team members whose efforts are well coordinated and supportive of each other. Using a sensory approach can create challenges for team members and organizations that are not accustomed to taking sensory needs into account, but a successful effort can transform lives.

Frequency of Service in the Ready Approach

Over the several years in which we were sharpening our understanding and skills related to sensory issues, one thing was always clear: The more sensory service we provided, the better the results we got. When the sensory services were started, therapy time was not integrated into the daily routine. Treatments were provided in isolated clinics; sessions typically lasted about 30 minutes, usually scheduled twice a week. Almost everyone served at the facility got occupational therapy because it was assumed that giving everyone some therapy was better than giving some individuals more and others none.

It was soon apparent that results from sensory services warranted more therapy time, so two decisions were made. One was that therapy services would be reorganized to provide more intensive treatment to fewer individuals. The second was that therapy staff would stop providing any service that could be provided by someone else. This would enable therapy staff to concentrate their efforts solely on sensory matters and intensify services for those who were considered the highest priority cases. A few receiving intensified service were seen as much as twice a day, sometimes for 45 minutes at a time, but this contact continued to occur in isolated clinics rather than in the clients' typical environments.

Once again, results indicated that more service was warranted. Progress was very evident with the sensory-oriented efforts. People were improving fast and in big ways, and everyone wanted to capitalize on the momentum. So, therapy staff were reorganized once again. This time, in an attempt to bring the therapy service into the natural setting, therapy staff members were scheduled for blocks of time in different work areas where several people with priority sensory needs were served. Again, people receiving more sensory services improved faster and more dramatically, and teams wanted even more intensive sensory service.

Finally, the largest day program of the institution, involving 90 clients, was restructured under the direct supervision of the therapy staff. To facilitate this change, it became more difficult for people who were not served in that day program to receive occupational therapy, although essential support services, requiring someone with occupational therapy expertise, continued to be available on a consulting basis. For people in the subject day program, however, the change meant being immersed in a totally sensory-oriented routine. There were no pull-out services and no isolated clinics, and therapy staff with sensory expertise were influential decision makers for all aspects of the program.

Each of the previous changes to intensify sensory services had yielded faster and bigger gains in the people served, but none of these results was anything like the gains achieved when the sensory service was fully integrated into someone's overall program. The full sensory orientation clearly resulted in the most impressive improvement for the largest number of individuals. In fact, after comparing what could be achieved through fully integrated service versus supportive or consulting service, all clinics and therapy equipment were given up for program areas in which there was a commitment to using sensory approaches, even with minimal support from occupational therapy.

Summary of What We Learned

1. All Behavior Must Be a Product of Sensory Processing.
If that were not the case, why would there be such a direct correlation between improved behavior and intensity of sensory-oriented service?

2. Sensory Approaches Foster Positive Dynamic Interactions.
Among the many changes that occurred as we shifted to a sensory frame of reference were increasingly positive interactions among the people associated with the programs: staff and clients. Staff became more client centered, more gentle and responsive with clients. Where relationships had formerly been characterized by the need to control, staff became much more accepting and respectful of client preferences and choices. Staff also became more respectful with each other, and some clients began to approach others for positive interaction.

3. People Achieve So Much More When They See the Value of What They Are Doing.
People who have severe sensory needs do not have time for team members to argue about territorial issues or matters of control. They need people working on their behalf who know how to share and release aspects of their expertise with and to other team members. Service providers who move from one place to another, seeing many different settings and people, have a very different experience from those who provide continuous service to the same group in the same setting, day after day. As therapy staff, we had never understood that as much as we did after we were assigned responsibility for a whole-day program unit. There is no substitute for being in the shoes of someone else, nor for on-site priming, than immediate feedback, correction,

or compliment one provider can share with another in the real work situation. What we accomplished in the 10th year, despite the layoffs and reorganization necessitated by downsizing, was truly incredible, something that would never have been possible if the majority of staff had not been similarly committed to making it work. The difference had to be related to their belief that we were finally on the right track, "in it together," doing something that made sense, and getting results that made the effort worthwhile. By the 10th year, most of the staff were quite familiar with what we understood about meeting sensory needs. No matter how much positive feedback we had provided, no matter how much administration recognized employees for outstanding achievement, no matter what kind of supervision they received, the real change in staff occurred when they saw, firsthand, the results they could achieve with sensory strategies.

4. Sensory Approaches Show Respect for Differences.

Interpreting the behavior of others from one's personal point of view is fraught with problems. The terrible toll of misunderstanding or misinterpreting someone's response, especially missing the sensory implication, is evident all around us (Masters & McGuire, 1994) and is poignantly described by those who can tell us what it feels like to be misunderstood—for instance, Anne, the narrator of the film *Learning About Learning Disabilities*.

It seems inconsistent to appreciate the power of the human brain without recognizing the effort it will expend to do things right. Those who have the most severe problems sometimes have the most remarkable abilities, abilities that we may not be able to see because they are hidden behind a mask of sensory issues. Meanwhile, their behavior may be so challenging that we fight exhaustion to get it changed. It is ironic that those who have the most severe problems do not stay awake at night trying to figure out ways to make our lives difficult, yet, when we do not understand, we may stay awake at night unintentionally figuring out ways to make their lives difficult by focusing on how to change their behavior. If our inclination is to interpret the behavior of others as something they do with motives we ascribe to them, then we will invariably put even more pressure on a nervous system that is already struggling. We would never insist that a paralyzed person in a wheelchair walk up a flight of stairs; yet, we may do something comparable to people whose symptoms of sensory processing problems we do not understand.

In their wonderful book about appreciating people who are different, Anne Donnellan, a behavioral psychologist, and Martha Leary, a speech and language pathologist, remind us that behavior does not automatically need to be changed just because it is different. They ask us to imagine what happens if we try to put ourselves in the other person's place, and they predict that we will begin to see the person as quite remarkable. Remarkable because this person may be struggling to stay in an interaction, to contain a behavior, or to keep from disturbing a situation with involuntary movements. With such a perception we begin to see our relationship to that person very differently. This is a person to learn from as well as to teach. This is a person to work with, not to work on. This is a person who has likely found strategies to accommodate for his or her differences and to keep disturbance to a minimum. Our job is to help expand and extend those strategies, not for the person but with the person. (Donnellan & Leary, 1995, p. 57)

For us to respect differences in people, we must accept that there are differences, differences we may not understand. Such acceptance helps us to interact with the person from a perspective that does not, in and of itself, become a limiting factor for us and one more barrier for those who are different from us.

When we use sensory approaches, instead of judging someone's behavior, we take into account that the responses we see may well be beyond a person's control. With a sensory perspective, we are much more likely to respond to the person rather than act on the person. With sensory-oriented eyes, we use a gentle approach, one that encourages, invites, and entices rather than one that demands, coerces, or controls. Imagine the relief that brings to a struggling nervous system!

5. Behavioral Technology Is Different From a Behavioral Approach.
Behavioral technology helps us to be objective, collect reliable data, and operationalize what we say to make it clearer. It is a must for monitoring progress and making valid treatment decisions. However, behavioral technology is not the same as using a behavioral approach. The first helps us to evaluate the results of our services. The latter is a clinical perspective that influences how we view people. By posing restrictions on our consideration of why behavior might be occurring, behaviorism becomes somewhat arbitrary. Why would anyone serving people with behavior-related needs not want to consider other explanations for the behavior, especially if behavioral interventions are not yielding results? Even if behavioral interventions get results, the issue may be less the results and more the cost of those results. What does the change in behavior mean for the person whose behavior was changed? What if the behavioral view turns out to be too limited, as asserted by two Nobel laureates, Gerald Edelman (1992) and Francis Crick (1994)? What if there is more to behavior than just learned responses?

6. There Is No Single Clinical Perspective That Is the Answer for Everyone.
Interdisciplinary teams, serving a wide variety of individuals, should be able to evaluate several options and alternative views to find what works best for specific individuals. Someone may do best by starting with services based on

one approach but, as improvement occurs, there may come a time when another approach will be more helpful. It is important to select the approach on the basis of the person's need rather than expect the person to fit the available or prevailing approach.

7. Programs That Try to Provide Something for Everyone Are Likely to Diminish Their Effectiveness With Anyone.

There are multiple ways to organize services and configure groupings for large numbers of people. Optimal results come with services that are focused to target specific kinds of needs for specific kinds of individuals. It is difficult and impractical to provide for several alternatives when groups are small, but when many people are being served, a single large program can be organized into several different subprograms to provide access to more specialized service.

8. Being a Good Therapist, Whatever Approach You Use, Involves Being a Good Problem Solver.

That means recognizing the difference between problems and solutions. We eliminate problems by figuring out appropriate solutions. If we figure out wonderful solutions but have not correctly identified the problem, we may not get the results we seek. Program planning, like treatment planning, can be only as effective as the accuracy with which one identifies needs.

Summary of Ideas Related to the Ready Approach

Ideas From the Neurosciences

1. All behavior is fundamentally a product of the neurobiology of the brain.
2. Brain efficiency is dependent on the effectiveness of various neural mechanisms involving brain centers and the neural circuitry and neurochemistry that enable them to communicate with each other.
3. Strong brain stem sensation has a profound and pervasive influence on brain chemistry and subsequently on the circuitry that enables multiple brain mechanisms to function properly.
4. Neural plasticity makes it possible for the brain to improve its own efficiency for the whole of its life span.
5. Disordered sensory processing may compromise the brain's ability to take full advantage of its many varied sensory opportunities.
6. The human brain thrives on sensation, particularly touch, movement, and body sensations. If it does not get enough of these important sensations, it may drive a person to engage in behaviors that produce the desired sensations.
7. The human brain does not drive a person to engage in self-injurious behavior or persistent self-stimulation unless there is something seriously wrong.

Ideas That Parallel Sensory Integration Theory

1. We can draw inferences about the efficiency and effectiveness of sensory processing by interpreting, from a sensory perspective, the products of brain activity—for instance, behavior, emotion, cognition, and motor responses.

2. Keeping in mind that everything the brain takes in is sensation, we can influence the efficiency of the brain by influencing what sensation the brain experiences.

3. The ultimate goal for efficient sensory processing is adaptive participation in functional activities that are meaningful to the person. There is no substitute for what can be achieved to improve brain efficiency through purposeful engagement in appealing activities and interactions.

Ideas Specific to the Ready Approach

1. There Are Four Different Sensory Processing Problems.
Each should be considered a separate problem, although some people display evidence of multiple problems, sometimes secondary to one or more that are primary. Primary problems should be treated first and, in the presence of more than one primary problem, there is a specific order in which the problems should be treated to achieve optimal results.

2. Readiness Is a Bridge Between Sensory Processing and Adaptive Behavior.
Being ready to respond means the brain is able to catch on to what is happening, generate adaptive responses, and keep up with new situational demands. When the brain has achieved a ready state, the person can participate in functional activities and interactions with just the right amount of challenges without becoming overwhelmed, confused, or distressed. When the brain is not ready, any sensory demand can be too much.

3. Sustained Optimal Arousal Eliminates Sensory-Driven Behaviors.
Small recurring doses of helpful sensation increase the probability that a challenged person will be able to maintain readiness and benefit from other available services without having to engage in sensory-driven socially maladaptive behaviors.

4. Adaptive Behavior Is Acquired in Natural Routines.
Sensory strategies, designed to enhance readiness, should be delivered in the context of the natural routine, provided that the setting is sensory sensitive—modified to lower sensory demands for overly challenged individuals. Nothing improves behavior, performance, interaction, or learning like the opportunity to participate in functional activities that have purpose and meaning for the individual—if the individual is ready.

5. Everyone Benefits.

All humans benefit from enriched sensory diets, not just people with disabilities, and everyone benefits when anyone with disordered sensory processing improves. The payoffs include more efficient use of resources and more productive and happier people—clients, family members, care providers, and service administrators.

The case examples at the beginning of this chapter illustrate the difference sensory approaches made for some of the adults served in one large state-operated institution. Every person in the examples had a primary diagnosis of profound mental retardation. All had been served at the same institution for at least 15 years. All had grossly impaired communication, with no reliable means of communicating and no consistent reliable responses to what was communicated to them. Severe behavior problems were well documented for each of them, and a variety of intensive behavioral interventions had been tried without success. Each person also had been prescribed a variety of strong medications, sometimes in combination. None had a history of seizures. All had shown little or no progress for many years. Since 1990, hundreds of adults have been served with sensory programs based on what is now being called the Ready Approach. This work has occurred in different states and involved multiple service providers in varied service settings. Many of the individuals served have improved in comparable ways to the case examples, some with even more dramatic results. Our experience with the Ready Approach has been encouraging, to say the least.

Successful intervention based on a sensory processing perspective requires an understanding of

- How the brain responds to sensation;
- The neurobiology of behavior, emotion, and consciousness;
- The four sensory processing problems;
- The power sensations and how they influence the brain; and
- How the power sensations can be used to enhance the neurobiology of the central nervous system.

This requires advanced expertise and keeping pace with the findings of neurologists, who are making new discoveries at an exponential rate. There is still much to be learned. In the past 10 years alone, scientists have learned more about the brain and how it influences and is influenced by experience than was known in all the years before that time (Kotulak, 1996).

With the Ready Approach, we are capitalizing on the incredible new insights of these scientists. It is possible that, like the imaging that now makes it possible to trace a thought through the brain, there may be some new technology on the horizon that will make the best and most current insights obsolete, just as our understanding today makes us wonder about the wisdom of so many of our practices of the past. However, for now, everyone involved in sensory-oriented services needs to understand how human brains need and use sensation to increase their efficiency. Without such understanding, it is difficult to make appropriate situational judgments related to what sensation is needed, how much, and how to provide it.

Issues related to sensory processing disorders are complex, and the details of the Ready Approach and how it works are beyond the scope of this chapter. Occupational therapy practitioners, however, can learn this approach and have access to advanced sensory-related expertise in a variety of ways. Most therapists are introduced to sensory integration theory in their basic training. That becomes an important foundation on which to build, but the evaluation and treatment of individuals who have severe sensory processing problems requires advanced specialist training.

Increased knowledge and technical proficiency related to sensory services can be obtained by working with therapists who are skilled in using sensory approaches. When looking for mentors, we must bear in mind that the measurement for success is in the outcome for clients. Impressive results are much more important than impressive programs. Many service providers welcome qualified therapists for work–study or mentorship programs. Continuing education activities can include formal courses in colleges and universities and courses designed and sponsored by organizations, such as the American Occupational Therapy Association, which offers several innovative and flexible choices to accommodate different learner styles and preferences. Several continuing education sponsors concentrate their efforts on training and on publications for those who are specifically interested in sensory issues, and there is an increasing number of Internet sites that enable people with this interest to network, share ideas, and learn from each other. The companies listed under "Continuing Education Resources" are especially concerned with sensory-oriented subject matter. Several publications are listed in the "Related Reading" section at the end of this chapter. Any one of them can be a good place to start.

Conclusion

In this chapter, we have talked about the challenges and potential benefits associated with viewing adults who have developmental disabilities from a sensory perspective. The development of a specific sensory-oriented frame of reference was described, and several examples were provided to illustrate the kinds of issues service providers might face, if they were to introduce a sensory processing frame of reference into a long-term-care program. It was shown that the specific sensory-oriented approach advocated for adults with severe behavioral challenges is based on, but different from, sensory integration theory. It was also shown that new information available in the neurosciences provides the scientific rationale for many features of the approach that builds on current understanding about the neurobiology of behavior, emotion, awareness, and cognition.

Sensory strategies associated with the Ready Approach can be an efficient, effective, and relatively permanent treatment for many adults who have not responded favorably to any other intervention alternative. Occupational therapy practitioners have a unique advantage in using the Ready Approach for two reasons: (a) their neurohabilitative background makes it possible for them to make differential diagnoses related to sensorimotor problems, and (b) they are experts at modifying and adapting environments and activities to match special needs. No one has background and training better suited for identifying sensory needs and designing intervention strategies, including sensory diets that take sensory needs into account. What a perfect match: occupational therapy practitioners and adults with developmental disabilities!

Acknowledgments

I referred to "we" throughout this chapter because of the many people who contributed to the evolution of the Ready Approach, but I particularly want to acknowledge our consultant, mentor, and colleague, Judith Reisman, PhD, OTR, FAOTA, who opened our eyes and taught us how to see.

References

Aoki, C., & Siekevitz, P. (1988, December). Plasticity in brain development. *Scientific American*, pp. 56–64.

Ayres, A. J. (1972). *Sensory integration and learning disorders*. Los Angeles: Western Psychological Services.

Bidabe, L. (1991). *M.O.V.E. curriculum for mobility opportunities via education program*. Bakersfield, CA: Kern County Schools.

Brocklehurst-Woods, J. (1990). The use of tactile and vestibular stimulation to reduce stereotypic behaviors in two adults with mental retardation. *American Journal of Occupational Therapy, 44*, 536–541.

Brodal, P. (1992). *The central nervous system*. New York: Oxford University Press.

Chopra, D. (1989). *Quantum healing*. New York: Bantam Books.

Churchland, P. (1993). *Neurophilosophy: Toward a unified science of the mind/brain*. Cambridge, MA: MIT Press.

Crick, F. (1994). *The astonishing hypothesis*. New York: Charles Scribner's Sons.

Damasio, A. (1994). *Descartes' error: Emotion, reason, and the human brain*. New York: G. P. Putnam's Sons.

Donnellan, A., & Leary, M. (1995). *Movement differences and diversity in autism/mental retardation*. Madison, WI: DRI Press.

Duker, P. C., & Rasing, E. (1989). Effects of redesigning the physical environment on self-stimulation and on task behavior in three autistic-type developmentally disabled individuals. *Journal of Autism and Developmental Disorders, 19*, 449–461.

Durand, V. M., & Crimmins, D. B. (1988). Identifying the variables maintaining self-injurious behavior. *Journal of Autism and Developmental Disorders, 18*, 99–117.

Durig, A. (1996). *Autism and the crisis of meaning*. New York: New York State University Press.

Edelman, G. (1992). *Bright air, brilliant fire: On the matter of the mind*. New York: Basic Books.

Fisher, A., Murray, E., & Bundy, A. (1991). *Sensory integration theory and practice*. Philadelphia: F. A. Davis.

Gazzaniga, M. (1988). *Mind matters: How mind and brain interact to create our conscious lives*. Boston: Houghton-Mifflin.

Gazzaniga, M. (1992). *Nature's mind: The biological roots of thinking, emotions, sexuality, language, and intelligence*. New York: Basic Books.

Gazzaniga, M. (Ed.). (1995). *Cognitive neurosciences*. Cambridge, MA: MIT Press.

Goleman, D. (1995). *Emotional intelligence*. New York: Bantam Books.

Grandin, T. (1992). Calming effects of deep touch pressure in patients with autistic disorder, college students, and animals. *Journal of Child and Adolescent Psychopharmacology, 2*(1), 63–72.

Greenspan, S. (1997). *Growth of the mind*. Reading, MA: Addison-Wesley.

Hobson, J. (1994). *Chemistry of conscious states: How the brain changes its mind*. Boston: Little, Brown.

Iwasaki, K., & Holm, M. (1989). Sensory treatment for the reduction of stereotypic behaviors in persons with severe multiple disabilities. *Occupational Therapy Journal of Research, 9*, 170–183.

Joseph, R. (1993). *The naked neuron*. New York: Plenum Press.

Kandel, E., & Schwartz, J. (1991). *Principles of neural science* (3rd ed.). New York: Elsevier Science.

Kandel, E., & Schwartz, J. (1995). *Essentials of neural science and behavior*. Norwalk, CT: Appleton & Lange.

Knickerbocker, B. (1980). *Holistic approach to the treatment of learning disorders*. Thorofare, NJ: Slack.

Kotulak, R. (1996). *Inside the brain: Revolutionary discoveries of how the mind works*. Kansas City, MO: Andrews & McMeel.

Kuno, M. (1995). *Synapse: Function, plasticity, and neurotrophism*. New York: Oxford University Press.

LeDoux, J. (1996). *The emotional brain*. New York: Simon & Schuster.

Levitan, I., & Kaczmarek, L. (1997). *Neuron: Cell and molecular biology*. New York: Oxford University Press.

Lovaas, I., Newsom, C., & Hickman, C. (1987). Self-stimulatory behavior and perceptual reinforcement. *Journal of Applied Behavior Analysis, 20*, 45–68.

Masters, R., & McGuire, M. (1994). *Neurotransmitter revolution: Serotonin, social behavior, and the law*. Carbondale: Southern Illinois University Press.

McGimsey, J. F., & Favell, J. E. (1988). The effects of increased physical exercise on disruptive behavior in retarded persons. *Journal of Autism and Developmental Disorders, 18*, 167–179.

Merrill, S. (1990). *Environment: Implications for occupational therapy practice*. Bethesda, MD: American Occupational Therapy Association.

Mosey, A. (1981). *Occupational therapy: Configuration of a profession*. New York: Raven Press.

Nicholls, D. (1994). *Proteins, transmitters, and synapses*. Cambridge, MA: Blackwell Science.

Nuland, S. (1997). *Wisdom of the body*. New York: Alfred Knopf.

Pearsall, P. (1996). *Pleasure prescription*. Alameda, CA: Hunter House.

Rahmann, H., & Rahmann, M. (1992). *Neurobiological basis of memory and behavior*. New York: Springer-Verlag.

Reed, K. (1984). *Models of practice in occupational therapy*. Baltimore: Williams & Wilkins.

Reisman, J. (1993). Using a sensory integrative approach to treat self-injurious behavior in an adult with profound mental retardation. *American Journal of Occupational Therapy, 47,* 403–411.

Reisman, J., & Hanschu, B. (1992). *Sensory Integration Inventory–Revised for individuals with developmental disabilities: User's guide.* Hugo, MN: PDP Press.

Reisman, J., & Hanschu, B. (1993). Using the consultative model to introduce sensory integration services for adults with developmental disabilities. *Occupational Therapy Practice, 4*(4), 38–46.

Rosenthal-Malek, A., & Mitchell, S. (1997). Effects of exercise on the self-stimulatory behaviors and positive responding of adolescents with autism. *Journal of Autism and Developmental Disorders, 27,* 193–202.

Royeen, C., & Lane, S. (1991). Tactile processing and sensory defensiveness. In A. Fisher, E. Murray, & A. Bundy (Eds.), *Sensory integration theory and practice.* Philadelphia: F. A. Davis.

Ruden, R. (1997). *The craving brain.* New York: HarperCollins.

Shepherd, G. (1988). *Neurobiology* (2nd ed.). New York: Oxford University Press.

Silver, L. (1993). *Dr. Larry Silver's advice to parents on attention-deficit hyperactivity disorder.* Washington, DC: American Psychiatric Press.

Tomporowski, P. D., & Ellis, N. R. (1985). The effects of exercise on the health, intelligence, and adaptive behavior of institutionalized severely and profoundly mentally retarded adults: A systematic replication. *Applied Research in Mental Retardation, 6,* 465–473.

Trott, M. (1993). *SenseAbilities: Understanding sensory integration.* Tucson, AZ: Therapy SkillBuilders.

Watters, R. G., & Watters, W. E. (1980). Decreasing self-stimulatory behavior with physical exercise in a group of autistic boys. *Journal of Autism and Developmental Disorders, 10,* 379–387.

West, T. (1991). *In the mind's eye: Visual thinkers, gifted people with learning difficulties, computer images, and the ironies of creativity.* Buffalo, NY: Prometheus Books.

Wilbarger, P., & Wilbarger, J. (1991). *Sensory defensiveness in children ages 2–12: An intervention guide for parents and other caretakers.* Santa Barbara, CA: Avanti Educational Programs.

Williams, D. (1996). *Autism: An inside-out approach.* Bristol, PA: Jessica Kingsley.

Related Reading

Ayres, A. J. (1979). *Sensory integration and the child.* Los Angeles: Western Psychological Services.

Baars, B. (1997). *In the theater of consciousness: The workspace of the mind.* New York: Oxford University Press.

Baron-Cohen, S. (1995). *Mindblindness: An essay on autism and theory of mind.* Cambridge, MA: MIT Press.

Bauman, M. (1991). Microscopic neuro anatomic abnormalities in autism. *Pediatrics, 78,* 791–796.

Bauman, M., & Kemper, T. (1995). *Neurobiology of autism.* Baltimore: Johns Hopkins University Press.

Cataldo, M. R., & Harris, J. (1982). The biological basis for self-injury in the mentally retarded. *Analysis and Intervention in Developmental Disabilities, 2,* 21–39.

Churchland, P., & Sejnowski, T. (1992). *Computational brain.* Cambridge, MA: MIT Press.

Comings, D. E. (1990). *Tourette syndrome and human behavior.* Duarte, CA: Hope Press.

Courchesne, E., Yeung-Courchesne, R., Press, G. A., Hesselking, J. R., & Jernigan, T. L. (1988). Hypoplasia of cerebellar vernal lobules VI and VII in autism. *New England Journal of Medicine, 318,* 1349–1354.

Davis, J. (1997). *Mapping the mind: The secrets of the human brain and how it works.* Secaucus, NJ: Birch Lane Press.

Grandin, T. (1992). An inside view of autism. In E. Schopler & G. Mesibov (Eds.), *High-functioning individuals with autism* (pp. 105–126). New York: Plenum Press.

Grandin, T. (1995). *Thinking in pictures.* New York: Doubleday.

Greenspan, S. (1995). *Challenging child: Understanding, raising, and enjoying the five "difficult" types of children.* New York: Addison-Wesley.

Hallowell, E., & Ratey, J. (1995). *Driven to distraction: Recognizing and coping with attention deficit disorder from childhood through adulthood.* New York: Touchstone.

Hartmann, T. (1993). *Attention deficit disorder: A different perception.* Grass Valley, CA: Underwood Books.

Hartmann, T. (1995). *ADD success stories.* Grass Valley, CA: Underwood Books.

Irlen, H. (1991). *Reading by the colors: Overcoming dyslexia and other reading disabilities through the Irlen method.* Garden City Park, NY: Avery.

Kinnealey, M., Oliver, B., & Wilbarger, P. (1995). A phenomenological study of sensory defensiveness in adults. *American Journal of Occupational Therapy, 49,* 444–451.

Ratey, J., & Johnson, C. (1997). *Shadow syndromes.* New York: Pantheon.

Reisman, J., & Gross, A. (1992). Psychophysiological measurement of treatment effects in an adult with sensory defensiveness. *Canadian Journal of Occupational Therapy, 59,* 248–257.

Sacks, O. (1970). *The man who mistook his wife for a hat.* New York: Harper & Row.

Sacks, O. (1995). *An anthropologist on Mars.* New York: Knopf.

Williams, D. (1992). *Nobody nowhere.* New York: Times Books.

Williams, D. (1994). *Somebody somewhere.* New York: Times Books.

Williams, M., & Shellenberger, S. (1994). *How does your engine run? The alert program for self-regulation.* Albuquerque, NM: Therapy Works.

Continuing Education Resources

The following organizations have offerings that are specifically geared to adults:

Developmental Concepts
(Courses, publications, and consultation related to the Ready Approach)
P.O. Box 31759
Phoenix, AZ 85046-1759
Phone: (602) 482-0572
(888) 287-3239 or (888) AT READY
Fax: (602) 482-9851
E-mail: atready@bitstream.net

Future Horizons
(Courses, conferences, and publications, including video- and audio-
tapes, all related to autism)
422 Lamar Boulevard East, Suite 106
Arlington, TX 76011
Phone: (800) 489-0727
Fax: (817) 277-2270
E-mail: edfuture@onramp.net

Professional Development Programs and PDP Products
(Courses, including defensiveness; publications, including the
Inventory; and products, all related to serving people with severe
developmental disabilities. PDP's annual symposium is considered
a must by many therapists working in the area of developmental
disabilities)
14398 North 59th Street
Oak Park Heights, MN 55082
Phone: (612) 439-8865
Fax: (612) 439-0421

CHAPTER 5

Low-Vision Intervention for Adults With Developmental Disabilities

T. Ann Williams, OTR/L

Introduction

The following chapter addresses visual dysfunction and the adult who is developmentally disabled, but it focuses primarily on the evaluation and treatment of visual dysfunction. It is intended to provide basic knowledge regarding the causes of vision loss, vision evaluation, and treatment of the functional problems that result. All daily living tasks can be affected by visual dysfunction, including self-care tasks, meal preparation, vocational tasks, and leisure activities. No matter what other disabilities the individual has, evaluation and treatment principles of vision loss are the same. As with any intervention used with the population with developmental disabilities, appropriate modifications should be made for individual cognitive and physical abilities.

Background

People with developmental disabilities encounter myriad obstacles in their attempts to adapt to their environment. These obstacles include a variety of chronic conditions manifested in childhood that include physical, psychological, and cognitive impairments. Impairments of the visual system occur with high frequency in this population. It has been reported that the rate of incidence ranges from 48 percent to 75 percent (Manacker, 1993). The most common disorders that affect these individuals include refractive errors, strabismus, amblyopia, and motility problems. The etiology of these disturbances can be categorized as congenital, genetic, infectious, and traumatic.

The *congenital* causes often include abnormal embryologic development that can affect the eye or visual pathways. The ophthalmic problems resulting from these types of disturbances include strabismus, nystagmus, optic nerve hypoplasia, and cortical visual impairment. These conditions are long-lasting and often irreversible.

Ophthalmic findings that result from *genetic* causes of visual impairment vary in their characteristics. Disability can range from total vision loss to mild impairment. For example, retinitis pigmentosa is a progressive disorder with no known intervention that can cause total loss of vision. On the other end of the spectrum, people with Down syndrome often experience nonprogressive visual disturbances, such as high refractive errors, strabismus, and cataracts, which are highly treatable conditions.

Examples of *infectious* processes that can occur at birth or in childhood include toxoplasmosis, cytomegalovirus, and herpes simplex. Retinal scarring resulting from these diseases is common. This scarring is permanent and sometimes progressive, causing significant visual impairment, especially when the macula (the area of best vision on the retina) or fovea (the most acute vision in the macula) is involved.

Traumatic injury is a leading cause of visual impairment and developmental disability in children. Direct injury to ocular or cortical structures and hypoxia are examples that induce damage. Individuals with developmental disabilities may suffer traumatic visual impairment that is caused by themselves (eye poking, head banging), their caregivers, or peers. Hypoxia is the primary cause of cortical visual impairment in children.

Visual impairments with congenital onset in a person with developmental disabilities should be evaluated and treated as early as possible to ensure the visual system's best chance to mature in a normal fashion. It is estimated that the human visual system matures between the ages of 6 and 7 (Manacker, 1993). Before this age, if there is visual deprivation or a disparity in the visual images that the two eyes receive, amblyopia can occur. *Amblyopia* is defined as subnormal visual acuity without a visible organic cause. It can be caused by visual acuity deficits due to asymmetrical refractive errors or by disparate images caused by strabismus. Treatment of the underlying causes, and the occlusion of the better eye, have proved to be successful in normalizing the acuity of amblyopic eyes in young children. After the visual system matures, amblyopia cannot be caused or cured. Because a high percentage of people with developmental disabilities experience the types of vision problems that can cause amblyopia, it is imperative that ophthalmological intervention begin early in life.

The occupational therapist working with the adult with developmental disabilities may be able to provide effective intervention for visual impairment even if it has been present since childhood. Adaptation of the person's environment using the principles presented below could prove beneficial, as could the use of adaptive equipment that would maximize the use of the client's remaining vision. In addition, as the person with a developmental disability ages, new vision impairment may occur that affects his or her ability to function at work or at home. Vision loss in the adult can occur as the result of many conditions. This loss may be due to

- Infectious diseases,
- Vascular abnormalities,
- Tumors,
- Traumatic injury, or
- Ocular diseases such as macular degeneration and glaucoma.

Functional implications depend on whether the vision loss is central or peripheral.

The visual system gathers information through central and peripheral fields. This information is processed by the central nervous system simultaneously. *Focal vision,* which uses the central visual field, is defined as the ability to perceive detailed information about an object. The macula and fovea are the ocular structures that constitute the central visual field. The *fovea* is the area of most acute vision in the eye. The *macula* is the 20° of visual field surrounding the fovea. Any area of decreased retinal function or blind spot that is within this 20° field is called a *scotoma* (Schuchard, 1995). Scotomas can be classified by their position on the retina (central or paracentral) and by their sensitivity to light (dense or threshold). Central scotomas are those that involve the fovea. The presence of a central scotoma forces the person to use an eccentric viewing position to view objects (Schuchard, 1995). Because the fovea is the area of best acuity, the person unable to use this area will require magnification to view small objects when using the chosen eccentric viewing position. A paracentral scotoma is one that is in the macula but does not involve the fovea. The person with a paracentral scotoma will continue to use the fovea as the primary viewing position but may miss visual information if it falls within the scotoma or blind spot. Dense scotomas are areas of the retina that do not respond to light at any intensity. Threshold scotomas are areas of decreased sensitivity that respond to light at high intensity but behave as blind spots in low lighting situations (Fletcher, Schuchard, Livingstone, Crane, & Hu, 1994). It is estimated that 83 percent of persons experiencing low vision have dense macular scotomas (Fletcher et al., 1994). These scotomas can cause the person to miss salient features when trying to identify objects; they can also cause distortion of the visual image that the person perceives.

The peripheral fields are used to gather information about the environment and the person's relationship to it. They work in conjunction with the vestibular and proprioceptive systems to provide balance and are important in maintaining orientation.

The therapist working with individuals who have experienced a decrease in visual function should know which type of vision (central or peripheral) is affected by each diagnosis and should be aware of typical problems that occur with each type of loss. Listed below are brief descriptions of some common causes of vision loss in the adult.

Common Causes of Vision Loss in Adults

Infectious Diseases

Histoplasmosis
This disease is caused by a fungus transmitted by spores found in the dried excrement of animals. It commonly affects vision and can be life threatening if not treated. Histoplasmosis causes scattered lesions on the retina in both the macular and peripheral areas. When the macula is affected, a decrease in visual acuity is present and color vision is often deficient. As with other conditions that cause macular scotomas, contrast sensitivity scores may also be reduced.

Toxoplasmosis
Toxoplasmosis is an intraocular infection caused by *Toxoplasma gondii*. It is transmitted through contact with infected animals or ingestion of raw meat. This disease causes retinal lesions, especially in the macular area. The disease is nonprogressive, although new lesions may develop over time. As in all other conditions that affect the macula, a loss in visual acuity, decreased contrast sensitivity scores, and deficient color vision may be present.

Acquired Immune Deficiency Syndrome
AIDS is caused by the human immunodeficiency virus (HIV) and predisposes the infected person to a host of other diseases that affect vision. People with HIV have an increased risk of retinopathy, especially from the cytomegalovirus. Both the macula and peripheral fields are affected. This disease can (and often does) cause complete vision loss in the AIDS patient.

Tumors and Traumatic Injury

Tumors and traumatic injury can cause visual impairment through a variety of means. Damage may be inflicted by direct or indirect injury to ocular or cortical structures. For example, the optic nerve can be directly injured through stretching by sudden deceleration during a traumatic head injury or by a direct penetrating injury to the nerve such as occurs with stab or gunshot wounds. Indirect injury to this same structure can occur by compression from edema, hematoma, or tumor.

The ocular structures and all parts of the central nervous system, including the brain stem, cerebellum, and cortex, are vital to the processing of vision.

The vision loss resulting from a traumatic injury or tumor depends on which structures are involved and the extent of the damage caused by such insults. Common problems include visual field loss, ocular motility problems, decreases in acuity, and paralytic strabismus.

Ocular Diseases

Macular Degeneration

Macular degeneration is any kind of ocular degeneration affecting the macula. The most common type is age-related macular degeneration (ARMD). This is a disease that primarily affects those ages 50 and older. It causes retinal deterioration in the central visual field, thus resulting in decreased acuity, contrast sensitivity, and color discrimination. Peripheral vision is spared in this type of disease process.

There are two types of ARMD: exudative and dry. The exudative type is characterized by neovascular structures that bleed or leak fluid into the space between the retina and underlying structures, thus causing macular swelling and death to the cells of the retina. The person with exudative ARMD can experience a gradual or sudden loss of vision, depending on the severity of the bleed. Laser treatments are used to seal off these neovascular structures, thus attempting to slow the progression of the disease. However, research has demonstrated that these treatments postpone the onset of severe vision loss only by approximately 18 months. This is because of the high rate of recurrent growth of new vessels. The dry type of ARMD is characterized by gradual onset and has no known treatment. The pigment epithelium is a layer of tissue just beneath the retina and provides nourishment to it. In the dry type of ARMD, the part of this layer that nourishes the macula dies, thus causing these retinal cells to degenerate or to die. The causes of macular degeneration are not known at this time.

Glaucoma

Adult onset of glaucoma can be of the primary or secondary type. "Glaucoma" is a generic term much like "cancer"; it refers to a group of disease processes in which the intraocular pressure is so high that it damages the tissues of the eye, resulting in vision loss. The most common type of glaucoma is primary, open-angle glaucoma. As with all other glaucomas, it is caused by insufficient outflow of the aqueous humor from the eye. The etiology of this condition is unknown. It causes peripheral visual field loss first. Thus, the person who has it may not be aware of a visual impairment until late in its progression, when visual acuity may be affected. People with glaucoma often experience a decrease in contrast sensitivity function and a "washing out" phenomenon when exposed to too much light. This phenomenon is one in which the image at which they are looking fades out when the illumination level is high.

Diabetic Retinopathy

Diabetic retinopathy is the leading cause of blindness in the United States (Gardner & Schoch, 1987). It occurs in those people who have diabetes mellitus, which is a systemic condition resulting from the lack of insulin in the bloodstream. There are two types of diabetes mellitus. Juvenile diabetes (onset before age 20) is the most severe and most difficult to treat. Onset of the disease after age 40 is considered mature diabetes and is generally controlled by oral medication and diet control. The complications from diabetes mellitus depend on the severity of the disease process and its onset. The ocular problems associated with this disease stem generally from changes in the blood vessels of the eye. However, some early signs of diabetes are the general loss of the ability to accommodate and a fluctuating refractive measurement.

There are two types of diabetic retinopathy: nonproliferative and proliferative. In nonproliferative retinopathy, the changes in the eye are confined to the retina. These changes include dilation of veins, hemorrhages, and edema or exudates in the retina. Proliferative retinopathy involves both the retina and the vitreous and has the worst prognosis. The most damaging feature of proliferative retinopathy is the growth of new blood vessels on the surface of the retina that sometimes extend into the vitreous. These new blood vessels can cause retinal detachment, as well as new hemorrhaging in the eye. Visual impairment depends on which area of the retina is affected and can vary from one hemorrhagic episode to the next. Fluctuating visual function is a common characteristic of diabetic retinopathy.

Evaluation

As an occupational therapist working with adults with developmental disabilities, one must be able to recognize signs that may point to visual dysfunction. Some common visual symptoms are

- Ocular pain,
- Blurred vision,
- Diplopia,
- Distortion of vision,
- Photophobia,
- Flashing lights,
- Halos around lights,
- Abnormal color vision,
- Visual hallucinations,
- Night blindness, and
- Inability to see details (Gardner & Schoch, 1987).

Many people with developmental disabilities are unable to accurately describe the symptoms they are experiencing. Therefore, observation by the occupational therapist is critical for early detection of visual problems experienced by this population. If a therapist believes that a client is experiencing visual problems, more formal testing will be necessary to determine the severity of the deficit.

Four areas of visual function that are commonly affected by disease and trauma include acuity, contrast sensitivity function, visual field, and oculomotor dysfunction (Giatnutsos, Ramsey, & Perlin, 1988; Rubin, 1989; Schlageter, Gray, Hall, Shaw, & Sammet, 1993). Deficits in these areas can affect all daily living tasks, including

- Self-care (applying toothpaste, eating neatly, selecting clothing),
- Meal preparation (measuring ingredients, cutting or chopping items, identifying foods),
- Housekeeping,
- Work tasks,
- Shopping (making change),
- Community activities (accessing transportation, recognizing acquaintances, negotiating curbs/steps), and
- Reading and leisure activities (card games, bingo).

Acuity

Conditions that affect the macula, such as macular degeneration, glaucoma, and many infectious diseases, can cause decreased acuity, as can trauma to the eye or central nervous system. The function of acuity is to ensure that a sharp image is focused on the retina. It depends on the transparency of all of the structures between the outside of the eye and the retina, on the length of the eyeball, on the closeness of the object, and on the integrity of the retina.

Measurement of acuity is simply the evaluation of the threshold for recognition of high-contrast materials at different distances (Lampert & Lapolice, 1995). It is most commonly written in a Snellen fraction (20/40), which in this case means that the examinee was able to see at 20 feet what a person with average normal visual acuity can see at 40 feet. This far distance acuity could affect the person in some mobility tasks and community interaction tasks but may not have any functional implications in the home or workplace. Because most activities of daily living are performed at near or intermediate distances (16 inches to 3 feet), it is important to measure the person's acuity at these distances (Colenbrander & Fletcher, 1992). Because of accommodation, the presence of myopia/hyperopia, and myriad other factors, the measurements gained at near and intermediate distances may very well be different from those obtained at a far distance.

Clinical observations that may indicate visual acuity problems include being unable to recognize faces and difficulty in seeing small objects or the salient features of larger objects. A more detailed list of clinical observations can be found at the end of this chapter (Appendix 5.C).

Formal evaluation of acuity can be performed with a variety of commercially available products. In adults, visual acuity is normally measured with eye charts using letters or numbers, such as the Pelli-Robson and Snellen charts. These tests require the person being tested to have the ability to recognize and name the characters presented. Some people with developmental disabilities have the ability to name letters and numbers, but many do not. Because of this fact, a test designed for acuity measurement in children may be more appropriate for use with this population. The Lea Symbols acuity chart is designed for individuals who are developmentally age 18 months and older. It uses four symbols and a variety of testing tools to allow evaluation of nonverbal and multihandicapped individuals. The test is easy to administer and gives acuity values for the viewing distance at which each chart is most commonly used (10 feet, 16 inches). For people who are developmentally below 18 months, acuity can be measured using grating acuity tests. Because of the skill required to accurately give this test, it is recommended that these people be evaluated by an ophthalmologist or optometrist familiar with grating acuity measurements. In this type of test, the person detects the presence of parallel lines of decreasing width. The gratings are defined by the numbers of pairs of black and white lines within one degree of visual angle. The examiner presents two targets to the individual. One has the parallel lines on its surface, and the other has a solid gray surface. The person being tested is more likely to look at the patterned surface if he or she can detect the lines, because there is more visual stimulation than on the gray surface. Acuity is calculated by noting the smallest distance between lines that the person appeared to be able to see.

Contrast Sensitivity

Decreased contrast sensitivity can cause significant functional problems in many daily living tasks, including facial recognition and mobility activities. *Contrast sensitivity function* is defined as the ability to differentiate objects of similar luminances (Hyvarinen, 1995). A white cup sitting on a white table is an example of a low-contrast situation. A person with impaired contrast sensitivity function would have difficulty seeing the cup, because its hue and luminance are only faintly different from the table's. Decreased contrast sensitivity can be an early indicator of glaucoma and diabetic retinopathy. It also occurs with many other conditions that cause vision loss, and its assessment should be a part of any vision evaluation.

Clinical observations that may indicate poor contrast sensitivity include
- Inability to accurately identify colors of similar luminance and hue,
- Difficulty in pouring liquids without spilling, and
- Decrease in performance when in dim lighting.

As with measurement of acuity, contrast sensitivity function should be measured at distances in which the person is required to perform functional tasks. Assessment tools for contrast sensitivity include the Pelli-Robson test and Lea Symbols Low Contrast Visual Acuity Test. The person's ability to recognize letters or symbols will determine which test is the most appropriate. There is also a grating test, the Cambridge Low Contrast Gratings, for those individuals who are not able to match or name letters/symbols.

One method the occupational therapist can use to determine if a client is experiencing contrast sensitivity dysfunction is to have the client perform a task in bright light and then perform the same task in dim lighting. The task can be as simple as matching colored pieces of paper. If the client is able to accurately match the colors in bright light but not dim light, a problem with contrast sensitivity is indicated. The therapist should ensure that the client's eyes have had time to adapt to the decrease in light level before performing the second portion of the observation. If the therapist is able to see the difference in the color of the paper prior to when the client can perceive it, this may be an indication that the client's eyes are deficient in their ability to adapt to changing light levels.

Visual Field Deficits

Visual field deficits are most commonly caused by postchiasmal pathway lesions, occipital lobe lesions, anoxia, central retinal artery occlusion, and glaucoma. The loss of visual field can cause changes in oculomotor behavior such as irregular and inaccurate saccades and changes in visual exploration of the environment (Warren, 1993). These changes result in many functional problems involving mobility and activities of daily living.

Evaluation of visual field losses include the quantification of the deficit and assessment of the functional problems that may result. Decreased performance during daily living tasks can provide the first evidence that a client has sustained a visual field loss. Observations that may indicate this type of vision loss are provided at the end of this chapter.

The occupational therapist can perform a confrontation test to screen clients suspected of having a visual field loss. Confrontation testing is a simple procedure that gives a gross approximation of the size and type of visual field loss. The examiner sits in front of the client and has the client fixate on the examiner's nose. The examiner then presents stimuli in opposite visual fields and has the client indicate if he or she can see the objects. Each of the four quadrants of visual field should be tested. If the client does not see the stimulus in any specific quadrant or hemifield, a visual field loss is indicated. The stimulus used is often the examiner's hands and fingers. However, other objects can be used, such as pencil toppers or brightly colored dots affixed to tongue depressors. Confrontation testing should be used only in conjunction with careful observation of the client during daily living tasks, because confrontation testing alone is only useful as a gross indication of the presence of a visual field deficit. This type of testing may miss more subtle visual field losses.

The most accurate method of testing for visual field loss is the use of computerized automated perimetry (Warren, 1993). If a therapist does not have an automated perimetry device in his or her clinic, referral to an ophthalmologist or optometrist can be made. In this type of testing, the person places his or her chin on a chin rest and fixates on a central target inside a bowl-shaped device. As the person fixates on the central target, lights are displayed inside the bowl. The person is asked to respond each time he or she sees the light by pushing a button. Perimetry evaluation can be of the kinetic or static type. In kinetic measurement, the test spot moves from the side toward the center of the visual field until it is noticed by the client. In static measurement, points of light are flashed in specific spots in the visual field, and the client indicates whether he or she sees them.

Some people with developmental disabilities may not be able to be reliably tested with automated perimetry examination because of motor or cognitive limitations. For these individuals, a tangent screen visual field evaluation could be more appropriate. Tangent screen evaluation can also be performed by an ophthalmologist or optometrist. A tangent screen is used mainly for evaluating for the presence of central field scotomas but can also detect the presence of a peripheral field loss. It does not provide results as accurate as an automated perimetry for peripheral field loss, but it is quick and the evaluator can control the pace of the test. In this evaluation, the person is asked to fixate on a central point on a black screen affixed to a wall. The screen measures approximately 57" × 57", and testing is performed at a distance of 1 meter. The examiner uses a black wand with a white light on the end and presents it in different portions of the visual field. The person being examined is asked to indicate when he or she is able to see the light. The examiner marks the screen with a pin at the spot where the client first perceives the light. The resulting pattern is an outline of the client's good visual field.

Oculomotor Dysfunction

The purpose of oculomotor function is to keep the image being viewed on the fovea (area of most acute vision) of each eye (Daroff, 1974). The accurate control of the eyes is dependent on the integrity of the ocular structures, extraocular musculature, brain stem, cortex, and cerebellum. Any damage to these structures can cause oculomotor problems.

One common cause of oculomotor dysfunction is trauma. In a study performed by Schlageter et al. (1993), it was found that 59 percent of traumatic brain injuries admitted to an inpatient rehabilitation hospital had problems with oculomotor function. These problems can occur as a result of damage to the structures of the central nervous system, laceration of an extraocular muscle, or entrapment of a muscle due to orbital fractures (Baker, 1991). Cerebrovascular accidents and vascular diseases such as diabetes, hypertension, and atherosclerosis can damage structures of the central nervous system that control the movements of the extraocular muscles. Other diseases that attack the central nervous system, such as Parkinson's, Huntington's chorea, Alzheimer's, and muscular sclerosis, can also damage these structures, thus causing paralysis or paresis in one or more of the extraocular muscles.

Paralytic strabismus is often the result of such damage. Strabismus is a noticeable deviation of one eye in relation to the other (Lavich & Nelson, 1993). This deviation can be in any direction, depending on which extraocular muscle has been affected. Characteristics of paralytic strabismus include diplopia and restriction of eye movement. Some common complaints resulting from strabismus are diplopia, eye fatigue, and headaches after a period of sustained viewing. More clinical observations are listed at the end of this chapter (see Appendix 5.C).

The evaluation of oculomotor dysfunction as a diagnostic tool requires experience and skill. It is recommended that if a therapist believes a client has experienced a recent onset of this type of problem, a referral be made to a qualified professional for detailed evaluation. However, the occupational therapist can perform a screening test to determine areas of functional deficits. This screening should determine whether the eyes work together and in what situations the visual system works the best and worst. To answer these questions, the testing should include measurement of eye alignment, range of motion, and the ability to locate and fixate on targets (Warren, 1993). It should be noted at this time that difficulties experienced in performing accurate saccades, pursuit patterns, and localization/fixation tasks could be attributed to visual field loss (central or peripheral) as well as oculomotor dysfunction. Visual field evaluation should be performed if problems are noted with these tasks.

Eye alignment can be measured by observation of the corneal light reflex. This test consists of asking the client to fixate on a penlight and then observing the reflection of the light on the corneas of both eyes. When the eyes are aligned, the reflection will appear in the same location on each pupil. If one eye is deviated inward, the corneal reflection will be located toward the lateral side of the pupil in that eye. If the eye is deviated outward, the reflection will be toward the medial side of the pupil. Vertical deviation will place the reflection toward the bottom or top of the pupil, depending on the direction of displacement (Lavich & Nelson, 1993). Another screening test for eye alignment is the cover test. The client is asked to fixate on a central target. One eye is then quickly covered, and the examiner observes the uncovered eye to determine if it moves to establish fixation. The test is then performed with the other eye. No movement of the eyes indicates that the eyes are aligned (Warren, 1993).

The purpose of a visual saccade is to place the image of the object being viewed onto the fovea. The individual's ability to accurately and quickly perform visual saccades can be observed by having the client alternate fixation on two objects held approximately 6 in. apart and 16 in. from the bridge of the nose (Warren, 1993). The client should be able to quickly and smoothly shift gaze between the two targets. The examiner should watch for difficulties in initiating the saccade and the accuracy with which the saccades are performed.

Smooth-pursuit eye movements can be measured by having the client fixate on a target that is moved through the nine cardinal gaze positions. Observation should be made with regard to speed, coordination, and range of motion of the eyes. The patient's ability to perform convergence movements should also be evaluated at this time. This skill is tested by having the client fixate on a central target that is moved toward the bridge of the nose. The examiner should note at what distance convergence is broken. In people with normal oculomotor control, the near point of convergence is approximately 3 in. from the bridge of the nose. Insufficiency in convergence can cause increased difficulty in performing tasks that require focusing at close distances.

Finally, the therapist should observe the client during localization and fixation tasks in different visual fields. The examiner should hold up a target in various locations and distances and ask the client to find and look at the object for a period of time. Observations made include the ability of the client to quickly find the object and the ability to maintain fixation on the object.

Adaptation Deficits/Glare Sensitivity

The ability of the visual system to function in different lighting levels can be affected by a variety of conditions and disease processes. Adaptation problems are common among the visually impaired population, as is sensitivity to glare (Lampert & Lapolice, 1995). Both conditions can cause significant functional difficulties, especially in mobility tasks.

The eye's ability to adapt to changing light levels is a function of the rods and cones, cells within the retina that are stimulated by light. Cones function best in bright light and provide color vision. They are more numerous than rods and are concentrated in the macula and fovea. Rods are extremely light sensitive and function best in low-lighting situations. They are most numerous in the periphery of the retina (Gardner & Schoch, 1987). When a person goes from a brightly lit area to an area with dim illumination, the eyes adjust within 10 to 15 minutes. During this time, the cones begin to decrease their activity and the rods respond by increasing theirs. If a person has a condition that has affected his or her peripheral vision, such as glaucoma, retinitis pigmentosa, or a visual field loss from trauma, his or her ability to adapt to low-lighting situations may be impaired. In some cases, as with retinitis pigmentosa, the loss of rods is progressive and the end result is night blindness. People with this condition have totally lost their ability to adapt to low lighting and essentially lose most vision under low light levels.

Adaptation to an increase in illumination occurs much more rapidly than to decreases in lighting. When a person enters a lighted environment from a dark one, he or she should be able to adapt in about 2 to 6 minutes (Jose, 1983). This adaptation occurs as the cones are stimulated by the increase in lighting level and the rods are bleached out by the same.

Clinical observations that may indicate a problem with light adaptation include the following:

- The person becomes hesitant, trips, or bumps into objects when entering an area of decreased illumination.
- When outdoors, the person has difficulty ambulating in areas that have alternating shade and sunlit areas and becomes fearful when in dimly lit areas.
- The person shields eyes or wants to wear sunglasses or a brimmed hat at all times and avoids windows.

Sensitivity to glare, as stated above, is a common complaint among people with visual system disturbances (Jose, 1983). Glare is generally caused by opacities in the ocular structures anterior to the retina, but it is also a complaint of those who have diseases that affect the retina. Cataracts often cause a scattering of light rays that results in a decrease in acuity and color discrimination, as do any corneal or vitreous opacities. Glare also decreases perceived contrast and can cause fatigue and strain. Clinical observations for glare sensitivity are similar to those made for adaptation problems.

Treatment Options

The treatment for visual dysfunction is the same as for any other disability. The goals are to minimize areas of weakness and to maximize strengths. These goals can be achieved through adaptation of the person's environment, through training in compensatory techniques and use of adaptive devices, or a combination thereof.

The effectiveness of any intervention will depend on the person's ability to understand his or her vision loss, his or her ability to follow directions and to remember instructions, and his or her basic ability to adapt. Whether the person with a developmental disability is living in a group home or with a parent or guardian, it is also vital that the caregivers understand the nature of the vision loss and the resulting functional implications.

The occupational therapists should first look to adapt the person's environment to maximize function, especially when working with an individual with a developmental disability. Three areas of critical importance in evaluating the impact of the environment on the person's ability to function with a visual loss are lighting, contrast, and pattern. After adapting the environment using these principles, magnification devices and training in compensatory techniques can be used if the client is still experiencing difficulties in performing functional tasks. Teaching compensatory techniques such as eccentric viewing or teaching the use of a magnifier may be difficult with this population because of physical and cognitive deficits. General information on treatment options is presented below, followed by specific problems and their possible solutions.

Lighting

The first step that the occupational therapist must take in assisting the person with visual impairment is to assess the lighting situation at his or her workplace or home.

The importance of proper lighting cannot be overemphasized when working with people experiencing vision loss of any type. Central visual field disruption will cause a decrease in contrast sensitivity, and peripheral field loss will cause problems with adapting to dim-lighting situations. Increased illumination can stimulate portions of the retina that have a decreased sensitivity to light, thus minimizing the effects of threshold scotomas and improving perceived contrast between objects. Therefore, adequate illumination is critical for maximizing the abilities of the client with vision loss to cope with his or her environment.

There are two categories of lighting that the therapist needs to be aware of: ambient illumination and directional or task illumination. Ambient lighting is provided by ceiling fixtures, torchiere lamps, table lamps, and so forth and provides basic room illumination. Some of the light rays from these fixtures are projected directly into the living space, and some bounce off of ceilings, floors, and walls. Proper ambient illumination is critical for mobility tasks. If it is not possible to increase the amount of ambient light by increasing the wattage of the bulbs being used or by adding more light fixtures to the area, changing the colors of the walls and ceiling to a lighter hue may brighten the areas enough for improved function. Task lighting is that which is pointed directly at the activity being performed. This type of illumination is best provided by a directional lamp with a solid shade that has a support that allows for flexibility in positioning. It should be directed over the shoulder of the eye with the best vision or opposite the working hand and close to the work being performed. Care should be taken to ensure that the light does not shine into the person's eyes and that shadows do not fall on the task being performed. Proper task illumination is critical for performance of activities that require detail vision.

The ability to adjust illumination levels is also an important consideration when working with people with visual impairment. Those individuals with glaucoma experience a washing out of images when the light level is too high, and bright lights can cause significant glare problems with people who have cataracts or corneal scarring. Trauma or diseases that affect the optic nerve such as multiple sclerosis can cause significant sensitivity to light. People with macular degeneration, diabetic retinopathy, or field deficits often complain of a "dimming" of images and require extra lighting. Adjustment of the amount of illumination can be achieved through the use of dimmer switches, higher or lower wattage bulbs, and the proximity of the light source to the targeted area.

The control of glare is an important consideration when adjusting illumination. Glare can come from the surface of the activity, reflecting light into the person's eyes, and from the light source itself. If a person consistently complains of glare after all appropriate adjustments have been made to illumination sources, the use of a visor or sun filters may be indicated. These devices will restrict the transmission of light into the person's eyes, thus decreasing the effects of glare.

Contrast

As defined above, contrast sensitivity is the ability to discriminate among objects of similar luminances. Many ocular conditions cause a decrease in this ability, resulting in a variety of functional problems. Contrasts that can be perceived by the individual with normal sight can be impossible for the person with poor vision to see. For the individual with a visual disturbance, enhancing contrast can be a vital component in improving the ability to perform certain tasks. One way to enhance contrast is by increasing the amount of light on the subject (discussed in more detail in the previous section). Changing the color of the background to a hue of higher contrast to the objects in the foreground is another way to assist a person with poor contrast sensitivity. For example, a person may have difficulty applying white toothpaste to a toothbrush with white bristles, especially if this task has a white sink or counter as its background. To improve this individual's ability to accurately perform this activity, a dark washcloth could be placed on the counter or sink to heighten the contrast between the bristles and its background. Taking this concept one step further, red or blue toothpaste can be used to provide higher contrast between it and the white bristles of the toothbrush. The use of yellow filters can also enhance contrast for some tasks, especially reading printed material.

Pattern

The presence of pattern often hinders the ability of the person with vision problems to perform functional activities. Pattern can be described as "background noise" affecting the eyes in ways similar to the way static on the radio affects the ability to hear. Tablecloths, place mats, bedspreads, and rugs that have printed designs are examples of objects for which patterns may interfere with a person's ability to perform certain activities of daily living. Pattern tends to "draw objects in" and makes locating foreground items very difficult for the person with visual dysfunction (Figure 5.1). These individuals may have difficulty locating items on their plate or at their place setting if these objects are presented with a patterned background. The clutter found in drawers and on desks is another example of pattern that makes it difficult to locate needed items. To improve the person's ability to function in his or her environment, the presence of pattern should be decreased. Solid-colored tablecloths, napkins, and plates can be used at the dinner table to make location of utensils and food items easier. In the workplace, solid-colored place mats, which define the person's work space, can be used if his or her table or desk has a patterned surface. Organization of drawers and desktops is also important in decreasing the detrimental effects of pattern at home and work.

Figure 5.1. The fork on the left is much harder to distinguish from the patterned background of the napkin than is the fork on the right, which is on a solid-colored napkin.

Magnification and Optical Devices

If the client with poor vision is still experiencing significant difficulties with a particular task after environmental adaptations are made, the use of magnification devices can be considered. The most common detail task that requires magnification is reading. However, some other activities such as crocheting, playing cards, or performing assembly tasks while on the job may also require magnification. There are several types and strengths of magnifiers on the market, each with its own advantages and disadvantages.

Magnification strength is measured in diopters. When light rays pass through a plain plate of glass, the rays travel in a straight line, remaining parallel. However, if that glass is curved, refraction or bending of the light rays occurs. A diopter is a measurement of the light-bending power of a particular piece of glass or lens. The diopter number is higher for lenses that have more light-bending power (Jose, 1983). As the curve of a magnifying lens increases, so does its strength. Because of this fact, the higher power lenses tend to be smaller and thus provide a smaller field of view. Strengths of convex lenses are given a plus diopter value, and concave lenses are given minus diopter values. The optical devices discussed here all have plus values (adds). To determine the strength of magnification required by the person, one must first measure the best-corrected acuity. The reciprocal of this measurement gives the minimum diopter power needed for accessing details approximately the size of newsprint. For example, if a person's visual acuity is 20/200, first reduce the fraction to its simplest term, in this case 1/10. The reciprocal of this fraction, 10/1, gives the minimum number of diopters needed in a magnifying device to allow the person to see details the size of newsprint. It should be noted at this time that this number is merely a starting point. The activity to be performed may require more or less magnification, depending on its size and contrast and the lighting situation.

Diopter measurement is converted to "X-power" for most magnifying devices. The exceptions are head-borne magnifiers and spectacles. The X-power of a magnifier is written as "3X" or "10X." This is the most common description of a magnifying device's strength at the retail level. To convert the X-power into diopters, merely multiply the number of Xs by four. For example, the diopter strength of a 3X magnifier is 12.

The type of magnification device used by the client is determined by the activity being performed; whether the person requires the use of both hands when performing the activity; and the client's motor, visual, and cognitive skills.

Listed below is an assortment of types of magnifiers and their advantages and disadvantages. Magnifying devices can be purchased at optical supply stores, but the strengths and styles found may be limited. More variety can be found in catalogs that specifically carry low-vision supplies. Some of these catalogs are listed in the "Resource List" at the end of this chapter. It is important that the magnifying device used by an individual with low vision is of the proper strength and style. Using an improperly prescribed device can be extremely frustrating. Until the therapist has adequate experience, it is recommended that he or she consult with other professionals who specialize in this area before dispensing magnifying devices.

Head-Borne Magnifiers/Spectacles (Figure 5.2)

These devices give the widest field of view and allow both hands to be free to perform an activity. They range in strength from +2 to +48 diopters. Binocular vision is possible to approximately +10 if prismatic lenses are used. These magnifiers require a close working distance, to which it is difficult for some individuals to adjust. Some head-borne devices can fit over the person's own glasses, allowing the person to use his or her own correction plus the magnification power of the device.

Handheld Magnifiers (Figure 5.3)

Handheld magnifiers are commonly sold in optical shops and retail stores. Some come with a built-in light source. These devices are portable and can be

Figure 5.2. Examples of head-borne devices and spectacles. Visor-style device (on right) can be worn over the patient's own prescription glasses. Note the prismatic-style glasses on left, in foreground. Prism allows for binocular vision up to +10 diopters in strength. Binocular-style glasses in the rear are used for distance viewing.

Figure 5.3. Handheld magnifiers in the foreground have built-in light to illuminate objects being viewed.

used with the client's own glasses. One hand must hold the magnifier, unless it is used with a mounting device. Prolonged viewing is often uncomfortable and may cause hand/arm fatigue. The person must hold it at the correct focal distance to achieve optimal magnification, and some people find this distance difficult to maintain. However, these are very good for spot-viewing tasks, such as looking at appliance dials, reading prices, or identifying money.

Stand Magnifiers (Figure 5.4)
Stand magnifiers are ones that provide a base on which the lens is mounted, which holds the lens at the proper focal distance from the object being viewed. These devices are awkward to use on nonflat surfaces and are most often used for reading. Stand magnifiers can come with their own light source, powered by either batteries or a transformer that plugs into a wall outlet. They can be very strong but provide a narrow field of view. Activities cannot be performed under most designs.

Architect-Style Light/Magnifiers (Figure 5.5)
This type of magnifying device has the lens mounted on a flexible or goose-neck-style arm that is set into a base or can be attached to a table. These magnifiers sometimes come with their own light source, often a fluorescent or high-intensity lamp. They provide a wide viewing area, and activities can be

Figure 5.4. Examples of stand magnifiers. Magnifiers in the rear have their own light sources. Light sources can be powered by a plug-in handle (on right) or a battery (on left).

Figure 5.5. Examples of architect-style lighted magnifiers.

performed under them. Magnification strengths are generally on the low end of the scale (+7 to +12 diopters). This style of magnifier is most often used with craft activities.

Telescopes

Telescopes are mainly used for viewing distant objects. These units are portable and are useful for such spot viewing as street signs and aisle markers. They may be very difficult to use for a person with low vision and require extensive training to ensure proper use. The field of view is limited when using these devices, which causes problems in locating the proper target. Balance problems can also be experienced, because peripheral vision is severely limited during its use.

Compensatory Visual Skills

Training in the use of compensatory visual skills for central or peripheral field loss may prove difficult for the therapist working with individuals with developmental disabilities. Success depends on the ability of the person who has sustained vision loss to cognitively override habits that have been established for a lifetime. The experience and knowledge of the therapist is also critical in achieving these goals. The following descriptions of these processes are meant merely to be introductions to the concepts presented. Therapists who wish to use compensatory visual skills training in their work should consult with other professionals who are more experienced in this area or seek further information from the references listed at the end of this chapter.

Central Visual Field Loss

When a person experiences a central visual field loss that affects the fovea, an eccentric viewing position is naturally and reliably established (Schuchard & Fletcher, 1994). This preferred retinal locus (PRL) is then used to perform visual tasks normally performed by the fovea (Schuchard, 1995). However, the person who experiences this is often unaware of how to quickly and accurately locate the PRL during activities of daily living. The goal of the therapist working with these individuals is to improve the ability of the client to use the PRL in functional tasks.

Observation of the client as he or she is attempting to see an object can assist the occupational therapist in determining where the PRL is located. A simple screening can be performed by the therapist in this determination. The examiner should sit directly in front of the client and ask him or her to look at the therapist's face. Observation should be made as to which direction the client's eyes move to view the examiner's face. This movement will be in the direction of the established PRL. The client should also be asked if he or she can see the examiner's entire face or if any part looks distorted or dim. Areas of distortion indicate where the field loss or scotoma is located.

Eccentric viewing training teaches the client with central visual field loss to use this PRL during functional tasks. Clients are first asked to locate objects with their PRL in different visual fields and then to maintain fixation as they perform functional tasks. The success of this training depends on the client's ability to follow directions and the ability to control eye movements. (More information on eccentric viewing training can be found in the LUV Reading Series, distributed by Mattingly International, listed in Appendix 5.A.)

Peripheral Visual Field Loss

The loss of peripheral visual fields greatly affects the person's safety in mobility tasks and ability to locate objects in the environment. These individuals generally use poor scanning strategies and also tend to overlook details in the affected field. When dealing with functional problems, the client should be taught proper strategies to compensate for these deficits in addition to environmental adaptations.

The therapists should first determine where the field loss is located. This can be achieved through the use of a confrontation screening and subsequent perimetry evaluation. Behaviors that use the individual's remaining vision to monitor the missing visual field then should be taught and reinforced through structured activities. The desired behaviors are wider head turns and saccades; faster eye and head movement; the use of an organized, efficient search pattern; and an increase in anticipatory behavior (Warren, 1993). Examples of activities that can be used for reinforcing these behaviors include card matching, searching for objects or colors in the environment, and balloon volleyball.

Specific Problems/Solutions

Eating

Problems

Difficulties encountered in eating include locating items on the table, identifying foods, cutting meat into bite-sized pieces, eating neatly, and handling certain food items such as peas or salad.

Solutions

To improve the client's ability to perform these tasks, the therapist should first increase the light level by moving the client close to a window or adding a directional light to illuminate his or her place setting. Decreasing the background pattern through use of solid-colored tablecloths, place mats, napkins, and plates can also be of assistance. Placing food items in separate dishes can help the client to manage some types of loose foods. Increasing contrast between the food and the dishes can allow the client to more easily see the food. Having the client lean over the plate when bringing food to the mouth can reduce spillage. Knocking over items on the table is a common problem for individuals with both peripheral and central field losses. If the client tends to knock over items when reaching for other objects, teach him or her to "trail" the fingers over the surface of the table when reaching. Using this technique, if an obstacle is encountered, the client will hit the base of the object instead of the top, thus decreasing the chance of knocking it over. Techniques used by the blind can be taught for cutting meat and handling foods if necessary.

Dressing

Problems
Locating items in drawers and closets is often a problem for people with vision loss in either the peripheral or central fields. For people with decreased contrast sensitivity, discrimination of colors can also be difficult.

Solutions
Add light to the area if possible. Battery-powered wall lights are easily installed in closets, and a directional light placed near drawers can illuminate their contents. If neither of these options is possible, the person may benefit from the use of a flashlight when searching for needed items. Improving the organization of the closets and drawers may also prove beneficial, provided the person is able to maintain the order. Hanging matching clothes together in the closet and using dividers in drawers for different colors can help. Clothing items that are similar in color and style can be marked with a simple system using brass safety pins. For example, dark blue pants can be marked with a single safety pin in the waistband, whereas black pants would have none.

Minor Hygiene

Problems
Putting toothpaste on a toothbrush, locating items needed for minor hygiene tasks, applying makeup, and performing hair care and nail care are all tasks that provide difficulties for people with poor vision.

Solutions
Once again, the therapist should assess the illumination level of the area in which these tasks are performed. If needed, the therapist can increase lighting by using higher wattage bulbs or adding lighting fixtures. The therapist can decrease the pattern present by organizing the area and using solid-colored place mats or towels as backgrounds for tasks. The contrast between foreground objects and the background can be increased by using light- or dark-colored place mats or towels as appropriate. To improve the client's

ability to find personal care items, the therapist can put brightly colored tape or stickers on them. To improve the client's ability to apply makeup or to shave, he or she can use a magnifying mirror with or without lights. Nail care is very difficult because of the poor contrast between the nail and the skin. Clipping or cutting nails can be dangerous, so the person should be on a regular schedule of filing his or her nails to ensure safety.

Meal Preparation

Problems
Activities of low contrast, such as measuring ingredients, pouring liquids, and cutting/chopping/slicing food items, are often difficult for people with visual dysfunction. Those tasks that require detailed vision, such as setting appliance dials and reading instructions or labels, are also problem areas.

Solutions
As in all other areas, the illumination level of the area in which meal preparation is performed should be assessed first. If the light level is low, lighting can be increased through the use of extra fixtures or the use of a flashlight (for illuminating appliance dials). Contrast levels should also be addressed. Contrast can be increased between the food being prepared and the cooking utensils by using black/white cutting boards when chopping or slicing and using dark cups/glasses when pouring light-colored liquids, and vice versa (Figure 5.6). Measuring can be done more easily if separate, different-sized

Figure 5.6. Use of contrast to improve ability to see the level of liquid in cups. Milk or light-colored liquids should be poured into dark cups (left) to maximize contrast between the liquid and its background.

cups are used instead of a glass cup with measurements marked on the side. Appliance dials can be marked with tactile cues or brightly colored stickers at the appropriate settings. Magnifying devices can also be used to read appliance dials or measuring utensils and to see the food items being cut or sliced.

Functional Communication

Problems

Reading and writing are often areas that are affected by vision problems. Reading can be classified as continuous and spot. Continuous text reading includes reading magazines, newspapers, and books. Spot reading tasks are those that supply readers with information about the task being performed. They include reading food labels, prices, money, telephone numbers, the thermostat, watches, and telephone dials. Writing tasks that are affected by poor vision can be as simple as signing documents or as complex as writing letters.

Solutions

As with all other problem areas, the lighting level should be assessed initially and appropriate adaptations made. Improvement of contrast levels is often difficult in reading tasks that are preprinted but can be increased in written information through the use of bold, felt-tipped pens instead of pencils or ball-point pens. Written communications should also be printed in large letters instead of written in cursive writing.

Enlargement of preprinted materials can assist the client experiencing poor vision to gain access to the presented information. Large-print books and magazines are available through many outlets for continuous text reading. Magnifying devices can be used to enlarge printed materials that are not available in large-print editions.

Spot reading appliance dials, money, prices in stores, food labels, and telephone dials can be performed most easily with handheld or head-borne devices. Large-numbered telephones are available in retail stores for clients who experience difficulties dialing the phone because of visual impairment (Figure 5.7). There are also adaptive devices with enlarged numbers to attach to existing telephones that can be purchased from low-vision catalogs. For time-telling, there are large-numbered digital clocks, talking timepieces, and large bold-faced watches and clocks available in many retail stores (Figure 5.7).

Writing tasks can be made easier through a combination of improved lighting, contrast, and enlargement of the task. Task lighting directed at the writing surface should be placed so that the writing hand does not cast a shadow on the page. Increased contrast can be achieved through the use of a

Figure 5.7. A large-numbered phone with high-contrast lettering (on right) can make dialing the telephone easier for a person with low vision. The same principles of object enlargement and improved contrast are also used in the clock (on left).

bold, felt-tipped pen and bold-lined paper. Head-borne devices or magnifying spectacles can sometimes enlarge the material enough to allow for accurate and legible writing.

Distance Viewing

Problems

Distance viewing problems mainly occur during community activities. Reading bus signs and street signs, seeing street lights, and reading aisle signs in stores are all examples of difficulties encountered by people with vision loss. Watching television is one of the main concerns of poor distance vision in the home.

Solutions

Enlargement of the target being viewed can be achieved through the use of a telescopic magnifier. If glare is causing the client problems during outdoor tasks, the use of colored sun filters can reduce this effect, thus allowing the client to more clearly view his or her surroundings. To assist the person in seeing the images on the television, head-borne devices are available for distance viewing, or the client can simply move closer to the set.

Mobility

Indoor Problems

Bumping into opened doors, door frames, furniture, and other obstacles is often a problem for individuals with vision loss. Difficulties may also be encountered when going up and down stairs as well as when adjusting to varying light levels in different rooms. Decreased contrast sensitivity, poor light adaptation, and peripheral field loss cause most indoor mobility problems in people with visual dysfunction.

Solutions

As with all other areas discussed, lighting should be evaluated first. Is the illumination of rooms and hallways adequate for safe ambulation? If not, additional fixtures should be added. As the person goes from one room to another, does the illumination level vary? For example, is there a significant difference in the lighting level of his or her room as compared to the hallway? People experiencing problems with light adaptation may find this difference debilitating as they move from one place to another. Lighting should be uniform throughout the environment.

If lighting is adequate, the addition of contrast to the environment should be considered. For example, if a hallway is well-illuminated and the client continues to have difficulties in safely navigating it, a runner that contrasts with the floor as a guide can be installed. Painting the baseboard with a color that contrasts with the wall and floor is another solution. Improving contrast can also make stairways safer for the individual with vision loss. The leading edge of steps can be marked with a nonskid tape that contrasts with their color. This allows the client to more readily see where the steps are located and the number of stairs to be navigated. If the person bumps into furniture, it may be the result of poor contrast sensitivity. A person may not be able to see the edges of furniture if the contrast between the furniture and its background is low. If this is the problem, the objects should be marked with a high-contrast material. For example, a brightly colored towel attached to the arm of a couch or chair can identify its location for the client with vision loss.

The resolution of mobility problems may require the incorporation of compensatory visual skills training in addition to the environmental adaptations listed above. If visual or tactile cues are added to the environment, the person must be trained in their effective use. The person may need to scan the environment more effectively and notice details he or she would normally overlook. He or she must then understand the purpose of those cues and how to use them as guides. As mentioned above, these compensatory strategies may be difficult to teach to some individuals with developmental disabilities.

Outdoor Problems

Difficulties encountered by people with visual dysfunction in outdoor mobility include the ability to safely navigate uneven terrain, seeing curbs, safely crossing streets, seeing street signs and stoplights, and seeing signs on buses. These problems can be caused by decreased acuity, poor contrast sensitivity, glare sensitivity, and visual field loss.

Solutions

The use of sun filters can sometimes improve the person's ability to perceive objects of low contrast such as curbs and subtle changes in the walking surface. Filters can also be used to decrease the effects of glare. Telescopes can provide magnification for reading assorted signs and seeing streetlights. If the person will be required to cross busy intersections or perform other tasks that could significantly compromise his or her safety, it is recommended that he or she be referred to an orientation and mobility specialist. These professionals are described below.

Professional Resources

There are many other professionals who can assist the occupational therapist in the evaluation and treatment of clients who have experienced vision loss. Some of these professionals are in the medical community, and others provide services within the framework of the national blindness system. This system is a network of services provided by state, federal, educational, and private organizations. Following are some of those professions and a description of the resources/services they provide.

Ophthalmologists

Ophthalmologists are medical doctors who complete a residency in ophthalmology. They are responsible for diagnosing and treating ocular diseases that cause vision loss. Some ophthalmologists specialize in the treatment of specific types of conditions. For example, there are retinal specialists, glaucoma specialists, and neuro-ophthalmologists. Most people with developmental disabilities are probably under the care of a general ophthalmologist.

Optometrists

Optometrists have a college degree and a doctorate of optometry. Optometrists are not medical doctors but specialize in a variety of areas. An optometrist who specializes in the treatment of low vision can be an important resource for the therapist working with an individual with vision loss. These professionals have experience in evaluation of visual function and training in compensatory techniques and in the prescription of optical devices.

Orientation and Mobility Specialists

Orientation and mobility (O&M) specialists are professionals who have a master's or baccalaureate degree and are trained in addressing the travel needs experienced by the person with vision loss. They work in a variety of settings, including schools and private and state organizations. The O&M specialist uses an assortment of methods for teaching safe and effective travel to low-vision or blind individuals. These tools include training in the efficient use of visual skills, optical devices, and a long cane, if appropriate. The O&M specialist can be an important resource for consultation regarding a client who is experiencing mobility problems due to vision loss.

Rehabilitation Teachers

Rehabilitation teachers have a college degree and specialize in addressing the functional problems in daily living tasks experienced by the person with vision loss. They use adaptive techniques and devices to increase independence in self-care, meal preparation, minor hygiene, and leisure activities. As with the O&M specialist, rehabilitation teachers work in a variety of settings and organizations. They are most often found in residential schools, independent-living centers, and state organizations.

References

Baker, E. (1991). Ocular motor abnormalities from head trauma. *Survey of Ophthalmology, 35,* 245–267.

Boyle, C. A., Decoufle, P., & Yeargin-Allsopp, M. (1994). Prevalence and health impact of developmental disabilities in U.S. children. *Pediatrics, 93,* 399–403.

Carter, K. (1983). Assessment of lighting. In R. Jose (Ed.), *Understanding low vision* (pp. 403–414). New York: American Foundation for the Blind.

Colenbrander, A., & Fletcher, A. (1992). Low vision rehabilitation: Visual acuity measurement in low vision range. *Journal of Ophthalmic Nursing and Technology, 11(2),* 62–69.

Daroff, R. B. (1974). Control of ocular movement. *British Journal of Ophthalmology, 58,* 217–223.

Dickman, I. (1983). *Making life more livable: Simple adaptations for the homes of blind and visually impaired older people.* New York: American Foundation for the Blind.

Drost, P. J., Archer, S. M., & Helveston, E. M. (1991). Measurement of low vision in children and infants. *Ophthalmology, 98,* 1513–1518.

Fletcher, D. C., Schuchard, R. A., Livingstone, C. L., Crane, W. G., & Hu, S. Y. (1994). Scanning laser ophthalmoscope macular perimetry and applications for low vision rehabilitation clinicians. In A. Colenbrander & D. C. Fletcher (Eds.), *Low vision and vision rehabilitation ophthalmology clinics of North America* (Vol. 7, pp. 257–265). Philadelphia: Saunders.

Gardner, T. W., & Schoch, D. E. (1987a). Diseases of the retina, choroid and vitreous. In *Handbook of ophthalmology: A practical guide* (pp. 149–162). New York: Appleton-Lange.

Gardner, T. W., & Schoch, D. E. (1987b). Loss of vision. In *Handbook of ophthalmology: A practical guide* (pp. 39–51). New York: Appleton-Lange.

Giatnutsos, R., Ramsey, G., & Perlin, R. (1988). Rehabilitative optometric services for survivors of acquired brain injury. *Archives of Physical Medicine, 69,* 573–578.

Hritcko, T. (1983). Assessment of children with low vision. In R. T. Jose (Ed.), *Understanding low vision* (pp. 105–137). New York: American Foundation for the Blind.

Hyvarinen, L. (1995). Considerations in evaluation and treatment of the child with low vision. *American Journal of Occupational Therapy, 49,* 891–897.

Jose, R. T. (1983). Optics. In R. T. Jose (Ed.), *Understanding low vision* (pp. 187–210). New York: American Foundation for the Blind.

Lampert, J., & Lapolice, D. J. (1995). Functional considerations in evaluation and treatment of the client with low vision. *American Journal of Occupational Therapy, 49,* 885–890.

Lavich, J. B., & Nelson, L. B. (1993). Diagnosis and treatment of strabismus disorders. *Pediatric Clinics of North America, 40,* 737–752.

Manacker, S. J. (1993). Visual function in children with developmental disabilities. *Pediatric Clinics of North America, 40,* 659–674.

Marx, M. S., Werner, P., Cohen-Mansfield, J., & Hartmann, E. E. (1990). Visual acuity estimates in noncommunicative elderly persons. *Investigative Ophthalmology & Visual Science, 31,* 593–596.

Rubin, G. (1989). Assessment of visual function in eyes with visual loss. *Ophthalmology Clinics of North America, 2,* 357–367.

Rubin, S. E., & Nelson, L. B. (1993). Amblyopia: Diagnosis and management. *Pediatric Clinics of North America, 40,* 727–735.

Schlageter, K., Gray, B., Hall, K., Shaw, R., & Sammet, R. (1993). Incidence and treatment of visual dysfunction in traumatic brain injury. *Brain Injury, 7,* 439–448.

Schuchard, R. A. (1995). Adaptation to macular scotomas in persons with low vision. *American Journal of Occupational Therapy, 49,* 870–876.

Schuchard, R. A., & Fletcher, D. C. (1994). Preferred retinal locus: A review with applications in low vision rehabilitation. In A. Colenbrander & D. C. Fletcher (Eds.), *Low vision and vision rehabilitation ophthalmology clinics of North America* (Vol. 7, pp. 243–256). Philadelphia: Saunders.

Warren, M. L. (1993). A hierarchical model for evaluation and treatment of visual perceptual dysfunction in adult acquired brain injury: Parts 1 & 2. *American Journal of Occupational Therapy, 47,* 42–66.

Appendix 5.A. Resource List

Optical Aids/Adaptive Equipment

AFB Product Catalog
American Foundation for the Blind
    Product Center
100 Enterprise Place
P.O. Box 7044
Dover, DE 19903
(800) 829-3299

Independent Living Aids, Inc.
Can-Do Products
27 East Mall
Plainview, NY 11803
(800) 537-2118
www.independentliving.com

Lighthouse Low Vision Products
    Consumer Catalog
36-20 Northern Boulevard
Long Island, NY 11101
(800) 453-4923
www.lighthouse.org

LS&S Group
P.O. Box 673
Northbrook, IL 60065
(800) 486-4789
www.lssgroup.com

Maxi-Aids
P.O. Box 3209
Farmingdale, NY 11735
(800) 522-6294
www.maxiaids.com

LUV Reading Series
(Eccentric Viewing)

Lighthouse Low Vision Products
    Consumer Catalog
36-20 Northern Boulevard
Long Island, NY 11101
(800) 453-4923
www.lighthouse.org

UV Filters
(Sun/Light Filters)

NoIR Medical Technologies
6155 Pontiac Trail
South Lyon, MI 48178
(800) 521-9746
www.noir-medical.com

Visual Function Assessments
Contrast Sensitivity Function

Lea Symbols/Numbers Test
Precision Vision
721 North Addison Road
Villa Park, IL 60181
(708) 833-1454
www.precision-vision.com

Lighthouse Low Vision Products
    Consumer Catalog
36-20 Northern Boulevard
Long Island, NY 11101
(800) 453-4923
www.lighthouse.org

Pelli Robson Chart
Clement Clark
3218-D East 17th Avenue
Columbus, OH 42319
(800) 848-8923

Acuity Measurement

Organizations

Colenbrander Meter Combined Low
  Vision Test Chart
Lighthouse Low Vision Products
  Consumer Catalog
36-20 Northern Boulevard
Long Island, NY 11101
(800) 453-4923
www.lighthouse.org

LeaSymbols Visual Acuity Test
  System
Precision Vision
721 North Addison Road
Villa Park, IL 60181
(708) 833-1454

Vision Associates
7512 Phillips Boulevard, #50-316
Orlando, FL 32819
(407) 352-1200

American Foundation for the Blind
15 West 16th Street
New York, NY 10011
(800) 232-5463
www.afb.org

Helen Keller International
90 Washington Street
New York, NY 10006
(212) 943-0890
www.hki.org

Appendix 5.B. Recommended Reading

Dickman, I. (1983). *Making life more livable: Simple adaptations for the homes of blind and visually impaired older people.* New York: American Foundation for the Blind.

Jose, R. D. (Ed.). (1983). *Understanding low vision.* New York: American Foundation for the Blind.

Mangold, P. (1980). *The pleasure of eating for those who are visually impaired.* Castro Valley, CA: Author.

Appendix 5.C. Visual Impairment Checklist of Pertinent Clinical Observations

Acuity

Ask the client to read a line of standard-size print in a newspaper:

___ complains of print looking fuzzy or blurry

___ complains of not being able to bring print into focus

___ continuously adjusts focal length of the page as if trying to bring the print into focus

___ complains of print being too small or too faint

___ brings the page of print in very close (less than 16 inches) to try to read it

___ shifts the page of print to one side of midline (up, down, left, right) to read it

___ views printed line out of the corner of the eye or by looking above or below the line of print

General Observations:

___ complains of inability to recognize faces

___ states can see better out of the corner of eye

___ states that vision fluctuates throughout day

___ uses a flashlight to view objects

Contrast Sensitivity Function

Ask client to fill a clear glass with water from the tap or a pitcher to within one-half inch from the brim of the glass:

___ complains that he or she can't see the level of water as it rises in the glass

___ overfills the glass

___ uses tip of finger over the brim of the glass to tactually determine the level of the water

___ moves in very close to the glass to view it as it fills

___ tilts the glass back and forth to create movement of the water in order to determine the level of the water in the glass

Ask the client to fill a black cup with milk to within one-half inch from the brim of the glass, and compare performance.

Observe the client ambulate in environments with low-contrast features such as unmarked curbs, subtle changes in the support surface (transition from carpet to vinyl flooring without a significant change in color), areas with poor illumination, furniture that does not contrast from surrounding features, door frames that do not contrast from doors, etc.:

___ hesitates when approaching curb or subtle change in support surface
___ misses curb or does not see it until directly on top of it
___ trips when transitioning between support surfaces
___ bumps into or comes very close to low-contrast obstacles (furniture, etc.)
___ uses hands to guide self around an obstacle

General Observations:
___ complains of inability to recognize faces
___ performance declines in dimly lit surroundings
___ complains of inability to see changes in color of light at a stoplight
___ unable to accurately distinguish colors of similar hues such as dark blue
    from black, purple from blue, white from beige, etc.
___ requests additional light when performing a task

Visual Field Deficit
Observe the client ambulate through crowded areas with moving obstacles:
___ collides or comes very close to obstacles consistently on one side in an
    unfamiliar environment
___ stares straight ahead at the floor immediately in front of him/her
___ consistently stares to one side
___ stays very close to one side of the wall when ambulating down a hallway
___ uses fingers to "trail" wall to tactually guide self
___ refuses to take the lead when ambulating—prefers to walk behind others
___ appears anxious/uncertain in crowded areas
___ stops walking when passing by another moving person or object until the
    object/person has passed by
___ complains of feeling off balance, particularly to one side

Ask the client to read a paragraph of 1 m print larger printed on an 8.5 × 11
inch piece of paper:
___ transposes words when reading by omitting or misreading letters on one
    side of the word(s)
___ abbreviates scan to one side when reading a page of print, omitting
    word(s) on a line
___ is only able to read print accurately if uses finger to trace line of print
___ consistently loses place on one side of the page when reading
___ hesitates when reading words, reads words slowly or misreads a word
    initially, then corrects self

General Observations:
___ reads only half of a wide sign
___ avoids crowds and crowded environments such as shopping centers
___ transposes numbers

___ displaces writing to one side when completing a form

___ handwriting drifts up or down when writing on line or addressing an envelope

___ complains of being unable to follow what is happening on television, particularly when viewing a dynamic sporting event (football, basketball, etc.) or a show with a lot of action

___ has difficulty accurately dialing a telephone; transposes numbers on dial and presses wrong number

___ complains of disorientation when riding in a car or a wheelchair

___ avoids obstacles in familiar environments but collides with obstacles in unfamiliar environments

Visual Inattention

___ only comments on objects or visual details on one side of a visual scene

___ initiates scanning pattern beginning on the right side of an array and scans only right side

___ hesitant to shift eyes across midline toward left side; inability to maintain fixation on an object placed to left of midline

___ reluctance to turn toward the left or an avoidance of left turns during ambulation

___ failure to search the environment for information needed to adapt, such as failure to look at a clock or a wristwatch when asked what time it is

___ failure to rescan or check work for errors when completing a complex task

___ reduced effort on tasks

___ easily distracted by motion occurring on right side

___ unable to maintain concentration on a task that requires sorting through visual information or attention to visual detail; forgets what he/she is looking for or makes mistakes in identification

Combination of Visual Inattention and Visual Field Deficit

___ failure to acknowledge or notice persons on one side

___ failure to pick up or notice an object on one side during a visual search for the object

___ places only one foot on wheelchair footplate or ear piece of eyeglasses on one ear

___ shaves or applies makeup on only one-half of face or combs hair only on one side

___ eats food on only one side of plate

___ veers off toward one side when using wheelchair or when ambulating

___ consistently bumps into furniture or objects on one side in familiar environments

___ misreads time on a clock and does not correct error

___ omits or misreads words and does not correct error

____ complains of clumsiness but uncertain as to reason for clumsiness
____ places both legs through one hole in underwear or pants
____ misplaces clothing or toiletry items when getting dressed
____ becomes disoriented when moving in environment; unable to locate needed landmarks

Oculomotor Dysfunction

____ complains of double vision, or blurring vision or a shadow when viewing objects: usually varies with focal length or direction of gaze; may be constant
____ complains of being unable to keep objects in focus when working at a near focal distance
____ complains of eye fatigue or eye pain (not eye irritation) after a period of sustained focusing on a task
____ complains that print begins to swirl on a page or move after a period of sustained focus
____ complains of blurring when changing focus from a near object to a distant object
____ assumes a consistent and deliberate head position when viewing objects
____ shuts an eye or turns head when viewing an object up close
____ squints when viewing objects
____ complains of onset of headache after a period of sustained viewing
____ complains of fatigue after a period of sustained viewing
____ excessive blinking when viewing objects not related to eye irritation
____ complains of nausea during ambulation or head movement; accompanied by sense that peripheral visual field is in motion
____ resists change in head position
____ reluctant to participate in activities presented at a specific focal distance or attempts to change the distance at which the activity is placed (for example, changes focal distance of reading materials)
____ eye(s) appear to turn in or out when viewing objects
____ muscle tone in neck or mandibular area increases when head or body is moved
____ complains of difficulty concentrating on tasks that require sustained focus at a near distance
____ complains of eye pain with movement of eyes

Miscellaneous Observations

____ complains of sensitivity to light or keeps eyelids partially closed in brightly lit areas
____ nystagmus in primary gaze

Reprinted with permission from M.L. Warren.

PART 3

Specific
Applications

CHAPTER 6

Equine-Assisted Therapy for Adults With Developmental Disabilities

Kathryn L. Splinter-Watkins, MOT, OTR/L, FAOTA

Introduction

Equine-assisted activities and therapy can enhance the quality of life for people with developmental disabilities. Opportunities abound to meet therapeutic needs and goals, provide recreational and leisure outlets, or develop supported employment. All people, but particularly the often-underserved population of people with developmental disabilities, deserve programs that promote a richer quality of life. The principles of occupational justice (Wilcock, 1998) state that resources should be made available to support quality of life for people with disabilities. Programs bringing adults with disabilities together with horses can contribute significantly to the physical, cognitive, emotional, and social well-being of that group of people.

This chapter discusses several ways that equine-assisted activity, or therapeutic horseback riding, and equine-assisted therapy can offer opportunities for personal growth and improved functioning for adults with developmental disabilities. Professionals from many disciplines and with a diversity of perspectives work in the broad field of therapeutic horseback riding. It is an evolving industry, and increasing amounts of research are being done to document its effectiveness (Splinter-Watkins, 2002–2003). My perspective is that of an occupational therapist with many years of horse experience and involvement in the therapeutic horseback riding industry.

Overview

Therapeutic horseback riding is the traditional umbrella term that is something of a misnomer—actual riding of a horse might or might not be involved. Thus the term *equine-assisted activity* is now preferred. In North America, particularly in the United States, therapeutic horseback riding is defined as "equine-oriented activities for the purpose of contributing positively to the cognitive, physical, emotional, and social well-being of people with disabilities" (North American Riding for the Handicapped Association [NARHA], 2003). NARHA is an international nonprofit organization that accredits programs for people with disabilities and offers education and guidelines for conducting safe and effective activities with horses. Adults and children with developmental disabilities can benefit from a spectrum of horse-related activities, depending on their personal goals and needs. And those activities can be on or off the horse. They can focus on learning riding skills, on achieving educational or therapeutic goals, or on establishing a relationship with a horse. They can occur in many environments associated with horses.

Equine-assisted activity is categorized according to the professionals involved and the goals of participation. It can encompass a range of applications, from recreational riding to education to therapy. The versatility of the well-trained horse lends itself to extensive therapeutic adaptation and application through cultural context, life skills, life roles and patterns, various activity demands, and specific client factors (American Occupational Therapy Association [AOTA], 2002).

Within NARHA, four basic, but overlapping, areas of emphasis were developed by the participants and professionals involved. They are education, therapy, sport, and recreation and leisure (NARHA, 1999). As represented by Figure 6.1, each area overlaps with the others. NARHA also has two special interest sections—one for therapists (currently being reorganized) and the other for mental health professionals (Equine Facilitated Mental Health Association [EFMHA]). There are three role-delineated special interest categories, one each for instructors, for administration, and for higher education (NARHA, 2003). Additionally, driving and vaulting are two new categories that are being developed.

The American Hippotherapy Association, Inc. (AHA) is a separate organization affiliated with NARHA specifically for occupational, physical, and speech therapy (AHA, 2004). The term *hippotherapy* comes from the Greek word *hippo* for horse, and AHA defines hippotherapy as "a physical, occupational, and speech therapy treatment strategy that utilizes equine movement" (AHA, 2004). There is thus a great variety of professional services and programs available involving the horse community.

Occupational Therapist Involvement

Generally, the person in charge of therapeutic riding or equine-assisted activity is the therapeutic riding *instructor*. There are three levels of expertise for therapeutic horseback riding instructors through NARHA: registered,

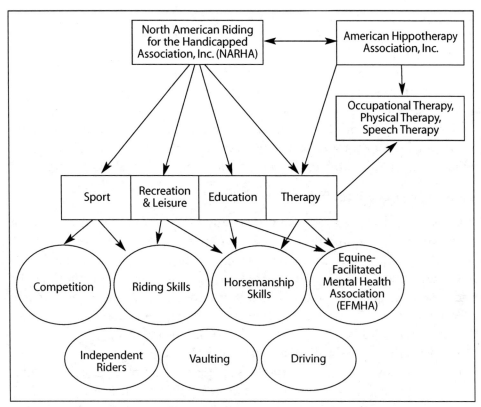

Figure 6.1. NARHA's four areas of emphasis. Developed by Kathy Splinter-Watkins, 2004.

advanced, and master instructor (NARHA, 2003). A riding instructor might consult with occupational, physical, recreational, or speech therapists or with special education teachers, although some instructors have dual credentials and are also therapists. Those instructors who hold therapy credentials often can provide more effective therapeutic activities during the participant's experience.

In contrast, for provision of equine-assisted therapy (including hippotherapy or equine-facilitated psychotherapy), the *therapist* is in charge of the session. In hippotherapy and in equine-facilitated mental health, a NARHA-registered therapeutic riding instructor and a credentialed horse handler assist the therapist.

Although therapeutic horseback riding or equine-assisted activity is intrinsically therapeutic, it is not billable as a therapy session. However, an occupational therapist might be paid for the initial screening and evaluation of participants for appropriateness and placement in a therapeutic riding program or for consultation to facilitate more effective handling, positioning, or adaptive equipment for a particular participant.

Many occupational therapists work as volunteers, consultants, evaluators, and teachers in therapeutic riding or equine-assisted activity programs, and one cannot discount to a client the value of referral to a high-quality therapeutic riding program. Clients who have developmental disabilities often receive tremendous benefit on many levels from their involvement with well-run, safe, and effective equine-assisted programs. The involvement of the occupational therapist might be through consultation with the therapeutic riding instructor, or the therapist could be certified as an instructor. An occupational therapist with horse experience and training as a therapeutic riding instructor is best equipped to use the horse environment to meet the variety of individual needs exhibited by adults with developmental disabilities.

Equine-Assisted Therapy

The specialized application of hippotherapy as a treatment strategy may be used within the occupational scope of practice and is billable and reimbursable. AOTA recognizes the use of hippotherapy as an occupational therapy intervention as long as it is based on an appropriate evaluation, goals, and treatment plan and assists in achieving the desired functional outcome (AHA, 2004; AOTA, 2002). Occupational therapy professionals who use horses in their work with people with developmental disabilities may also work through equine-facilitated mental health programs (EFMHA, 2003). It is critical, however, that the therapist is thoroughly trained and comfortable using these interventions. Specialized education and training workshops are available in hippotherapy and equine-facilitated mental health. For the most updated information, the Web sites of AHA (www.americanhippo therapyassociation.org) and EFMHA (www.narha.org/secefmha/) are valuable resources.

Therapists charge for their services through private payment, on a contractual basis, or through consultative services, depending on the services requested and needed. The arrangement of third-party reimbursement for hippotherapy is the same as would be reimbursement for any other occupational therapy treatment offered within a private or institutional practice. However, the formidable additional costs of extra personnel needed and for keeping, leasing, or training a horse should be a consideration within the billing constraints for usual and customary fees. More specific information on billing and reimbursement is available from AHA (AHA, 2004).

The occupational therapist's job is to determine whether a client or client group requires occupational therapy interventions and if that client or group would benefit from referral to a therapeutic riding program as a recreational outlet. The type of involvement for a person with developmental disabilities in any program with horses is based on that client or client group's needs and goals.

For occupational therapists who work with that population, horse-related connections can be used in several ways: in hippotherapy, in equine-facilitated mental health, in therapeutic riding or equine-assisted activity programs, and in prevocational and supported-employment opportunities. The direction of involvement will depend on the particular therapy needs and goals of the individual or client group. An occupational profile can help focus the priorities and directions for therapy and determine the appropriateness for connections with horses.

Hippotherapy

Occupational therapy might be requested for someone who has functional mobility problems or difficulty with sensory integration. Hippotherapy could be the treatment strategy of choice within the treatment plan.

The actual movement of the horse can be an effective treatment for improving neuromusculoskeletal function. The treatment strategy emphasizes posture, balance, and mobility. Treatment occurs with the client astride a horse and can include many positions on the horse to facilitate postural responses and development. Riding a specially trained horse "provides sensory input through movement, which is variable, rhythmic, and repetitive" (AHA, 2004). An effective hippotherapy treatment session would include off-horse and other activities that integrate the benefits from the movement of the horse with functional life activities. In some cases hippotherapy will prove the most effective and beneficial portion of a treatment plan.

Case Study: Wil

Wil, shown in Figure 6.2, is a 54-year-old man with mild left hemiplegia, developmental delays, and mental retardation. He presents with difficulties in speech, drooling, poor bilateral coordination and motor planning, and impaired posture and balance. He has been referred for occupational therapy because he often bumps into people or objects when he walks down hallways, and he has injured himself frequently. He has expressed an interest in cowboy culture he has seen on television.

Wil is brought to the barn and introduced to the horses. A general evaluation is performed to identify his strengths and areas of weakness. He is eager to get on a horse and ride, but first he is shown how to work around horses from the ground—respecting their space, acknowledging their "safe zones," and learning about positioning himself appropriately. Proprioceptive activities of grooming the horse, carrying the horse equipment, and sweeping the hall are incorporated during the next few sessions. A regular routine is developed for his time at the barn.

Wil learns to mount a horse from the mounting block step by step, with attention to sequencing and body position. While on the horse, Wil is seated in the forward position (facing forward). He wears a cowboy kerchief to help with drooling. The hippotherapy sessions consist of work at the walk in

Figure 6.2. Wil taking part in a hippotherapy treatment session. Photo by Kathy Splinter-Watkins.

various configurations to help with balance and posture. Speech is facilitated with commands of "Walk on" and "Whoa" at the appropriate times, along with facilitated conversation during the session. He is not taught riding skills in hippotherapy—instead he concentrates on actively maintaining his balance through the various school figures. After dismounting, Wil is again asked to groom the horse and put the tack (equipment) away, thus showing his respect for the space of others. After improvement is noted and documented, Wil "graduates" to the therapeutic riding program, in which he acquires riding skills and learns to guide his own horse in the arena.

Results of eight hippotherapy sessions included improved posture and balance, a more even gait while walking, increased body awareness and awareness of others' space, decreased drooling, and improved speech. His caregivers state that Wil is proud of his ability to "ride a horse like a cowboy" and that he runs into objects and people less frequently. He continues to participate in the therapeutic riding program, and his quality of life is enhanced through this active interest.

Equine-Facilitated Mental Health

EFMHA promotes equine-facilitated psychotherapy and equine-facilitated experiential learning (EFMHA, 2003) as specialty areas to include the use of horses within psychotherapy. Equine-facilitated mental health is based on cognitive and reflective insight and can include "mutually respectful equine activities such as handling, grooming, longing, riding, driving, and vaulting" (EFMHA, 2003). Generally, a licensed, credentialed mental health professional works with the equine professional to facilitate the sessions, but some professionals are credentialed in both fields.

Participation in equine-facilitated mental health programs can contribute to an individual's psychosocial development. Horses naturally provide a nonjudgmental, noncompetitive basis of interaction for people with various developmental disabilities. Frequently, a bond develops between the individual and the horse he or she rides or cares for. The human–horse bond often can be described as affectionate, friendly, and companionable. The human–horse bond is a great motivating factor to learn appropriate ways of relating first to the horse and then to other riders or participants.

Case Study: Marla

Marla, shown in Figure 6.3, is a 43-year-old woman with developmental disabilities. She presents as painfully shy and anxious, and she has limited social skills that prevent her from active participation in many daily activities.

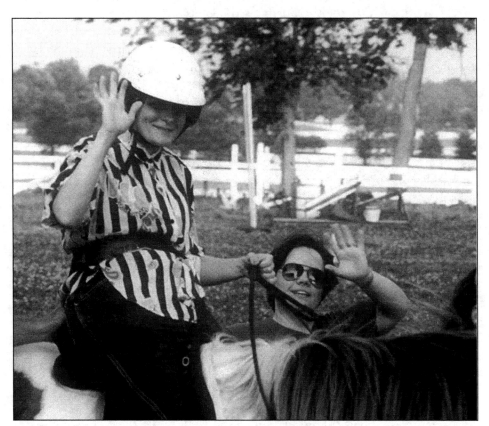

Figure 6.3. Marla taking part in an equine-facilitated mental health program session. Photo by Kathy Splinter-Watkins.

Marla is introduced to the horse world by letting her observe the horses freely roaming in the paddock. She is asked to pick which horse she likes best or feels friendship with. She chooses Sarah, a small chestnut mare. Through guided introductions and coaching about horses, Marla eventually begins to speak to Sarah, to the horse handler and volunteers, and to the therapist about various horse-related topics. After a few sessions of groundwork with the horse, then grooming, and finally group activities with the horses, Marla participates in therapeutic riding lessons with the group from her home.

Marla is able to express pride in her achievements. Her caregivers say that she is now able to talk with others at the group home about her experiences with the horse and that this has led to increased communication in all facets of her life.

Equine-Assisted Activity

Equine-assisted activity or therapeutic horseback riding involves learning riding skills, working on therapeutic goals, and forming healthful connections with the horse and with peers in a group. Participants generally enjoy learning about horses and often apply what they learn to the situations of daily life. Activities within the therapeutic riding class can be competitive or noncompetitive, parallel or interactive. Guiding the horse, for example, can facilitate right–left discrimination, bilateral and unilateral motor planning, postural stability, and the ability to cross midline. Riding an obstacle course influences the ability to sequence tasks, improves coordination, and strengthens visual-perceptual skills. Performing exercises to music while on horseback assists in isolating movements, maintaining balance, and reducing stress. Games can incorporate supportive and interactive activities, such as calling out names as a ball is tossed to each person or passing a ring from one rider to another as horses are guided beside one another. A big booster of self-esteem comes from winning a ribbon at the end of the riding session for completing specific tasks.

Equine-assisted activity includes more than just being on a horse. Enhanced learning in many dimensions is possible through a variety of activities within the equine environment. Activities such as grooming or bathing the horse can become a point of analogy for use in learning better self-care. Grooming especially addresses upper-extremity range of motion and eye–hand coordination, with proprioceptive, kinesthetic, and tactile senses all affected. For those who need deep, centering proprioceptive input or heavy work activities, such opportunities can be had in cleaning stalls, sweeping the barn aisle, climbing the mounting block, picking a horse's hooves, or lifting feed sacks.

Feeding involves caretaking and responsibility for the well-being of the animals. The different textures and smells of feed—from oats to sweet feed to hot bran mash to alfalfa or timothy hay—offer a sensory smorgasbord. Measuring out appropriate portions can be a great learning tool, and motor planning and visual-perceptual skills are reinforced in the task of carrying the feed to the stalls or to the fields. During holidays it is fun to follow a recipe to make seasonal horse treats: Halloween treats, Christmas or Hanukkah mash, or even a birthday carrot cake. Who doesn't smile with delight as the horses nicker their anticipation of feed at one's presence!

Tacking up or "dressing" the horse can help people with developmental disabilities meet various sequencing and self-dressing goals. Just as one must put on socks before shoes, so too does the blanket need to be on before the horse can be saddled. The acts of lifting and straightening the blanket, and then adding the heavier saddle in just the right place, require visual-perceptual skills, strength, and coordination. Buckling the girth and tying a knot in the lead rope to secure the horse provide opportunities for eye–hand coordination, problem solving, and learning activities of daily living skills that are important for self-dressing. The very act of carrying the equipment from the tack room adds coordination and proprioceptive input.

Children and adults with developmental disabilities often are fascinated by the daily needs and bodily functions of a horse. This can be a teaching and learning stimulus for improving awareness of one's own body and life functions—as well as a primer on what constitutes socially acceptable behavior.

Riding skills involve individual development as well as group awareness and social connection with the others in a class. Riding a horse improves physical strength, coordination, balance, posture, body awareness, visual tracking, and motor planning. All of the senses are stimulated and can be affected therapeutically. In the case above, Wil was able to learn right–left discrimination by learning how to guide his horse. Cognitive improvements are possible too as the rider learns about horses. This teaching can be in the form of questions and answers, games, or specific activities geared to address specific therapeutic challenges. For example, simply counting the number of legs on one's horse or number of horses in the ring can facilitate elementary math skills. Learning the various colors and breeds of horses may involve new information and memory skills.

Prevocational Skills and Vocational Opportunities

Many barn activities promote skills that can be generalized to daily life occupations or prevocational skills. Mastering the chores of the barn—mucking stalls, sweeping the hall, cleaning buckets, or moving bales of hay—can promote a sense of responsibility and occupational development. Just as people are needed to maintain a school, so too do people work to keep a barn and its surroundings in good order.

Barns and fences are in constant need of repair, and those chores can present a wonderful opportunity through which to learn general carpentry skills: hammering nails, sawing boards, and painting fences or gates. Fields sometimes need to be checked for rocks and holes and for weeds that cause illness in horses. This activity can be fun if made into a game or challenge, but it also is a necessary visual-observational task that includes the physical challenge of walking the fields, picking up rocks and weeds, and filling holes.

Tasks such as cleaning tack or equipment (e.g., saddles, bridles, blankets, and brushes) can be generalized to learning how to clean one's own clothes or dishes. In a therapeutic riding center participants also can help by stuffing envelopes for fund-raising, counting supplies, or making signs. These can be great prevocational activities.

The horse environment also can be a source of supported employment for those with developmental disabilities. A job coach might be needed to facilitate and train participants initially and to provide periodic checks, but many levels of skill generally can be accommodated beneficially within the barn environment. The process of developing a résumé and interviewing for a stable hand's position can offer an excellent opportunity to acquire job-seeking skills. Horses must be fed, groomed, and turned out on a regular schedule. Horse care thus is a repetitive daily activity that is readily learned and that provides useful training for those in need of habituation and consistency in their daily routines. A sense of productivity and the satisfaction of completing tasks (e.g., cleaning stalls, raking the hallway) are other benefits of employment.

Other Considerations

The most critical factor of any equine-assisted therapy program is its attention to *safety* at all times. There should be assurance that there has been extensive training for horses, volunteers, therapists, and participants. It is important in terms of professional liability to seek out programs that are accredited by NARHA or a similar organization; to maintain accreditation, the centers must adhere to the accrediting body's policies and procedures (NARHA, 2003). It is the therapist's responsibility to check out any center before sending clients to be involved with horses. If one's own facilities are being used, again, safety is the first consideration. It is crucial that the staff have a thorough knowledge of horses and their instinctive behaviors and that horses are trained in their responses to wheelchairs, assistive devices, loud or unusual noises, and the movements of the program participants.

Knowledge of the precautions, contraindications, behaviors, and skill levels of the clients must come before participation begins. An evaluative occupational profile to determine a client's skills, behaviors, and sensorimotor abilities should be performed before the client begins any activity. Precautions and contraindications for being in the horse environment or astride a horse can include but are not limited to allergies, impulsive or aggressive behavior, obesity, severely impaired balance, substance abuse, tendency to run away, history of physical abuse to animals, the presence of a heart condition, and scoliosis in excess of 30 degrees. A more complete list of precautions and contraindications is available from the NARHA Health and Education Committee (NARHA, 2003).

Special mention needs to be made here of the importance of assessing a client's height-to-weight ratio, balance, and behavior before offering a riding activity (Splinter, 1999). Although the untrained eye can see riding-stable horses as strong and placid, horses can develop back problems from carrying large, unbalanced riders. In some cases, the animals are unable to continue their jobs as therapy partners. Sidewalkers (volunteers who walk alongside a horse during a therapeutic riding session) cannot be expected to physically support a very large or tall rider or to safely and quickly dismount a rider in an emergency. Large clients who might not be good candidates for a riding program might do quite well helping in the stable or on the grounds.

Although many maladaptive behaviors can decrease with client involvement in the horse environment, some clients will exhibit behaviors that cannot be tolerated around horses. Unpredictable harmful behaviors toward volunteers, horses, or authority figures can be dangerous to all participants. Although horses can be very tolerant of unusual behaviors, they are also sensitive and will react to painful stimuli. For this reason, it is important to create an environment that is safe for all involved.

Resources

Therapists who work with adults who have disabilities must seek out programs that offer a safe environment that meets therapeutic goals. The occupational therapist might serve in various roles within an established program. The most comprehensive and up-to-date list of those programs is available on the NARHA Web site, http://www.narha.org (NARHA, 2003), which lists NARHA-accredited programs throughout North America. A list of therapeutic horseback riding facilities in other countries may be found through the Federation of Riding for the Disabled International at http://www.frdi.net (Federation of Riding for the Disabled International, 2003).

There are various resources to develop one's horse skills. NARHA offers educational workshops for therapeutic riding instructors and an annual national conference. The Association for Horsemanship Safety and Education (CHA, previously known as the Camp Horsemanship Association) (Association for Horsemanship Safety and Education, 1985) also trains and certifies riding instructors, focusing on summer camps and other riding programs for children. Other organizations that provide basic horse experience and training for young people include the Pony Club (Harris, 1994) and 4-H Clubs, which are accessible through state extension offices. The Equine-Assisted Growth and Learning Association (EAGALA) is another nonprofit organization that offers education on working with horses and humans in the psychoeducational realm (EAGALA, 2003). It cannot be stressed enough that people who are interested in using horses in therapeutic settings must have both the education and experience to deal competently with people who have specific types of disabilities and an in-depth understanding of how to work with horses.

Developing a program and facility oneself can be an exciting challenge for the entrepreneur. AHA is a resource for further education or connections to those providing hippotherapy within their practices. To set up your own practice for inclusion of hippotherapy, it is important to find an appropriate location, one that is clean and well maintained and that allows for the flexibility necessary to meet clients' needs. Healthy and well-trained horses are a must. Teaming up with a horse professional can be the best way to go about securing, training, and maintaining a good selection of animals. Equine-assisted therapy programs acquire horses through donations, leases, or purchases. Various workshops for training therapists are available through AHA, NARHA, and EFMHA as well as through college and university programs to train people for this specialized area of practice. One university, Western Michigan University in Kalamazoo (http://www.wmich.edu/hhs/ot/hippo/index.html), offers a graduate certificate program in hippotherapy through its Department of Occupational Therapy.

Conclusion

Occupational therapists will find a wealth of therapeutic value in the horse world. Areas of occupation, performance skills, and patterns are readily accessed through the use of equine-assisted activities. During evaluation, client factors within the occupational profile might indicate potential benefits for becoming involved in horse-related activities. Within a series of occupational therapy treatment sessions one might choose, for example, to incorporate hippotherapy to address sensory or physical impairments of an individual, equine-facilitated mental health techniques to concentrate on developing self-confidence, therapeutic riding to enhance daily life and social skills, or prevocational activities at the barn to develop potential supported employment.

During equine-assisted activities, well-trained horses generally respond with sensitivity and patience. Therapists guide this interpersonal interaction with the horse and with other individuals in the group, developing clients' skills in relating to one another and to their horses. Specific ways to facilitate appropriate behaviors occur naturally through the relationship with the horse and therapist. Unacceptable or unsafe behaviors around horses are not tolerated, but the horse is a great facilitator for, and responds to, appropriate behaviors.

Riding a horse can be an equalizing activity. Abnormal vocalizations or movements and facial or body irregularities are accepted by the horse and by the other people involved. Abilities, not disabilities, are emphasized. During a riding activity, the horse and rider often are seen as one being. Thus, unusual physical features are accepted, and many maladaptive behaviors become less frequent or are extinguished while riding.

By touching the human spirit, horses can produce feelings of freedom from life's challenges and impart enhanced self-concept and increased self-esteem. Many riders, regardless of disability, feel more powerful when sitting on a horse. A sense of elation and accomplishment is produced just from the fact of sitting high above other people. Successful participation in equine-assisted activities produces pride in oneself and often brings praise and recognition from family members, caregivers, and others. Participation in equine-assisted activities provides feelings of belonging, pride, and independence. By enhancing the occupational opportunities for those with developmental disabilities, equine-assisted activity and therapy can provide an avenue to an improved quality of life.

References

American Occupational Therapy Association. (2002). Occupational therapy practice framework: Domain and process. *American Journal of Occupational Therapy, 56*, 609–639.

American Hippotherapy Association. (2004, January). *What is hippotherapy?* Retrieved January 4, 2004, from http://www.americanhippotherapyassociation.org/aha_hpot.htm.

Association for Horsemanship Safety and Education. (1985). *Riding instructor manual*. Tyler, TX: Author.

Equine-Assisted Growth and Learning Association. (2003, October). Retrieved October 10, 2003, from http://www.eagala.org.

Equine-Facilitated Mental Health Association. (2003, December). Retrieved December 27, 2003, from http://www.narha.org/secefmha.

Federation of Riding for the Disabled International. (2003, November). *FRDI website*. Retrieved November 1, 2003, from http://www.frdi.net.

Harris, S. E. (1994). *The United States Pony Club manual of horsemanship*. New York: Howell Book House/Macmillan.

North American Riding for the Handicapped Association. (1999). *NARHA guide*. Denver, CO: Author.

North American Riding for the Handicapped Association. (2003, September). Retrieved September 15, 2003, from http://www.narha.org.

Splinter, K. L. (1999). Weight considerations for therapeutic horseback riding. *NARHA Strides, 5*(1), 5–6.

Splinter-Watkins, K. L. (2002–2003). Research: Past and future. *NARHA Strides, 8*(4), 22–25.

Wilcock, A. A. (1998). *An occupational perspective on health*. Thorofare, NJ: Slack.

CHAPTER 7

Let's Do Lunch: A Comprehensive, Nonstandardized Assessment Tool

Susan Bachner, MA, OTR/L, FAOTA, CEAC

Introduction

Let's Do Lunch is a nonstandardized assessment tool based on mealtime activities. The chapter first relates this assessment tool to the managed care environment, an environment that increasingly dominates the provision of health care and related services. Adults with developmental disabilities or the therapists working with them are not immune to the need for cost-containment and outcomes accountability, hallmarks of the managed care movement.

Next, the sociological attributes of food-related activities, important to the understanding of the Let's Do Lunch assessment tool, are described, providing an overview of the thousands of years of culture, custom, attitudes, and values that are intertwined with all aspects of food. This should help readers understand why lunch, in particular, is used as the vehicle for this structured observation.

Finally, the Let's Do Lunch assessment tool is presented. Although the author recommends reading the entire chapter as presented, some may wish to immediately proceed to the last section ("Let's Do Lunch—A Tool to Study the Interaction Among Social, Psychological, and Biological Determinants"), which describes the assessment tool in detail, provides illustrative case examples, and discusses the value of using such a tool (see Appendix 7.A for a blank copy of the task analysis assessment tool).

Service Delivery in a Managed-Care Environment

Managed care, in its various formats, now dominates the current health care market. *Managed care,* which emerged in response to spiraling costs of health care for industry, government, and the public, has been defined by Inglehart (1994) as a system that integrates the financing and delivery of health care through selective contracting with providers who agree to provide comprehensive health care services to enrolled members for a predetermined premium. An additional feature is the modification of provider behavior through financial incentives to reduce the utilization of and access to services.

Managed care, therefore, places primary emphasis on the value of services delivered and, in effect, defines *value* as the ratio of quality to costs. At present, the highly competitive and profit-driven managed care marketplace emphasizes cost containment and may be described as a price-driven free fall. However, growing consumer backlash and government interventions are causing demands for higher levels of accountability and a renewed concern for quality of care.

This renascent quality initiative has merged with several other trends to produce a new interest in health care outcomes management and research. These other trends include

- The work of John Wennberg and his colleagues at Dartmouth University, demonstrating profound variations in regional practice without demonstrable differences in patient outcomes (Wennberg, 1991);
- The studies of David Eddy, demonstrating uncertainty about the value of widely accepted medical therapies (Eddy, 1991); and
- The efforts by the RAND Corporation and others, demonstrating high frequencies of unneeded and inappropriate care (Chassin, 1996).

Process and Outcome

These initiatives have culminated in a growing interest on the part of managed care organizations, providers, the academic community, health care agencies (both public and private), and the government to link the structure and process of health care to definable and measurable patient outcomes (Donabedian, 1988; Ellwood, 1988). In this context, an outcome may be considered to be the result of a process or treatment (Joint Commission on Accreditation of Healthcare Organizations, 1994). According to Rogers and Holm (1994), "The focus on functional outcomes is critical because it targets attention appropriately on the patient" (p. 871). Rogers and Holm referred to Relman's article in the *New England Journal of Medicine* and share his belief that the public's growing concern over the quality and cost of American health care make this an era of "assessment and accountability" (Relman, 1988, p. 1220). To rephrase in terms of process and outcome, *process* is the attempt to do things the "right way," and *outcomes* emphasize doing the "right thing."

Occupational therapists, like other health care professionals, must be accountable for what they do, why it is being done, what the outcomes are, and what resources are required.

Outcomes Defined by Different Constituencies

Outcomes may reflect clinical events, patient experience, or administrative or fiscal attributes. An occupational therapy outcome is the functional result for the client of therapeutic actions provided by an occupational therapist. However, in the marketplace at large, it is important to understand that conventional measurements of outcomes have been based on the five Ds:

- Death,
- Disease,
- Disability,
- Discomfort, and
- Dissatisfaction.

These categories may be partially mapped to five basic dimensions:

- Clinical results,
- Functional status,
- Well-being,
- Satisfaction, and
- Cost.

These dimensions are emphasized differently, depending on the point of reference. Payers tend to focus on cost, practitioners on clinical results, and consumers on functional status and well-being.

In selecting outcomes for clients or patients, occupational therapists need to settle on those that carry a reasonable expectation of change—change that is functional and subscribed to by the individual engaged in the treatment process. Let's Do Lunch enables the therapist to observe behavior and understand it (in part, as a manifestation of the underlying performance skills); to evaluate behavior within the context of what has meaning and value to the client (as described in sociological and psychological terms); and, finally, to arrive at mutually agreeable goals or outcomes. It is easier, perhaps, for occupational therapists to collaborate on goals or outcomes that are meaningful to the client than it is for other medical specialists, because of the profession's emphasis on function. As Wetzler (1994) suggested, individuals are concerned with their own functional status and well-being.

Occupational Therapy Outcomes

With occupational therapy services, the "outcome is the functional consequence for the patient of the therapeutic action implemented by an occupational therapist" (Rogers & Holm, 1994). Within the occupational therapy profession, Forer (1996) spoke about occupational therapy evaluation and outcome and noted there is

> the temptation of many practitioners to use refined clinical measures, such as range of motion, muscle strength as measured by a dynamometer, endurance, lifting and reaching capacity, rather than

measuring the actual functional outcome [that is, independence in activities of daily living, return to work or former lifestyle, quality of life, and general health perception]. Although increased ROM, muscle strength and endurance, sensory and motor function, and cognitive and psychosocial function are all important, the key question is, What is the patient able to do as a result of these increased skills? Furthermore, if an increase of 10 percent in ROM does not appear to make any difference in a patient's ability to dress or feed himself or herself, then the intervention may not be perceived as cost-effective by those paying for services. Care should be taken in identifying the expected outcomes and measures for occupational therapy. (p. 4)

Let's Do Lunch is a tool to quickly assist the therapist in this process, for it

- Gives a snapshot of all the performance skills working or not working in synergy for adaptive responses,
- Reflects lifelong cultural issues, and
- Offers a built-in list of appropriate outcome items.

Distinguishing Between Clinical and Client-Referenced Outcomes

The need and importance of knowing client values and preferences are well documented in the literature and directly influence the likelihood of achieving patient satisfaction outcomes. Concern with quality-of-life issues is finding center stage. However, it is important to clarify that there are, indeed, two discrete paradigms in the spotlight, and each reflects a distinction between clinical and patient-referenced outcomes. In their 1995 presentation in the *Journal of the American Medical Association* of a conceptual model of patient outcomes, Wilson and Cleary (1995) described two different models: one held by clinicians and basic science researchers and the other by social scientists. "The models of these two academic traditions differ in purpose, methods, and intellectual history" (Wilson & Cleary, 1995). For instance, in the clinical or biomedical paradigm, the focus or outcome is framed in biological, physiological, and clinical measurements. "In contrast, the social science paradigm, or the quality of life model, focuses on dimensions of functioning and overall well-being, and current research examines ways to accurately measure complex behaviors and feelings" (Wilson & Cleary, 1995). These models of health have their foundations in sociology and psychology. However, the concept of quality of life, although related, can be distinct.

Silberman (1991), in "From the Patient's Bed," referred to the patients who are often misjudged by the professionals who "treat" them. "Such misjudgments are rooted in an enormous gulf between the way physicians think about disease and the way patients experience it" (Silberman, 1991). To illustrate the point, he presented the *Merck Manual*'s definition of *multiple sclerosis* as "a slowly progressive CNS disease characterized by disseminated patches of demyelination in the brain and spinal cord, resulting in multiple and varied neurologic symptoms and signs, usually with remissions and exacerbations" (as cited in Silberman, 1991). The response of someone who has multiple sclerosis is illustrative:

> What I experience every day is not the demyelination in the white matter of the nervous system. . . . The ongoing and seemingly relentless diminishment of physical abilities which is surely, but gradually, eroding my independence. . . . For me, multiple sclerosis is the constant effort to overcome my body's resistance so that I can carry out the most mundane activities, the frustration of not being able to do the simplest of things, . . . and the anguished uncertainty of a perilous future. (Silberman, 1991)

In listening to this narrative, one is struck by the two-pronged description of multiple sclerosis. Yet, the medical definition of multiple sclerosis juxtaposed with the human experience is a challenge occupational therapists face routinely, regardless of the populations served. Occupational therapists come to the marketplace with a studied understanding of the significance of function and independence in daily living as well as a medical orientation. In establishing occupational therapy outcomes, the clinical reasoning process must accommodate both.

Need for Determining a Course of Action for Individuals With Profound and Multiple Developmental Disabilities

In working with adults with developmental disabilities that range from severe and profound to mild, how does the therapist, an agent for change, determine a course of action that produces a functional outcome having relevance to the client, as well as to the other outcome dimensions of

- Clinical results,
- Functional status,
- Well-being,
- Satisfaction, and
- Cost?

If the client (who may have significant cognitive deficits) is also nonverbal or hampered by any number of communication impairments, what then? How are we therapists to get a quick glimpse into his or her value system, customs, attitudes, and preferences that are the substratums for quality-of-care outcomes? Information gleaned from medical histories, physical exams, range of motion, and so forth is readily available. Often, the problem is to identify what constitutes an individual's quality of care and client satisfaction determinants. Assessing that information quickly and accurately is the task.

Value in Nonstandardized Assessment Tools

Standardized tests for adults with developmental disabilities do not yield the information needed for a variety of reasons. By definition, a standardized test works with criteria and parameters that have been carefully established with rigid rules during test development. To determine what it would take in the form of cues to move a client to a higher level of expression and performance, the therapist cannot maintain the testing atmosphere and environment for which the scores were referenced. For example, it might be necessary for a therapist to provide additional cues, adaptations, and time to elicit optimal performance; these accommodations would violate the standard procedures and compromise the standard scores. In addition, standardized tests do not allow for individual client expression about the social qualifiers that identify a person's uniqueness.

Caplan and Shecter (1995) took the position that there is a critical difference between testing and evaluation: *Testing* is viewed by them as essentially a mechanical enterprise. . . .

> *Evaluation* is, by contrast, an art applied on an individual basis that involves not only testing skills, but also professional creativity, observational expertise, flexibility, and ingenuity in the service of developing a multidimensional understanding of patients—their abilities and deficits, their emotional state, self-regulatory functions, the impact of environmental variables on test performance, and so forth. (Caplan & Shecter, 1995)

In their chapter on "The Role of Nonstandard Neuropsychological Assessment in Rehabilitation: History, Rationale, and Examples," they attempt to enlighten clinicians so as to "avoid this kind of psychometric showdown by viewing the evaluation process in a less constrained manner" (Caplan & Shecter, 1995). They refer to Lezak's (1983) text that "noted that two particular patient populations, the elderly and 'the severly handicapped patient,' might require special testing procedures" (Caplan & Shecter, 1995). It is of interest that, although they feel that adjustments might appear in the neuropsychological testing procedures, they believe it is still possible to adhere to the essential standardized features of the test. Although I personally have not found that to be the case when working with individuals having severe and pervasive deficits, these and other authors represent that viewpoint. Perhaps some of the differences in opinion relate to disparate testing and evaluation goals, dissimilar consumer presentations, severity of deficits, or locus of client dysfunction, that is, impairment versus disability. Rogers and Holm (1994) referred to *impairment* as a "dysfunction at the level of an organ or system," whereas *disability* is defined as "dysfunction in task performance." Lisette Kautzmann (1997) built on this conceptualization, stating that symptom status or impairment-level problems (performance components) may lead to a disability or disturbance in functional status (performance areas) that may, in turn, lead to a handicap or social role disruption, affecting a person's overall quality of life.

Let's Do Lunch—A Model for Combining Quality of Care, Client Satisfaction, and Payer Acceptance

Why concentrate on mealtime in an occupational therapy screening or evaluation? When one considers some of the inherent qualities that begin with the ability to understand the human biological drive for food, as well as the large cultural domain that reflects complex systems of significance, rituals, and meaning, the answer becomes clear. People, indeed, must eat to survive. Their concerns about food, however, expand and assume considerably more than the biological reality (Maurer & Sobal, 1995).

Let's Do Lunch, a nonstandardized assessment for adults with developmental disabilities administered during mealtime, was devised to deal with the challenges of combining quality of care, client satisfaction, and payer acceptance. It is based on structured observation of the human abilities that combine in a variety of ways to form the foundations for occupational performance. The facets are sensory, perceptual, neuromuscular, motor, cognitive, and psychosocial.

In addition, Let's Do Lunch simultaneously allows for freedom of expression to address the social and cultural issues that can have a profound effect on the client's overall satisfaction. "Interestingly . . . lower levels of functional status are not necessarily related to lower levels of satisfaction" (Wilson & Cleary, 1995). It cannot be overemphasized that the two areas of concern—the performance skills and the human experience—must merge at the time of assessment. Both functional status and level of satisfaction must be addressed. Let's Do Lunch, despite its simplicity in design, is one way to accomplish this objective.

Relating the Sociology of Food to the Occupational Therapy Treatment Arena

To gain a more complete understanding of the Let's Do Lunch assessment tool, it is appropriate to explore the sociology of food. The cultivation, preparation, and consumption of food involve thousands of years of culture, custom, attitudes, and values that can be analyzed in terms of division of labor, power, or gender roles, not to mention celebrations, culinary choices, rituals, dietary rules, and so forth. It becomes a very long list.

Performance Skills That Emerge at Mealtime

Mealtime behaviors include and are partly driven by sensory, perceptual, neuromuscular, motor, cognitive, and psychosocial skills. As Judith Goode

(1992) wrote, "Food is both physically manipulated to feed us and intellectually manipulated to refer metaphorically to important aspects of existence. The unique, incorporative nature of eating makes food an important sacred and social symbol." While a person's sensory, cognitive, physical, and emotional state interact with what occurs at mealtime, these individual components are always in a dialogue with tradition and animate and inanimate props in the surrounding environment. These props, with their range of calming to noxious elements, exert their own powerful influences. It is through a discussion of some of the mixtures of these essential ingredients associated with mealtime that Let's Do Lunch takes on its significant linkage to functional outcomes and managed care, including the setting of purposeful goals, quality services, and cost containment.

Social Status Demonstrated at Mealtime

One of the areas of interest to sociologists is social status and how it is conveyed in cultures. Of issue here is the awareness that food items can reflect a particular social status and are often selected accordingly. Pheasant under glass or certain wine selections speak to one end of the spectrum, and a soup may represent the opposite. Whereas Goode (1992) spoke about certain food items as conveyors of status, my experience within facilities serving people with developmental disabilities suggests that status is perhaps marked more frequently by the individual's ability to communicate and exercise opportunities for additional portions or choices. Additionally, there are customs intertwined with pecking-order rules that dictate the proper approach for acquiring additional food. It is of interest that "in Denmark, it is customary to ask for more, in Ireland second helpings are a must, in Bulgaria you are warned to take small portions and will be expected to eat several" (Marshall, 1995). In institutional settings, people sometimes grab additional portions when customs, communication, and other problems, such as inability to inhibit or poor impulse control, dominate the moment.

Gender- and Age-Related Issues Expressed at Mealtime

Selection is also influenced by gender and age. A study referenced by Goode (1992) indicated that, in public settings where food choices were open, men's and women's choices differ distinctly. In family restaurants, food choices reportedly cluster to age.

Cognitive Functioning Observed at Mealtime

Level of cognitive functioning, I find, is also a factor in some behavioral responses observed at mealtime. Similarly, more complex levels of food presentation (dishes, meal structures, and cycles) engaged in by "higher level" clients transmit noteworthy social and cultural messages.

Mealtime exhibits a temporal aspect. One often observes a client whose functioning is punctuated by intrusions from profound problems yet who is still able to anticipate an upcoming meal or snack. Ordinary meal cycles mark regular activity and leisure cycles. In *Food Choice and the Consumer,* David Marshall (1995) noted, "While there is a broad range of content negotiation within the meal, the format remains fixed, and it appears the structure per se is actually more important in the choice process than the contents." Goode (1992) spoke of the significance of special food events that historically mark major breaks in productivity: weekends, harvests, and successful hunts. Well-known, too, are get-togethers at Sunday brunch, special parties, banquets, and other events. These and other celebratory temporal markers are certainly present in day programs, residential settings, group homes, sheltered workshops, and virtually any environment that serves people with or without developmental disabilities.

Organizational Skills—Teasing Out the Scripted Cultural Rules vs. Individualized Choices

How foods and meals are organized, and the individual's involvement in the "doing," provide insight into mealtime activities. There are rules for appropriate compositions of a meal; dishes must be organized in time sequences or spatial arrangements to constitute a meal. Meals and, indeed, feasts follow a scripted sequence. In what order are dishes presented? If presented simultaneously, as in a cafeteria, does that order persist? Soups first and sweets or nuts last finds expression in the cliché "from soup to nuts." If an individual undergoing evaluation eats dessert first as a deliberate choice, then that may be noteworthy. I have witnessed this many times and noted it as an aberration to convention. Although it is difficult to make conclusions about the causes, some possible reasons warranting further investigation might include sensory preferences (taste), cultural factors (lack of socialization to rules), or cognitive factors (sequencing deficits). The therapist documenting this information might best use it later, when reviewing patterns of scoring, to identify and prioritize areas of concern and decide whether anything, if at all, is necessary for remediation.

Rules About Eating Utensils vs. Using One's Hands

Eating with the hands is generally discouraged in Western society. According to David Marshall (1995), "In cultures where it is practised it becomes an art form in its own right signifying informality and social intimacy." He said later, "These unspoken rules about how food should be eaten are found across cultures, and they can be a source of embarrassment for the uninitiated—eating is also about etiquette."

Social Boundaries Conveyed by Food "Rules"

Relationships between individuals and groups can be viewed as being controlled by rules for food; they have the ability to define inclusion, encourage discipline, and assist with the maintenance of social boundaries. It is the rare adult with developmental disabilities, no matter how low the IQ is, who does not understand that there is a "staff" break room that is "off-limits." Whether the door is locked or not is of little significance; there is an awareness that staff enters freely and clients do not.

Food transactions describe a great deal; the food-giving and food-receiving relationships are notches of position in the food chain. The "haves" and "have-nots" in a total system are clearly defined by a variety of symbols. This is true for any such system, whether it be an institution serving adults with developmental disabilities, the army, or any other setting that has the capability or responsibility for total care. The holder of the key to the kitchen is in a position of power, whereas KP duty is interpreted as low status or punishment.

Messages Conveyed Through Diets, Food Consistency, and Preferences

Across cultures, children's food tends to be easy to chew and digest. What messages are imparted when adults are given pureed foods? It cannot be assumed that a person with profound cognitive deficits has no awareness of what another is served. I have witnessed disdain, envy, anger, and agitation when one individual notices and covets another's meal. The recognition of the differences between his or her own and the others' meal carries meaning. Further, the study of food preferences has been well researched, with consistent results showing that food preferences have a distinct foundation in sensory preferences. It is entirely possible that someone with pureed food at a table with another eating a regular diet may begin to demonstrate negative behaviors associated with (a) dissatisfaction over the recognition that things are different and (b) the deprivations caused by pureed foods that starve the individual's sensory diet of tactile, olfactory, or gustatory input.

Ethnicity and Food Preparation

Whereas it is almost common knowledge to remark that food items are associated with ethnic groups, it is perhaps more significant and less well known that ethnicity is revealed by the complex rules for how to prepare the items and when to eat. "Many people in the United States eat as many bagels as Jewish-Americans or as much pasta as Italian-Americans, but they do not follow the rules for how to prepare these foods, when and with whom to eat them, and how they should be served" (Goode, 1992). In working with clients in a cooking group who were born and raised in the mountain culture of eastern Kentucky, I found it was not enough to have eggs and bacon and margarine. To be true to the mountain culture, lard and biscuits were essential ingredients in this "All-American" breakfast meal.

Significance and Power of Timing and Belief Systems Associated With Mealtime

Controlling when one should actually begin eating, the pace of eating, and how much one consumes—all these can communicate messages about personal traits, previous experiences, and group affiliations.

The power of believing can surface in and around mealtime. If one believes that he or she will be healed, be sickened, or find comfort by ingesting certain food items, it may well happen. The following was overheard in Harlan County, Kentucky: "You know, turtles have all kinds of meat in 'em—chicken, duck, fish, cow, hog, and every kind of meat there are—and make awful good eating" (Bronner, 1986). To others from another locale, this diet would be considered inedible or worse! Refusal to eat certain foods or, alternatively, craving for certain foods may be traced to the power of believing. The therapist should consider this during the evaluation stage.

Placement of Food Items as an Indicator

The positioning of food items reflects still more rules. For those who have difficulty in or reluctance to moving their hands across their bodies at midline, customary positioning of foods becomes dysfunctional. Self-styled modifications will give insights into sources of difficulties or demonstrate a level of adaptability.

Mealtime Communications—Verbal and Nonverbal and Subtle Role Definitions

During the act of eating, whether defined as a "power lunch," "tea for two," "dinner dance," or "potluck dinner," there is an opportunity to communicate appropriate role behavior. In our roles as participants and therapists, we are able to engage in this communication. We are able to learn through listening and observing and interacting. Nonverbal communication speaks the loudest. In the preface to *Mealtimes for Persons With Severe Handicaps*, the editors (Perske, Clifton, McLean, & Stein, 1986) recounted a mealtime during which they were to simulate being "handicapped" for the duration:

> I learned that it's hard eating my meals when I couldn't do it myself. It's harder when I'm not able to speak for myself: to tell others what I want to eat next, what I don't want to eat, and to say, "Slow down!" It could be maddening when a certain movement of hands, arms, lips, jaws, tongue, or swallowing mechanism began to trip over itself and mess up what was intended to be a beautifully orchestrated sequence of actions. It ripped at everything I am or could be when the person helping me eat was uptight

and rushed. Once I received a little respect from my "feeder." He never knew I didn't respect him either. On the other hand, it might not be a picnic helping me to eat. Mealtimes like this can be tough on everybody. (p. xix)

Relationship of Quality of Life to Mealtime

Of note here is Perske et al.'s (1986) estimation that in excess of 80 percent of people with severe handicaps do not experience relaxed, human communion types of meals comparable to those described by individuals without handicaps. For each culture, there is an ideal mealtime experience. Many of us could provide a clear description of one that incorporates our own values, rules, customs, and parameters for sensory equilibrium. Whereas Perske et al.'s statistics describe an alarming percentage of people who represent deviation from the ideal, it is perhaps incumbent on us, as occupational therapists, to offer the managed care health market a wake-up call about what we can offer to quality-of-life issues. Mealtime, in particular, is laden with issues that directly relate to quality of life or client satisfaction. Occupational therapists have the professional training to examine a mealtime and to modify it to achieve desired outcomes, to look at variations from the norm, and to analyze those differences in terms of a person's handicapping condition. The functional status, therefore, can be jeopardized by either internal or external challenges, or both; the ever-present social overlays influence outcome as well.

Let's Do Lunch—A Tool to Study the Interaction Among Social, Psychological, and Biological Determinants

"To study a person's food-related behavior is to study the interaction of a person's social, psychological, and biological needs" (Axelson & Brinberg, 1989, p. 2). The researchers continued with a discussion of how a social psychologist views the effect of culture on behavior (the beliefs, preferences, and attitudes of the individual), whereas an anthropologist views culture as a direct determinant or explanation of an individual's behavior.

An occupational therapist, with the Let's Do Lunch assessment, is able to merge the two positions, to see people as expressing their individual histories and narratives as well as reflecting a cultural legacy through their behavior. At mealtime, the therapist is able to observe behaviors, rules, gender, age, and other issues that are passed down from previous generations or significant others. This is what the sociologist and social psychologist address. Paradoxically, to observe and study environment and culture as determinants of behavior is what the anthropologist views as important. The expression "institutionalized behaviors" is an example of the anthropological frame of reference.

Another dimension is created when the occupational therapist uses his or her unique training to analyze a client's occupational performance and underlying skills. Learning the client's patterns of living and needs and wants and identifying barriers to performance are critical in this process. Let's Do Lunch is a tool that structures observations and quickly permits the therapist to tease out, within the evaluation process, the individual's unique presentation as both a cause for and result of behavior, as well as to understand the significant influences of underlying performance skills. What comes to mind is a recipe that might read as follows:

- Mix an individual's unique presentation that is the sum of interactions from his or her physical and psychological history.
- Place this into a mold in the shape of current surroundings.
- Position it in living space and leave at room temperature, to enable a pattern of synergies to occur.
- Meanwhile, set the table for a dialogue between therapist and client.
- When ready, subject the product to a "taste test."
- Decide what would improve the ingredients, conditions, process, and taste, articulating some functional outcomes.

Context in Which Let's Do Lunch Was Developed

Adults with developmental disabilities come in all textures and, although all have needs and wants, only some are able to effectively express them. If all could find the words to relate their vestibular needs, their visual deficits, and their wonderment at the ramifications of cause and effect, assessments would indeed be a "piece of cake." Yet, the reality is that many juggle elements of physical, emotional, motor, visual, and other sensory deficits that are, in part, not self-comprehended nor offered to the team in a neat package. The kaleidoscopic patterns of presentations require a professional to properly identify the contours and significance of the various performance factors. The occupational therapist's eye, having been structured and trained to observe both the individual elements and the gestalt, is able to simultaneously assess the participant's strengths and needs and establish functional outcomes with enduring capabilities.

Let's Do Lunch captures the client's strengths and needs in perceptual, neuromuscular, sensorimotor, psychosocial, and physical areas. The surrounding mealtime issues—already described—provide the stage on which the areas of occupation and contextual components present themselves and interact.

In the preface to *Mealtimes for Persons With Severe Handicaps,* Perske et al. (1986) noted,

> It had to be written, this book on mealtime experiences for seriously handicapped persons. Too many voices across the nation have said so. This may come as a surprise to those who wouldn't expect such a subject to be interesting reading. . . . They [the contributors to this book] recalled that mealtimes weren't seen as heroic or

interesting at institutions where they worked. That was the time when almost all of the institution's staff left the grounds to fill the community's restaurants, leaving "the ignoble task of feeding" to a few aides. Or it was the time when the community professionals stayed away from the homes because, as one nurse stated, "There wasn't anything therapeutic about that hectic time." But a new interest in these mealtimes is emerging. There is an upsurge in training opportunities that can lead to increased mealtime sensitivities and skills.

Although in complete agreement with Perske et al.'s (1986) insights regarding training opportunities at mealtime, Let's Do Lunch is based on the expanded belief that evaluation opportunities exist at mealtime. These opportunities are as varied and satisfying as an extravagant smorgasbord. Sensory development, social and emotional growth, self-help skills, fine and gross motor development, and decision making, flavored by culture, values, and all the other elements of a sociological perspective, offer a feast of material that meets the criteria associated with managed care, functional outcome, and quality care within a time-specific period.

Why Mealtime Is the Perfect Activity for Evaluation Purposes

For the occupational therapist, mealtime is one of those "perfect" activities—everything needed in a comprehensive evaluation is available to the trained eye and ear. For the client, the evaluation is synonymous with the everyday activity of lunch. Any anxieties associated with testing or assessment situations are rare or nonexistent. The client usually views the interaction as a social one—after all, we're "doing lunch!"

There are times, nonetheless, when a therapist may choose to remain outside of direct interaction with the client, because the individual, so starved for attention, processes the contact in an all-consuming manner. The client's riveting reaction can skew and overshadow the usual behaviors available for observation and could easily become counterproductive to the ultimate goal of the assessment. The therapist would do well to borrow the "participant–observation" methodology from the anthropologist's repertoire.

Participant–Observation Methodology

Participant–observation is rooted in an 18th-century technique that assumes it is possible for a person to be able to enter into, explore, and understand the distinctive experiences of others. The investigator participates as a member of the group being studied. Participant–observers are sometimes known by the group members to be observers, although they join in the activity as well as assume the obligations of a member. In other situations, the observer is thought to be an ordinary member, and the group members are simply not aware that they are being observed. This concept was introduced in 1925 by E. C. Lindeman in his book, *Social Discovery*.

Because we cannot truly enter into the mind or body of another person, the observer must bring to the encounter a skill level and focused inquiry that differentiates him or her from the casual observer; that is to say that the therapist–observer must have the perspective and capability to ask the significant question(s). Let's Do Lunch is an example of this approach for the following reasons:

- It structures and prompts the therapist to be an observer.
- It enables the therapist to ask the significant questions relating to performance components and environment.
- It enables the therapist to enter into a nonverbal dialogue.
- It enables the therapist to move from total participation to separation, in a wax-and-wane pattern, to find the "just-right" distance that allows for both an empathic and objective position.

In other words, the therapist must assume a position as close to center stage as possible, without a disruption of the authenticity of the environment. The environment, rules, and expectations are certainly familiar; a meal is something that the clients know they can count on. It is the rare resident who does not know how to find the dining room or is unaware that food is available if certain sequences can be mastered. Variations on the theme of food procurement are what becomes "food for thought" to the observing therapist.

In defining *food-related behaviors,* they can be described simply as what people do: their actions toward food. "People can consume food, sell food, buy food, throw food, use food as a weapon, and perform a host of other actions toward foods" (Axelson & Brinberg, 1989, p. 2).

Application of Clinical Reasoning

Observing client behaviors becomes the basis of a chain of critical-reasoning steps. The therapist's trained eye begins to analyze, make inferences, check them out for their reproducibility, and understand which circumstances result in which behaviors. The therapist gathers evidence to identify and record what influences (biological or social) configure with the observations noted as significant. Throughout the entire process of the Let's Do Lunch assessment, the underlying concern of the therapist is to attempt to determine what it takes to facilitate optimal functioning in each of the performance skills. What type of cueing or "seasoning" will it take to produce in an individual an outcome showing less restriction or a higher level of performance? As discussed at the outset of this chapter, in a managed care environment, the social science or quality-of-life model operates with attributes of functioning—the little things that constitute a foundation for higher levels—and our value, as clinicians, is to quickly ascertain for the record what those attributes are for each client in our care. Under what circumstances will the client be less at risk for injury and more likely to achieve health? What information can be passed along to others in this person's support system that describe the personal textures as well as needs and wants? Delegating routine and nonskilled treatment strategies to others is cost-effective, but plans must be clearly presented.

Changing the Conditions to Improve Performance

Joan Toglia (1993) discussed "The Dynamic Interactional Approach" and assessment in her chapter on attention and memory. She described the approach as seeking "to examine the extent to which task performance can be changed by determining which conditions increase or decrease symptoms." Further, she "emphasizes how the individual goes about performing the task rather than the task itself. In contrast, conventional standardized tests are designed to identify and quantify the deficit." During an assessment, the dynamic interactional approach, similar to participant–observation, has attributes of awareness questioning, strategy investigation, task grading, and response to cueing.

These concepts are at the core of Let's Do Lunch. Because this is a nonstandardized tool, it is perfectly acceptable and indeed desirable to interact, to cue, to suggest, to experiment, to experience pleasure, to find something mutually amusing and, if possible, to laugh. Remember Perkse et al.'s (1986) statistic that only about 20 percent of people with handicapping conditions find mealtime at all pleasurable! Besides, with defenses down, reliable information flows.

A Description of Let's Do Lunch

The residential facility where I worked and where I developed the Let's Do Lunch tool serves 180 adults with developmental disabilities. Their diagnoses range from mild to severe retardation, and many carry dual diagnoses. Everyone is ambulatory, some with mobility aids, and no one is on feeding tubes. Let's Do Lunch is a task analysis of 60 steps that follows a person from the starting point of entering the dining room to the end point of locating the exit to leave. Most everyone exhibits a variety of conditions; no one has challenges limited to only cognitive deficits. The 60 steps track mealtime at this facility. The task analysis, if it is to be of value to others in different environments, can be constructed to reflect alternative settings.

Scoring the Assessment

In addition to the "personalized" task analysis, there is a rating system of 0 to 3, for which 0 signifies independence and 1–3 indicates the type of cueing or assist required:
- 1 for verbal,
- 2 for physical, and
- 3 for total assist.

Not applicable, or NA, is always an option. If used, however, a clarifying statement is appropriate. For instance, Item 9, "Sees Food Items," may score NA if the client is blind or has marked visual deficits.

Lets Do Lunch is scored subjectively by the therapist, who uses observational skills to examine and note an individual's responses to each subskill. It is a time to comment on the individual's functional status and quality-of-life issues.

Each of the six scoring codes represents one of the following six performance skills:

- Sensory
- Perceptual
- Neuromuscular
- Motor
- Cognitive
- Psychosocial.

Performance skills are checked selectively and reflect, in the final analysis, an assessment of strengths and needs. It is entirely possible that summary recommendations from the assessment may lead to referrals for services with others on the team, such as an ophthalmologist, physical therapist, or neurologist. A therapist's comments on any item can be noted in the space below the action, and therapists are urged to use this space to describe how a client performs. If a client displays some dysfunction, whether or not the task is completed, a score is given. There are situations when performance skills need not be marked, such as if the task item is completed or the functional outcome achieved. However, narrative comments entered below the item are often helpful and are factored into the final summary.

Sometimes I have paused in a deliberation over the significance of an observation. Should it be recorded? Is it part of an unfolding pattern, or simply an insignificant aberration? Is it merely a quirk that has no ultimate significance? It is a hard call until all the data are in. Sometimes, the entry of a question mark is used, instead of a check, under a performance component. This simply reflects that the therapist feels uncertain about the area that underlies the difficulty or inability to perform the task. All these notations and marks contribute to the picture that comes together at the end.

My overall experience suggests that it is far easier to disregard superfluous information in the final analysis than it is to try to reconstruct subtle points that occurred along the way. There should be adequate information to allow the therapist to synthesize and summarize. Checks in the performance component columns are summarized to indicate specific areas in which the client shows both strengths and needs. Patterns of strengths, deficits, and question marks are noted, and these contribute to the analysis of the patterns of scoring. The component(s) that received the most checks, because of difficulty in execution, may become a ready-made "functional outcome" for needs-driven goal setting. Question marks may be factored into the final analysis and carry weight as well. Notations in the form of 0 scores, indicating independence, or narrative comments about strengths are extremely helpful when the time comes to identify strengths onto which treatment strategies are built.

It is important to reiterate that, in almost each of the 60 items listed, there are elements of all performance fundamentals. The therapist needs to note those task items that are problem areas so that further investigation and outcome formulations may be initiated. Clarifications are always helpful in the execution of the recording. For example, if a client had difficulty entering the dining room, it might be helpful to indicate whether it was

- A cognitive problem, in which the client was new to the facility and did not know where to enter;
- A visual-perceptual problem, in which the client could not locate the door handle;
- A neuromuscular problem, such as inadequate strength to open the heavy door; or
- A psychosocial issue, such as the dining room was very crowded, and the client expressed a preference to return when it was less congested.

Patterns of deficits and strengths are of great importance. There is really no rule that says that a certain number of check marks is required in a column for the area of occupation to gain significance. Patterns are the key to understanding the generalized ripple effect on a person's functional status.

The case examples that follow illustrate only some of the infinite permutations inherent in the Let's Do Lunch tool. In these examples, readers also will see how it is possible for someone to complete the tasks independently but still demonstrate problem areas that require a critical pathway to prevent injury. In deciding whether it is appropriate to pursue a critical pathway or not, the therapist may ask some questions. Will the problem have an impact on health? Safety? Relationships? Quality of life? The presence of affirmative answers suggests that intervention should follow and, in turn, the functional outcomes be negotiated and defined by the client and therapist. Treatment strategies will build on the client's strengths, noted during the observation. The strengths become the foundations to support the bridges leading to the desired outcomes.

Case Example 1: Julie—Using Let's Do Lunch as an Assessment Tool and Blueprint for Low-Cost Interventions

When a client, who shall be referred to as Julie, and I did the Let's Do Lunch assessment, the following information was obtained (see Figures 7.1a–7.1d). Each time Julie entered the crowded dining room, she dropped to the floor.

Resident: _JULIE_   Therapist: _S. BACHNER, OTR/L_ Date: _1/29/97_

"Let's Do Lunch" Assessment Tool
Task Analysis: Eating in the Lodge

Scoring Codes:
S=Sensory= tactile, proprioceptive, vestibular, visual. auditory, gustatory, olfactory
P=Perceptual=stereognosis, pain response, body scheme, visual perceptual, visual acuity
N=Neuromuscular=reflex, ROM, muscle tone, endurance, postural control
M=Motor=gross coordination, crosses midline, laterality, praxis, oral motor control
C=Cognitive Integration=level of arousal, attention span, initiation, problem-solving
p=Psychosocial=social conduct, self-expression, self-management

TASK 0=independent, 1=verbal cue, 2=physical assist, 3=total assist	S	P	N	M	C	p
1. Enters Dining Room (0) 1 2 3 ELBOWS & KNEES FLEXED – HOLDING WASH CLOTH IN © HAND	?	?				
2. Locates End of Line 0 1 2 3 DROPS TO FLOOR BEFORE LOCATING END OF LINE	✓					
3. Stands on Line 0 1 2 3 REFUSES TO STAND. SITS ON FLOOR ; BODY IN FLEXION	✓					
4. Collects a Tray N.A. 0 1 2 3 STARTS TO SCREAM	✓					✓
5. Puts Tray on Counter 0 1 2 3 N.A.						
6. Faces Correct Direction 0 1 2 3 N.A.						
7. Moves "Forward" 0 1 2 3 N.A.						
8. Balances on Two Feet 0 1 2 3 N.A.						
9. Sees Food Items 0 1 2 3 N.A.						
10. Reaches for Food Items 0 1 2 3 N.A.						
11. Inhibits Impulse to Take All Food 0 1 2 3 N.A.						
12. Makes Food Choice Decisions 0 1 2 3 N.A.						

Figure 7.1a

			S	P	N	M	C	p
13. Holds Loaded Tray with Two Hands *N.A.*	0 1 2 3							
14. Navigates Turn Off of Line to Seating Area *N.A.*	0 1 2 3							
15. Ambulates Efficiently with Tray and Contents *N.A.*	0 1 2 3							
16. Visually Scans Room *APPEARS TO LIMIT* *SCANNING TO APPROX. 5 FOOT RADIUS*	0 1 2 (3)							
17. Visually Targets an Available Seat *GUIDED TO TABLE*	0 1 (2) 3	✓	✓					
18. Visually Targets an Available Seat with Friends *N.A.*	0 1 2 3							
19. Gets to a Targeted Seat	0 1 2 (3)							
20. Puts Tray on Table *STAFF DID THIS*	0 1 2 (3)							
21. Pulls Chair Out	(0) 1 2 3							
22. Sits Down and Positions Legs Under the Table	(0) 1 2 3							
23. Achieves Good Upper Body Posture in Seat	(0) 1 2 3							
24. Achieves Good Lower Body Posture in Seat	(0) 1 2 3							
25. Aligns Self with Tray at Midline *DONE BY STAFF* *AS TRAY PLACED ON TABLE. UNCLEAR IF SHE HAS* *'SHUT DOWN'*	0 1 2 (3)	?				?	
26. Acknowledges Peers at Table (or nearby) *JUST LOOKS*	(0) 1 2 3	?	?			?	
27. Visually Attends to Tray /Contents	0 (1) 2 3							
28. Reaches for Utensils (Wrapped in Napkin)	0 (1) 2 3							

Figure 7.1b

		S	P	N	M	C	p
29. Uses Two Hands to Unwrap Utensils CONTINUES TO HOLD CLOTH IN (L) HAND; USES (R) TO SEARCH FOR UTENSILS	0 1 2 3	✓					
30. Places Napkins in Lap — NO	0 1 2 3						
31. Uses Bilateral Hand Movements to Open Packets WON'T RELEASE WASH CLOTH	0 1 2 (3)	✓					
32. Seasons Food with Salt and Pepper	0 1 2 (3)						
33. Holds Knife by the Handle DOESN'T USE KNIFE	0 1 2 3						
34. Spreads Butter with Knife	0 1 2 3						
35. Cuts Food with Knife	0 1 2 3						
36. Grasps Eating Utensils with Functional Grip (R) or L) RAG/CLOTH IN (L)	0 1 2 3						
37. Visually Targets Desired Food Items	0 (1) 2 3						
38. Initiates Movement of Utensils Toward Food Item	0 1 2 3						
39. Loads (Spoon) Pieces with Fork SEEMS TO SPOON FOOD; EYE-HAND COORDINATION (? DEVELOPMENTAL)	(0) 1 2 3						
40. Contains Food Items on Plate/Bowl HAS DIFFICULTY. GIVEN HI-SIDED DISH. RESULTS BETTER	0 1 2 3						
41. Brings Food to Mouth with Utensil	(0) 1 2 3						
42. Closes Lips to Contain Food in Mouth FOOD SPILLING ONTO CLOTHES	0 (1) 2 3			✓			
43. Chews Bolus with Teeth	(0) 1 2 3						
44. Swallows Bolus	(0) 1 2 3						
45. Safe Chewing and Swallowing	(0) 1 2 3						

Figure 7.1c

		S	P	N	M	C	p
46. Wipes Mouth as Needed	0 (1) 2 3		✓				
47. Targets Drinking Glass	(0) 1 2 3						
48. Crosses Midline (R/L) with Hands as Needed NO	0 1 2 3						
49. Reaches/Grasps/Lifts Glass to Mouth	(0) 1 2 3						
50. Drinks Liquid with a Safe Pace and Adequate Swallow	(0) 1 2 3						
51. Finishes All Food Items on Plate	(0) 1 2 3						
52. Pushes Chair Back	0 (1) 2 3						
53. Sitting to Standing with Adequate Balance ARMS RETURNED TO TOTAL ELBOW FLEXION. FLEXED POSTURE	0 1 (2)(3)	✓		✓			
54. Reaches to Table and Picks up Tray REFUSES	0 1 2 3						
55. Realigns Body for Ambulation FLEXED BODY. FEET HIT FLOOR HARD, eg. MARCHING	0 1 2 (3)	✓					
56. Carries Tray without Spilling N.A. REFUSES. SEEMS TO NOT WANT TO ASSUME NEEDED BODY POSTURE	0 1 2 3	✓					
57. Determines Where to Return Tray SEEMS TO FOCUS ON IMMEDIATE SURROUNDINGS; WANTS TO PROTECT SELF	0 1 2 3	✓					
58. Reaches Location for Tray Deposit NO - WANTS TO GO TO EXIT DOOR	0 1 2 3						
59. Deposits Tray in Return Window N.A.	0 1 2 3						
60. Locates Exit Door from Dining Room LEAVES	(0) 1 2 3						

Summary of Components:

	S	P	N	M	C	p
Needs (Least Functional)		✓	?	?	✓	
Strengths (Most Functional)				✓		✓

Item Numbers Identified for TX: #2 - 15

COMMENTS: SAFE AMBULATION · GOOD STRENGTH. "P" & "N" NOT YET DETERMINED (LITTL
EVIDENCE OF EYE-HAND COORDIN.) "N" BREAKS DOWN FROM PROTECTIVE BODY POSTURE. DOESN'T
CROSS MID-LINE. "C", SEEMS NOT TO IMPACT POSIT/NEGAT ON OUTCOMES

Figure 7.1d

This behavior was recorded in Items 2 through 15. It was my opinion that she essentially shut down when confronted with a sensory bombardment; sitting on the floor was her way of expressing this overload. Julie is nonverbal. Other interpretations among team members included "attention-seeking motivations" and wanting food brought to her rather than obtaining it herself. Whereas Items 16 through 60 further corroborated the assumption regarding a dysfunctional sensory processing system, the items also highlighted problems with performance. It also became obvious that a desirable and functional occupational therapy performance outcome would have to revolve around sensory modulation strategies, because whatever strengths she exhibited, they quickly seemed to become nonfunctional as a result of a sensory system overload. With the intention of increasing her ability to handle the dining room stimulation, therapy should enable her to locate the end of the line (Item 2) and, moreover, stand on line (Item 3). In turn, she should be able to make her own food choices and let go of the seemingly negative behaviors, so as to enjoy and participate more fully in the mealtime process. These are quality-of-life issues. There are cost factors here as well. Items 4 through 15 would bring Julie to a position of greater independence, freeing a staff person from dealing with her obstructive positioning on the floor, as well as another staff person who customarily brings a meal to the table where Julie is brought by staff on getting up from the floor.

The particular "flavor" of Julie's therapy should reflect the therapist's ability to assume the participant–observer's role and all that is implicit in that. Because I viewed her dysfunctional behavior of dropping to the ground when on overload, I checked "S" for sensory issues and tackled the outcomes based on a sensory modulation approach. The most practical and immediate intervention was to arrange for Julie to come to the dining area when the line was about to open, reducing the visual and auditory stimulation, which only grew as mealtime progressed. She was positioned and ready to obtain her meal before the others. After getting through the line, during which she made her food selections, she was provided with a tactile and proprioceptive focus for attention—that is, she was given a trolley that could substitute as a walker and tray-holder to carry and roll her meal. Julie was taught how to hold on to the handlebars and push the trolley to her seat of choice, without concern for spills on the tray, loss of balance, or colliding with another individual. This simple intervention, the trolley and tray-holder, at an approximate cost of $130, has been successful. Training was minimal, and her comfort level clearly improved. Further, in an attempt to facilitate sensory processing changes, her direct-care service provider, at the programming site, was empowered by the OTR to begin a series of sensory-based activities that graded the amount of stimulation deemed acceptable by the client. This work continues and is monitored, upgraded, adjusted, and documented on a routine basis by the OTR. Because the OTR operates in a consultative model, the professional costs are minimized.

Case Example 2: Steve—Using the Tool to Identify Additional Areas for Examination

Let's Do Lunch may also be used to flag problem areas requiring additional examination (see Figures 7.2a–7.2d). For example, when a young man, Steve, stood in line facing the servers, he was observed touching and holding the wall above his head with his left hand. This was noted on Steps 6 and 7, and later Step 14. Even as he reached for the food from the servers with his right dominant hand, he maintained contact with the wall. After moving forward along the line, he again caught my attention by giving himself extra proprioceptive feedback, as he leaned the left side of his body into the room divider, while navigating the turn to the left off the line to the seating area. Later, after he was seated, it was noted that he unconsciously positioned his body so that his tray was mostly to the right of his midline (Item 25). Although there were other noteworthy items, those points formed a cluster and indicated that further assessment of his left-sided sensory responsiveness was indicated. This extra attention showed that his visual response time to stimuli on his left was significantly slower (or nonexistent) than the visual response time to the same stimuli on his right. One might ask, "So what!" After a review of previous accident reports, it was discovered that he had sustained an injury at his programming site when he tripped over an object on the ground that was to his left as he was running. Let's Do Lunch highlighted a functional vision problem. A further clinical assessment pinpointed the problem, and his injury history demonstrated the need to teach compensatory skills to prevent or reduce risk of further injuries. This information was imparted to Steve and his team. Although he had learned to compensate well in obtaining his food and other self-care activities, it was evident that he needed additional training to compensate for visual-perceptual and processing deficits peculiar to his left side.

Case Example 3: Helen—Discovering Her Narrative Over Lunch

Helen further illustrates the evaluation potential in Let's Do Lunch (see Figures 7.3a–7.3d). Helen was admitted to the facility with multiple problems, including mental retardation and physical anomalies (the extent or etiology of which were not known at admission) and a minimal amount of background information, because she had been "discovered" by a county social services worker living in a sibling's shack with no amenities or regard for developmental needs. Because she was nonverbal, glimpses into her pre-admission world were obtained only through current observations.

By using Let's Do Lunch, it was possible to identify a serious visual

Resident: _STEVE_   Therapist: _S. BACHNER, OTR/L_ Date: _6/12/96_

"Let's Do Lunch" Assessment Tool
Task Analysis: Eating in the Lodge

Scoring Codes:
S=Sensory= tactile, proprioceptive, vestibular, visual, auditory, gustatory, olfactory
P=Perceptual=stereognosis, pain response, body scheme, visual perceptual, visual acuity
N=Neuromuscular=reflex, ROM, muscle tone, endurance, postural control
M=Motor=gross coordination, crosses midline, laterality, praxis, oral motor control
C=Cognitive Integration=level of arousal, attention span, initiation, problem-solving
p=Psychosocial=social conduct, self-expression, self-management

TASK 0=independent, 1=verbal cue, 2=physical assist, 3=total assist	S	P	N	M	C	p
1. Enters Dining Room ⓪ 1 2 3						
2. Locates End of Line ⓪ 1 2 3						
3. Stands on Line ⓪ 1 2 3						
4. Collects a Tray ⓪ 1 2 3						
5. Puts Tray on Counter ⓪ 1 2 3						
6. Faces Correct Direction ⓪ 1 2 3 USES Ⓛ HAND TO HOLD WALL ABOVE HEAD	✓	✓				
7. Moves "Forward" ⓪ 1 2 3 CONTINUES TO USE Ⓛ HAND FOR TACTILE INPUT	✓	✓				
8. Balances on Two Feet ⓪ 1 2 3 HOLDS ONTO WALL c̄ Ⓛ HAND	✓	✓				
9. Sees Food Items ⓪ 1 2 3						
10. Reaches for Food Items Ⓡ HAND ⓪ 1 2 3 Ⓛ HAND MAINTAINS CONTACT c̄ WALL	✓	✓				
11. Inhibits Impulse to Take All Food ⓪ 1 2 3						
12. Makes Food Choice Decisions ⓪ 1 2 3						

Figure 7.2a

		S	P	N	M	C	p
13. Holds Loaded Tray with Two Hands	(0) 1 2 3						
14. Navigates Turn Off of Line to Seating Area LEANS (L) SIDE OF BODY INTO PARTITION AS TURNS	(0) 1 2 3	✓	✓				
15. Ambulates Efficiently with Tray and Contents	(0) 1 2 3						
16. Visually Scans Room	(0) 1 2 3						
17. Visually Targets an Available Seat - STRAIGHT AHEAD	(0) 1 2 3		✓				
18. Visually Targets an Available Seat with Friends ?	0 1 2 3						
19. Gets to a Targeted Seat	(0) 1 2 3						
20. Puts Tray on Table	(0) 1 2 3						
21. Pulls Chair Out	(0) 1 2 3						
22. Sits Down and Positions Legs Under the Table	(0) 1 2 3						
23. Achieves Good Upper Body Posture in Seat FUNCTIONAL	(0) 1 2 3						
24. Achieves Good Lower Body Posture in Seat	(0) 1 2 3						
25. Aligns Self with Tray at Midline TRAY POSITIONED MOSTLY TO (R) OF MIDLINE	(0) 1 2 3		✓				
26. Acknowledges Peers at Table (or nearby)	(0) 1 2 3						
27. Visually Attends to Tray /Contents	(0) 1 2 3						
28. Reaches for Utensils (Wrapped in Napkin)	(0) 1 2 3						

Figure 7.2b

		S	P	N	M	C	p
29. Uses Two Hands to Unwrap Utensils	(0) 1 2 3						
30. Places Napkins in Lap	0 (1) 2 3						
31. Uses Bilateral Hand Movements to Open Packets	(0) 1 2 3						
32. Seasons Food with Salt and Pepper N.A.	0 1 2 3						
33. Holds Knife by the Handle	(0) 1 2 3						
34. Spreads Butter with Knife N.A.	0 1 2 3						
35. Cuts Food with Knife	(0) 1 2 3						
36. Grasps Eating Utensils with Functional Grip (R) or L)	(0) 1 2 3						
37. Visually Targets Desired Food Items TRAY REMAINS POSITIONED (R) OF MIDLINE	0 1 2 3		✓				
38. Initiates Movement of Utensils Toward Food Item	(0) 1 2 3						
39. Loads Spoon/Pieces with Fork	(0) 1 2 3						
40. Contains Food Items on Plate/Bowl	(0) 1 2 3						
41. Brings Food to Mouth with Utensil	(0) 1 2 3						
42. Closes Lips to Contain Food in Mouth	(0) 1 2 3						
43. Chews Bolus with Teeth	(0) 1 2 3						
44. Swallows Bolus	(0) 1 2 3						
45. Safe Chewing and Swallowing	(0) 1 2 3						

Figure 7.2c

		S	P	N	M	C	p
46. Wipes Mouth as Needed	(0) 1 2 3						
47. Targets Drinking Glass	(0) 1 2 3						
48. Crosses Midline (R/L) with Hands as Needed	(0) 1 2 3						
49. Reaches/Grasps/Lifts Glass to Mouth	(0) 1 2 3						
50. Drinks Liquid with a Safe Pace and Adequate Swallow	(0) 1 2 3						
51. Finishes All Food Items on Plate	(0) 1 2 3						
52. Pushes Chair Back *TURNS TO (R)*	(0) 1 2 3		?✓				
53. Sitting to Standing with Adequate Balance *?APPEARS TO TAKE RAPID, SMALL STEPS IN PLACE TO BALANCE SELF*	0 1 2 3	?✓	?✓				
54. Reaches to Table and Picks up (Tray) *= (R) OF MIDLINE*	(0) 1 2 3						
55. Realigns Body for Ambulation	(0) 1 2 3						
56. Carries Tray without Spilling	(0) 1 2 3						
57. Determines Where to Return Tray	(0) 1 2 3						
58. Reaches Location for Tray Deposit	(0) 1 2 3						
59. Deposits Tray in Return Window	(0) 1 2 3						
60. Locates Exit Door from Dining Room	(0) 1 2 3						

Summary of Components:

		S	P	N	M	C	p
Needs (Least Functional)		✓	✓				
Strengths (Most Functional)				✓	✓	✓	✓

Item Numbers Identified for TX: _____

COMMENTS: *INVESTIGATE & RULE-OUT (L) SIDED VISUAL RESPONSE DEFICITS*
CLIENT'S (L)-SIDED SENSORY-IN-PUT NOTEWORTHY.

Figure 7.2d

Resident: *HELEN*   Therapist: *S. BACHNER, OTR/L* Date: *11/13/96*

"Let's Do Lunch" Assessment Tool
Task Analysis: Eating in the Lodge

Scoring Codes:
S=Sensory= tactile, proprioceptive, vestibular. visual, auditory, gustatory, olfactory
P=Perceptual= stereognosis, pain response. body scheme, visual perceptual, visual acuity
N=Neuromuscular= reflex, ROM, muscle tone, endurance, postural control
M=Motor= gross coordination, crosses midline, laterality, praxis, oral motor control
C=Cognitive Integration= level of arousal, attention span, initiation, problem-solving
p=Psychosocial= social conduct, self-expression, self-management

TASK 0=independent, 1=verbal cue. 2=physical assist, 3=total assist	S	P	N	M	C	p
1. Enters Dining Room 0 1 ②3	✓	✓				
2. Locates End of Line 0 1 2 ③	✓	✓				
3. Stands on Line ⓪1 2 3						
4. Collects a Tray 0 1 2 ③		✓			✓	
5. Puts Tray on Counter 0 1 2 ③		✓			✓	
6. Faces Correct Direction 0 1 2 ③						
7. Moves "Forward" 0 ① 2 3						
8. Balances on Two Feet ⓪1 2 3						
9. Sees Food Items 0 1 2 ③ ?		✓				
10. Reaches for Food Items 0 1 2 ③		✓		✓		
11. Inhibits Impulse to Take All Food ⓪1 2 3						
12. Makes Food Choice Decisions 0 1 2 ③ *N.A.*					✓	

Figure 7.3a

	S	P	N	M	C	p
13. Holds Loaded Tray with Two Hands 0 1 2 (3)					✔	
14. Navigates Turn Off of Line to Seating Area 0 1 2 (3)		✔			✔	
15. Ambulates Efficiently with Tray and Contents 0 1 2 (3)	✔	✔				
16. Visually Scans Room 0 1 2 (3) ONLY RESPONDS TO STIMULI IN CENTRAL VISUAL FIELD		✔				
17. Visually Targets an Available Seat 0 1 (2) 3 GUIDED TO TABLE c̄ AVAILABLE SEAT						
18. Visually Targets an Available Seat with Friends 0 1 (2) 3 STANDS BESIDE CHAIR PER ESCORT #17						
19. Gets to a Targeted Seat 0 1 (2) 3						
20. Puts Tray on Table 0 1 2 (3)						
21. Pulls Chair Out 0 1 2 3 REFUSES						
22. Sits Down and Positions Legs Under the Table 0 1 2 3 REFUSES TO SIT						
23. Achieves Good Upper Body Posture in Seat 0 1 2 3 N.A.						
24. Achieves Good Lower Body Posture in Seat 0 1 2 3 WANTS TO EAT WHILE STANDING						
25. Aligns Self with Tray at Midline 0 1 2 3 CONTINUES TO RESIST SITTING IN CHAIR						
26. Acknowledges Peers at Table (or nearby) 0 1 2 3 SMILES AT PEERS IF IN HER CENTRAL VISION (20°-30° CENTRAL)	✔					
27. Visually Attends to Tray /Contents 0 1 2 (3) MOVES VISUAL TARGET TO 4" FROM EYES						
28. Reaches for Utensils (Wrapped in Napkin) 0 1 2 (3)						

Figure 7.3b

	S	P	N	M	C	p
29. Uses Two Hands to Unwrap Utensils ⓪ 1 2 3 *IF GIVEN TO HER*						
30. Places Napkins in Lap 0 1 2 3 *STILL STANDING — N.A.*						
31. Uses Bilateral Hand Movements to Open Packets 0 1 ② 3 *FINE-MOTOR OK. — DOESN'T COORDINATE c̄ EYES*						
32. Seasons Food with Salt and Pepper 0 1 2 3 *N.A.*						
33. Holds Knife by the Handle ⓪ 1 2 3 *ONLY USES SPOON*						
34. Spreads Butter with Knife 0 1 2 3 *N.A.*						
35. Cuts Food with Knife 0 1 2 3 *N.A.*						
36. Grasps Eating Utensils with Functional Grip (Ⓡ or L) ⓪ 1 2 3 *ONLY BRIEFLY — PREFERS TO USE FINGERS*						
37. Visually Targets Desired Food Items 0 1 2 3 *SEEMS TO NEED HIGH CONTRAST, CENTRAL 20°-30°, 4" FROM EYES*						
38. Initiates Movement of Utensils Toward Food Item ⓪ 1 2 3 *PREFERS FINGERS FOR FOOD EXPLORATION*						
39. Loads Spoon/Pieces with Fork ⓪ 1 2 3 *CAN USE SPOON BUT LIKES FINGERS*						
40. Contains Food Items on Plate/Bowl 0 1 ② 3 *GIVEN HI-SIDED PLATE TO ASSIST c̄ CONTAINMENT — DID BETTER*		✓				
41. Brings Food to Mouth with Utensil ⓪ 1 2 3 *HOLDS BOWL AT 4" FROM FACE c̄ Ⓛ HAND*		✓				
42. Closes Lips to Contain Food in Mouth ⓪ 1 2 3						
43. Chews Bolus with Teeth 0 1 2 3 *NEEDS MECHANICAL-SOFT/GROUND MEAT FOR SAFETY*						
44. Swallows Bolus ⓪ 1 2 3						
45. Safe Chewing and Swallowing — *NOT WHEN* 0 1 2 3 *EATING REGULAR DIET (CONSISTENCY)*						

Figure 7.3c

		S	P	N	M	C	p
46. Wipes Mouth as Needed	(0) 1 2 3					✓	
47. Targets Drinking Glass *HAVING TROUBLE LOCATING IT*	0 1 2 (3)		✓				
48. Crosses Midline (R/L) with Hands as Needed	(0) 1 2 3						
49. Reaches/Grasps/Lifts Glass to Mouth *NEEDS TO PLACED IN HER HAND*	0 1 2 (3)		✓				
50. Drinks Liquid with a Safe Pace and Adequate Swallow *DOESN'T TIP HEAD BACK. ? WHY*	(0) 1 2 3						
51. Finishes All Food Items on Plate *REQUIRED VERBAL & PHYSICAL PROMPTS TO LOCATE FOOD*	0 1 2 (3)		✓				
52. Pushes Chair Back *N.A.*	0 1 2 3						
53. Sitting to Standing with Adequate Balance	(0) 1 2 3						
54. Reaches to Table and Picks up Tray	0 1 2 (3)						
55. Realigns Body for Ambulation	(0) 1 2 3						
56. Carries Tray without Spilling	0 1 2 (3)						
57. Determines Where to Return Tray	0 1 2 (3)		✓			✓	
58. Reaches Location for Tray Deposit	0 1 2 (3)						
59. Deposits Tray in Return Window	0 1 2 (3)						
60. Locates Exit Door from Dining Room	0 1 2 (3)						

Summary of Components:

Needs (Least Functional)   *LACK OF FAMILIARITY* ✓   ✓

Strengths (Most Functional)   ✓   ✓ ✓   ✓

Item Numbers Identified for TX: _____

COMMENTS: *IF BOWL REMAINS ON TRAY, CLIENT STRETCHES HEAD FORWARD-OBVIOUS MUSCLE STRAIN, TENSION. TENSION DISAPPEARED WHEN BOWL LIFTED 4" FROM EYES/MOUTH. NEEDS EYE EXAM. ? PREVIOUS SOCIALIZATION TO PEOPLE/OBJECTS*

Figure 7.3d

deficit and further appreciate the impact of her previous deprivations. For instance, she clearly had difficulty with Items 16 to 18:

- Visually scans room
- Visually targets an available seat
- Visually targets an available seat with friends.

Here, a differentiating question was whether this inability could be attributed to the newness of her arrival and absence of friends, or whether it was perhaps visually based. Things became more revealing when Helen refused to sit down in the chair at the table. She was visibly agitated when staff efforts to have her sit persisted. Therefore, Items 21 through 24 recorded these behaviors. Problems with using the chair at the dinner table were reproducible at all meals. Upon further investigation, it became evident that Helen also resisted lying in her bed. Helen's narrative was being told; her responses to tables, chairs, and even her bed provided much-needed messages to staff about her previous existence. Her story of extreme deprivation was coming through loud and clear, as she communicated nonverbally about her early impoverished environment, one in which she never had available for her use any furniture for sitting or sleeping. While eating—and she was indeed very hungry—she placed the bowl or dish within 4 inches of her eyes and only showed visual attention to items in her central vision (approximately 20 degrees to 30 degrees central) (Items 26 and 37). Peers at the table who were in her peripheral fields were not acknowledged. This observation was juxtaposed to Helen's outgoing personality. Although she demonstrated awareness of how to use a spoon, other utensils such as a knife and fork seemed unfamiliar. In fact, Helen had a distinct preference for using her fingers to get food from her dish to her mouth. This information was recorded in Items 38 though 41.

Helen had some teeth for chewing but not a full set. She had problems with Item 43, chewing bolus with teeth, and Item 45, safe chewing and swallowing. This evidence enabled the occupational therapist to contact both the facility physician and dietitian to arrange for a mechanical soft or ground diet to ensure Helen's safety. She had no problem crossing her midline (Item 48) but demonstrated a unique pattern for drinking liquids (Item 50): She would not tip her head back. Through further observation, this drinking style appeared to be rooted in a reluctance to move her eyes rather than a dysfunctional swallowing pattern. Diminutive Helen had the appetite of a lumberjack, and yet she would leave food on her plate. If she were directed to the food with verbal prompts, however, she quickly went after it for consumption!

Based on the highlighted items, I was able to submit a report that spoke to Helen's needs with limited visual fields, including

- Her seeming inability to perceive anything in her periphery, up or down
- Her need to hold items for viewing within 4 inches of her eyes

- Her need for chewing and swallowing precautions
- Her need for assistance with safe ambulation, due to apparent low vision
- Her impoverished cultural and experiential background, as re-enacted through her unfamiliarity with common eating tools and furniture.

Similarly, strengths were noted in neuromuscular and psychosocial areas, comfort with sensory input, ease with gross and fine motor tasks, and potential for cognitive growth through familiarization and cultural assimilation. Based on this input to the team, she was sent for an ophthalmological consult and found to have bilateral cataracts. Plans for surgery were made. Occupational therapy functional outcomes were delayed until the surgery was completed.

Let's Do Lunch as a Template

If one chooses, Let's Do Lunch may serve as a template for Let's Do *Anything*. All that is needed is a detailed task analysis. In fact, the task analysis format lends itself to infinite settings, situations, and tasks. The same principle of providing a structured observation is the key. Yet, I am hard-pressed to come up with another activity that enables a therapist and client to meet under such motivating conditions; an activity that is part of everyday living; an activity that is so culturally laden, so critical to survival; and one that has the potential to elevate the quality of life for someone with handicapping conditions.

Value in Using the Technique

From occupational therapy students to senior clinical staff, the technique works. Students at the facility like the simplicity of following the course of action step-by-step. It minimizes writing and allows for additional time to focus attention on the observations.

Senior clinicians report the same ease as well but place a greater value on the results. For the experienced clinician, there are the memories of those early days of practice, when one's mission was to juggle all the events and somehow triage presenting issues and conditions that, to the neophyte, all look like foreground. The environment, the components, the interactions, the critical questions, the observations, the "so whats"—these are the issues bombarding the therapist. The experienced clinician has digested these ingredients in evaluation settings so many times and knows in his or her gut the format for a reasonable sequence.

Examining the setting, the client, the deviations, the problem solving, the flavors, the aromas, the culture—it all becomes possible in short order. Wherever the observer is on the experience continuum, the tool has simplicity, logic, and inherent value. It enables the therapist to quickly get a taste of what is happening and to work within the confines of a managed care environment to arrive at functional outcomes critical to daily living, expression of self, and quality of life. It enables the therapist to describe a client's functioning—the levels of significance that are interpreted as strengths and the potentials that can be tapped—as well as definitions of need that will require a clinician's expertise in designing or conducting a program with measurable, functional outcomes. It's all there!

The value of a service delivery, as mentioned at the outset of this chapter, can be determined by the ratio of quality to cost. Let's Do Lunch, with a menu of performance skills available for selection, blends a biomedical model with the social sciences and quality-of-life model and produces the opportunity for measurable outcomes that have relevance and interest to all consumers: the client, the third-party payer, and the staff. Let's Do Lunch is both a process and a facilitating device for the establishment of relevant outcome.

According to Donabedian (1988),

> Much of what we call the art of medicine consists in almost intuitive adaptations to individual requirements in technical care as well as in the management of the interpersonal process. Another element in the art of medicine is the way, still poorly understood, in which practitioners process information to arrive at a correct diagnosis and an appropriate strategy of care. As our understanding of each of these areas of occupation improves, we can expect the realm of our science to expand and that of our art to shrink. Yet, I hope that some of the mystery in practice will always remain, since it affirms and celebrates the uniqueness of each individual.

Acknowledgments

Acknowledging people for the creation of a product is sometimes risky, for the author takes the chance that important people inadvertently remain unmentioned. With that in mind, I would like to thank my friend and colleague Valnere McLean, MA, OTR/L, FAOTA; my coeditor Mildred Ross, MS, OTR/L, FAOTA; and my husband Paul Bachner, MD, FCAP, for their respective patience, clarity in thinking, and willingness to review the chapter yet another time. Ruth Huebner, PhD, OTR/L, and her students from Eastern Kentucky University, individually and collectively, influenced the chapter's outcome, and I am most appreciative. Thank you, too, to those many people who provided encouragement and to those family members—two- and four-legged—who often waited for dinners long overdue without complaint.

References

Axelson, M. L., & Brinberg, D. (1989). *A social–psychological perspective on food-related behavior*. New York: Springer-Verlag.

Bronner, S. (1986). *Grasping things: Folk material culture and mass society in America* (pp. 160–179). Lexington: University Press of Kentucky.

Caplan, B., & Shecter, J. (1995). The role of nonstandard neuropsychological assessment in rehabilitation: History, rationale, and examples. In L. Cushman & M. Scherer (Eds.), *Psychological assessment in medical rehabilitation* (pp. 359–391). Washington, DC: American Psychological Association.

Chassin, M. R. (1996). Improving the quality of care. *New England Journal of Medicine, 335*, 1060–1063.

Donabedian, A. (1988). The quality of care: How can it be assessed. *Journal of the American Medical Association, 260*, 1743–1748.

Eddy, D. M. (1991). Oregon's methods: Did cost-effectiveness analysis fail? *Journal of the American Medical Association, 266*, 2135–2141.

Ellwood, P. M. (1988). Shattuck lecture—Outcomes management: A technology of patient experience. *New England Journal of Medicine, 318*, 1549–1556.

Forer, S. (1996). *Resource guide on outcome management and program evaluation for occupational therapy*. Bethesda, MD: American Occupational Therapy Association.

Goode, J. (1992). Food. In R. Bauman (Ed.), *Folklore, cultural performances, and popular entertainments* (pp. 232–245). New York: Oxford University Press.

Inglehart, J. (1994). *Health Policy Report, 331*, 1167–1170.

Joint Commission on Accreditation of Healthcare Organizations. (1994). *A guide to establishing programs for assessing outcomes in clinical settings*. Oakbrook Terrace, IL: Author.

Kautzmann, L. (1997). *Health-related quality of life status* [Unpublished handout]. Richmond: Eastern Kentucky University, Department of Occupational Therapy.

Lindeman, E. C. (1925). *Social discovery: An approach to the study of functional groups*. New York: Republic.

Marshall, D. (1995). *Food choice and the consumer*. Glasgow, Scotland: Blackie Academic & Professional.

Maurer, D., & Sobal, J. (Eds.). (1995). *Eating agendas: Food and nutrition as social problems*. New York: Walter de Gruyter.

Perske, R., Clifton, A., McLean, B., & Stein, J. I. (Eds.). (1986). *Mealtimes for persons with severe handicaps*. Baltimore: Paul H. Brookes.

Relman, A. S. (1988). Assessment and accountability: The third revolution in medical care. *New England Journal of Medicine, 319*, 1220–1222.

Rogers, J., & Holm, M. (1994). Accepting the challenge of outcome research: Examining the effectiveness of occupational therapy practice. *American Journal of Occupational Therapy, 48*, 871–876.

Silberman, C. (1991). From the patient's bed. *Health Management Quarterly, 13*(2), 12–15.

Toglia, J. (1993). Attention and memory. In C. B. Royeen (Ed.), *AOTA self-study series: Cognitive rehabilitation* (pp. 22–32). Bethesda, MD: American Occupational Therapy Association.

Wennberg, J. E. (1991). The road to guidelines. *Health Management Quarterly*, 2–7.

Wetzler, H. (1994, July/August). Outcomes measurement: A way to measure value. *Healthcare Forum Journal*,

Wilson, J., & Cleary, P. D. (1995). Linking clinical variables with health-related quality of life: A conceptual model of patient outcomes. *Journal of the American Medical Association, 273*, 59–65.

Appendix 7.A

Resident: _____ Therapist: _____ Date: _____

"Let's Do Lunch" Assessment Tool
Task Analysis: Eating in the Lodge

Scoring Codes:
S=Sensory= tactile, proprioceptive, vestibular, visual, auditory, gustatory, olfactory
P=Perceptual=stereognosis, pain response, body scheme, visual perceptual, visual acuity
N=Neuromuscular=reflex, ROM, muscle tone, endurance, postural control
M=Motor=gross coordination, crosses midline, laterality, praxis, oral motor control
C=Cognitive Integration=level of arousal, attention span, initiation, problem-solving
p=Psychosocial=social conduct, self-expression, self-management

TASK 0=independent, 1=verbal cue, 2=physical assist, 3=total assist	S	P	N	M	C	p
1. Enters Dining Room 0 1 2 3						
2. Locates End of Line 0 1 2 3						
3. Stands on Line 0 1 2 3						
4. Collects a Tray 0 1 2 3						
5. Puts Tray on Counter 0 1 2 3						
6. Faces Correct Direction 0 1 2 3						
7. Moves "Forward" 0 1 2 3						
8. Balances on Two Feet 0 1 2 3						
9. Sees Food Items 0 1 2 3						
10. Reaches for Food Items 0 1 2 3						
11. Inhibits Impulse to Take All Food 0 1 2 3						
12. Makes Food Choice Decisions 0 1 2 3						

	S	P	N	M	C	p
13. Holds Loaded Tray with Two Hands 0 1 2 3						
14. Navigates Turn Off of Line to Seating Area 0 1 2 3						
15. Ambulates Efficiently with Tray and Contents 0 1 2 3						
16. Visually Scans Room 0 1 2 3						
17. Visually Targets an Available Seat 0 1 2 3						
18. Visually Targets an Available Seat with Friends 0 1 2 3						
19. Gets to a Targeted Seat 0 1 2 3						
20. Puts Tray on Table 0 1 2 3						
21. Pulls Chair Out 0 1 2 3						
22. Sits Down and Positions Legs Under the Table 0 1 2 3						
23. Achieves Good Upper Body Posture in Seat 0 1 2 3						
24. Achieves Good Lower Body Posture in Seat 0 1 2 3						
25. Aligns Self with Tray at Midline 0 1 2 3						
26. Acknowledges Peers at Table (or nearby) 0 1 2 3						
27. Visually Attends to Tray /Contents 0 1 2 3						
28. Reaches for Utensils (Wrapped in Napkin) 0 1 2 3						

	S	P	N	M	C	p
29. Uses Two Hands to Unwrap Utensils 0 1 2 3						
30. Places Napkins in Lap 0 1 2 3						
31. Uses Bilateral Hand Movements to Open Packets 0 1 2 3						
32. Seasons Food with Salt and Pepper 0 1 2 3						
33. Holds Knife by the Handle 0 1 2 3						
34. Spreads Butter with Knife 0 1 2 3						
35. Cuts Food with Knife 0 1 2 3						
36. Grasps Eating Utensils with Functional Grip (R or L) 0 1 2 3						
37. Visually Targets Desired Food Items 0 1 2 3						
38. Initiates Movement of Utensils Toward Food Item 0 1 2 3						
39. Loads Spoon/Pieces with Fork 0 1 2 3						
40. Contains Food Items on Plate/Bowl 0 1 2 3						
41. Brings Food to Mouth with Utensil 0 1 2 3						
42. Closes Lips to Contain Food in Mouth 0 1 2 3						
43. Chews Bolus with Teeth 0 1 2 3						
44. Swallows Bolus 0 1 2 3						
45. Safe Chewing and Swallowing 0 1 2 3						

		S	P	N	M	C	p
46. Wipes Mouth as Needed	0 1 2 3						
47. Targets Drinking Glass	0 1 2 3						
48. Crosses Midline (R/L) with Hands as Needed	0 1 2 3						
49. Reaches/Grasps/Lifts Glass to Mouth	0 1 2 3						
50. Drinks Liquid with a Safe Pace and Adequate Swallow	0 1 2 3						
51. Finishes All Food Items on Plate	0 1 2 3						
52. Pushes Chair Back	0 1 2 3						
53. Sitting to Standing with Adequate Balance	0 1 2 3						
54. Reaches to Table and Picks up Tray	0 1 2 3						
55. Realigns Body for Ambulation	0 1 2 3						
56. Carries Tray without Spilling	0 1 2 3						
57. Determines Where to Return Tray	0 1 2 3						
58. Reaches Location for Tray Deposit	0 1 2 3						
59. Deposits Tray in Return Window	0 1 2 3						
60. Locates Exit Door from Dining Room	0 1 2 3						

Summary of Components:

Needs (Least Functional) _____

Strengths (Most Functional) _____

Item Numbers Identified for TX: _____

COMMENTS: _____

_____

CHAPTER 8

Structurally Based Manual Therapy and Improved Function

Lynn D. Simpson, OTR/L

Introduction

Adults with mental retardation are often not considered for therapeutic intervention in the same light as other populations because many of the dysfunctional behaviors displayed by them have been labeled "mental retardation" and are presumed, therefore, to be untreatable. Such labeling tends to preclude examining other reasons for these behaviors, such as physical or physiological. Traditionally, in this population dysfunctional behaviors are viewed as being fixed, systemic, and psychologically based entities in which the behaviors themselves rather than their causes are treated.

In this chapter, dysfunctional behaviors—motor, self-injurious, perceptual, and social—are regarded as symptoms of structural dysfunction. *Structural dysfunction* refers to a disruption in the normal balance of the body's framework of bones/joints, muscle, and fascial connective tissue. Structurally based therapy (Greenman, 1989; Mitchell, Moran, & Pruzzo, 1979; Upledger & Vredevoogd, 1983; Weiselfish & Kain, 1990) is presented and discussed here as a means to improve functional performance. The premise of this therapeutic approach is that structural, biomechanical stresses within the body framework interfere with function and establish a pattern of maladaptive behaviors (Simpson, 1996) based on lowered tolerances to stimuli. To alleviate these stresses and improve one's potential for function, manual therapy techniques are used. These techniques are briefly described, and the structural approach is differentiated from traditional functional approaches, such as sensorimotor therapies. To elucidate the underlying theories and concepts of structurally based therapy, four case histories are presented of adults diagnosed with mental retardation and other developmental disabilities.

It is important to consider that dysfunctional behaviors may be signs and symptoms of structural dysfunction that place the individual at a disadvantage to respond or react to his or her environment. Recognizing the interplay between structure and function (Barral, 1991; Greenman, 1978, 1989; Heinrich, 1991; Korr, 1978; Mennell, 1992; Upledger, 1987; Upledger & Vredevoogd, 1983) is necessary so an individual can receive the best therapeutic intervention to optimize function. The specific goal of manual therapy is to realign and rebalance the neuromusculoskeletal systems. Using these therapy techniques results in enhanced movement and ameliorated tolerances to internal and external stimuli and, consequently, maximizes functional performance.

Manual Therapy

What Is Structurally Based Manual Therapy?

Structurally based manual therapy is a part of manual medicine—osteopathy—an approach to health that views the nervous, muscular, and skeletal systems as major components of both physiological and physical/structural health. These three systems can be considered together as a unit (the neuromusculoskeletal system), or two of the systems can be considered together (neuromuscular and musculoskeletal). The evaluation and treatment processes use the therapist's hands to manually assess, through palpation, the function and dysfunction of different body tissues—arthrodial, muscle, and fascia—that constitute the neuromusculoskeletal system. It is possible to have impaired structural balance within a single tissue, such as a muscle spasm, or to have imbalance between different tissues, such as fascial adhesions interfering with muscle function. Further, a disruption in the balance of the neuromusculoskeletal system has the potential to disrupt function in other systems and vice versa (Barral, 1989, 1991; Barral & Mercier, 1988; Upledger & Vredevoogd, 1983). For example, the passage of the subclavian vein (circulatory system) around the clavicle and first rib (neuromusculoskeletal system) in the thoracic inlet may lead to compromised blood flow if the clavicle is depressed and impinges on this vein (Figure 8.1).

Structurally based manual therapy is established on a dynamic perspective that views the body as a biomechanical entity in which the "lever and pulley system" must be in good working order for the individual to function well. This implies that there is an optimal structural/postural alignment that allows for maximal functioning. Any departure from this alignment produces an imbalance in the system and creates stresses throughout the total structural framework. Such stresses result in a chain reaction of adaptive responses

Figure 8.1. The thoracic inlet is vulnerable to neuromusculoskeletal dysfunction with subsequent problems in, for example, the circulatory system (see text for more detail).
From S. Goldberg, *Clinical Anatomy Made Ridiculously Simple,* MedMaster 2004. Reprinted with permission.

(compensations), as in a complex system of interconnecting levers and pulleys; the body does, however, reach a point at which it no longer has any reserve to compensate—it is decompensated (Figures 8.2 and 8.3).

Overall, then, manual therapy assesses structural integrity: postural alignment, articular balance of both bony and soft-tissue interfaces, and mobility. According to this perspective, and to achieve maximum benefit from therapy (namely, to fulfill possibly untapped potentials), one needs to look first at structure and then at function.

Structurally Based Manual Therapy Treatment Techniques

General Considerations
The techniques addressed in this chapter are
- Muscle energy,
- Myofascial release,
- Visceral manipulation,
- Neurofascial release,
- Craniosacral therapy,
- Cranial osteopathy,
- Strain and counterstrain, and
- Zero balancing.

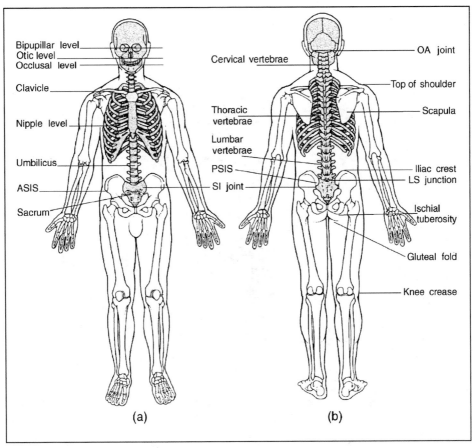

Figure 8.2(a)(b). Normal posture in which structural alignment in the coronal plane is assessed by comparing the height or level of (a) anterior structures, such as the eyes, ears (otic level), and the anterior superior iliac spine, and (b) posterior structures, such as the iliac crests, the tops of the shoulders, and gluteal folds. Alignment in a transverse plane is assessed by comparing some of the same structural landmarks but relative to anterior–posterior displacement. ASIS: anterior superior iliac spine. LS junction: lumbosacral junction. OA joint: occipitoatlantal joint. PSIS: posterior superior iliac spine. SI joint: sacroiliac joint.
From *Human anatomy and physiology,* by J. W. Hole, Jr., 1993, (6th ed.) p. 186, Wm. C. Brown Publishers. Reprinted with permission of the McGraw-Hill Companies.

Each technique has its own view of function/dysfunction; assessment protocol; and required, specialized treatment skills. All, however, are concerned with alleviating hypomobility and its effect on health and well-being.

Certain techniques are known to be more effective for treating certain tissue dysfunctions than others: myofascial release (Greenman, 1989; Weiselfish & Kain, 1991) and neurofascial release (Davidson, 1992) for fascial restrictions; visceral manipulation (Barral, 1989, 1991; Barral & Mercier, 1988; Kain, 1996; Weiselfish, 1996) for fascial restrictions interfering with visceral position and mobility; muscle energy (Breuer, 1989a, 1989b; Greenman, 1989; Mitchell et al., 1979; Summerfelt, 1991; Weiselfish, 1994) for

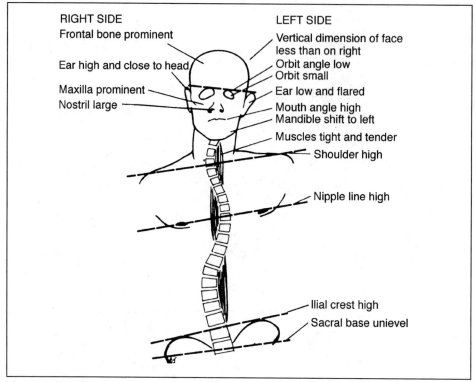

Figure 8.2(c). Abnormal posture.
From "Structural influences in temporomandibular joint pain and dysfunction," by J. O. Royder, 1981, *Journal of American Osteopathic Association, 80,* p. 465. Reprinted with permission.

articular imbalance at joints and for muscle spasms; strain and counterstrain (Jones, 1981) for both peripheral protective muscle spasm and central hypertonicity (Weiselfish, 1994; Weiselfish & Kain, 1993); craniosacral therapy (Upledger, 1987, 1990; Upledger & Vredevoogd, 1983) and cranial osteopathy (Hruby, 1994, 1995) for cranial suture restrictions and for intracranial and spinal dural membrane tensions; and zero balancing (Brown, 1993, 1994; Smith, 1986, 1996) for energetic restrictions in the bony skeleton. All techniques screen the entire body because the site of pain may not be the origin or cause of pain. Pain is often referred, and habits of movement and positioning that are taken on to avoid initial pain(s) may set up areas of secondary pain that eventually may be stronger.

To avoid confusion for those who may further explore these techniques, it is necessary to clarify "structural" versus "functional" techniques. In this chapter, I refer to all the above-mentioned techniques as "structurally based manual therapy techniques" because they all look for postural and musculoskeletal bases of structural imbalance. In distinction, functional techniques (Weiselfish & Kain, 1990) view the performance of an activity and focus on

Figure 8.3. (a) Normal posture in which structural alignment in the sagittal plane is assessed by evaluating the degree of deviation of the spinal curves (cervical, thoracic, and lumbar) from a posteriorly placed plumb line; the distances in centimeters give the normal distances in different areas of the spine. The body should touch the plumb line at the occiput, thoracic kyphosis, and buttocks. There is another plumb line that is drawn to be slightly anterior to the lateral malleolus of the ankle, posterior to the hip joint, and in line with the shoulder joint and external acoustic meatus of the ear. From this latter plumb line, one can observe, for example, placement of the head over the trunk, retraction or protraction of the shoulder, and anterior or posterior tilt of the pelvis. (b) An example of undesired structural alignment in which postural compensations are made to maintain the eyes parallel to the ground: exaggerated cervical, thoracic, and lumbar curves; anterior tilt of pelvis; flexion of hip and knee; dorsiflexion of the ankle; forward head posture (decreased suboccipital space); shortened anterior neck muscles; depression of the jaw; and flattened sternum and rib cage.

From "A proposed chronology of events for forward head posture," by M. W. Darnell, 1983, *CRANIO: The Journal of Craniomandibular Practice, 1,* p. 50. Reprinted with permission.

improvement in function without focusing on the causes of malfunction. However, in formal presentations and in the manual therapy literature, "strain and counterstrain" is considered a functional technique. This is done to differentiate between direct and indirect (functional) technique styles within the field of manual therapy itself. To find out more about the distinction between structural and functional manual therapy techniques, refer to Greenman (1989, p. 101) and Tehan (1980, pp. 94–96).

Based on my experience working with adults and children with developmental disabilities, muscle energy is the most challenging technique for achieving success because the client needs to perform isometric muscle contractions. However, the muscle energy protocol also provides the strongest foundation to begin to understand structure and the significance of disruption of structural balance.

Muscle Energy

The muscle energy protocol (Greenman, 1989; Mitchell et al., 1979) assesses postural balance and biomechanical dysfunction (articular balance). Bony landmarks, such as tops of shoulders; iliac crests; anterior superior iliac spines; and soft-tissue landmarks, including nipple-level and gluteal and knee creases, are assessed for alignment and symmetry (Figures 8.2 and 8.3). Along with this static assessment of postural alignment, movement is assessed for range of motion and quality of motion. Then it is determined if postural malalignment is due to muscle weakness, structural dysfunction, or both.

Treatment for muscle weakness enlists isotonic contractions, whereas treatment of structural dysfunction uses isometric contractions. Isometric contractions, along with specific and graded positioning of the appropriate body part, reduces the tone of hypertonic muscles. Relaxation of tone allows the muscle to lengthen and, subsequently, allows realignment of the skeletal framework.

Strain and Counterstrain

This assessment (Jones, 1981; Jones, Kusunose, & Goering, 1995) examines movement and determines the presence of tender points. (These tender points are different from Travell's trigger points [Ramirez, Haman, & Worth, 1989], which are located in muscle, tendon, ligament, or fascia.) They are areas that are edematous and hypersensitive to touch, and they indicate the presence of articular (joint) compression or protective muscle spasm. Protective muscle spasm and articular compression may develop from chronically shortened muscles (as occurs, for example, with long-standing poor posture) or from reflexive muscle strain. In both poor posture and reflexive strains, the neuromuscular reflex that reports muscle tension to the central nervous system is maintained in an abnormal state of hyperactivity and thus perpetuates the strain and poor posture (i.e., shortened state of muscles).

To simplify an explanation of how tender points develop, I avoid the use of the words *agonist* and *antagonist* to describe muscles and spell out the different types of strains encountered when using strain and counterstrain as a frame of reference.

Tender points can develop from several different situations (Jones et al., 1995; Jones & Wendorff, 1994), including

- Trauma,
- Repetitive motion (overuse syndrome),
- Panic reaction,
- High load effort (such as lifting something too heavy for oneself),
- Emotional stress, and
- Chronic poor posture (Weiselfish & Kain, 1993).

What is important to know and to keep in mind is that the tender point develops in a muscle that is (a) shortened and chronically maintained in this state, or (b) shortened, then abruptly stretched, then reflexively shortened.

Let us look at a situation that is likely to occur in adults with developmental disabilities. The example is one in which a client with poor head control is being assisted in feeding. The client's chin rests down toward the chest, thus shortening the anterior neck muscles and stretching the muscles in the back of the neck. The well-intentioned aide abruptly lifts the head to position it for feeding. This "lifting," because of its suddenness, strains (stretches) the anterior neck muscles, which then causes the muscles to rebound back to a shortened state. This sudden and abrupt stretch effectively acts like stretching a rubber band that, when released, rebounds to a shortened state. The suddenness of the stretch starts a series of reflex responses by the nervous system, placing the anterior muscles in protective muscle spasm and triggering the development of tender points. If, however, the muscles had been slowly or methodically stretched, a reflex reaction would not be forthcoming and tender points would not develop.

Strains are produced by

- Overstretching;
- Long-standing stretch (i.e., postural strain);
- Excessive and long-standing tension in a shortened muscle; and
- Sudden, unplanned stretch to a shortened muscle (e.g., panic reaction).

In the language of strain and counterstrain, there are two different types of strain: real strain and false (reflexive) strain. In the above example, the muscles that were originally maintained in a stretched position are those that develop real strain; they are the muscles at the back of the neck, stretched because the head hangs down on the chest. The shortened anterior neck muscles that were abruptly stretched and then rebounded are the ones that develop false strain. It is in these latter muscles that the tender points develop. Although the abrupt stretch (false strain) is released, the nervous system continues to report it as strain and, thus, the reason for referring to it as "false." The strain of "strain and counterstrain" refers to the false, reflexive strain.

The muscles that were abruptly stretched, then released, and reporting the false strain acquire an abnormally shortened resting length because they are in protective muscle spasm. Therefore, movements that normally would not stretch these muscles—which are now in spasm—perpetuate false strain. This situation results in limitation of range of motion and pain.

Thus, pain is due to three conditions:

1. Real strain (e.g., long-standing stretch)
2. Articular compression
3. False strain (i.e., movement away from the abnormal resting length).

Pain of a tender point is pain that one is aware of only upon palpation.

Treatment focuses on the alleviation of false strain by turning down the hyperactive neuromuscular reflex. This results in muscle relaxation, thus allowing the muscle to return to its normal resting length and relieving articular compression. Following these changes, range of motion of the joint normalizes and pain subsides. To achieve muscle relaxation during treatment, the client's body is passively positioned to maximally shorten the muscles reporting false strain; this position is called "counterstrain." By passively shortening the muscles and then returning the body slowly to a neutral position, the muscle spasm is relieved. Counterstrain is a position of comfort, whereas any movement in the opposite direction that abruptly stretches the muscle reporting false strain results in pain.

Both muscle energy and strain and counterstrain rely on neuromuscular reflexes based on gamma and alpha motor nerve outputs to explain muscle hypertonicity and the return of muscle to its normal resting length following treatment.

Myofascial Release

Myofascial release (Greenman, 1989; Weiselfish & Kain, 1991) assesses structural balance by observing static and dynamic posture, as does muscle energy. When imbalance is found, the next step is to determine if fascial dysfunction is a contributing factor. Fascial mobility (Upledger & Vredevoogd, 1983; Weiselfish & Kain, 1991) is assessed in areas of postural imbalance, and then myofascial mapping (Weiselfish & Kain, 1991) is performed to locate more discrete areas of fascial dysfunction (malalignment and inflexibility). Fascia responds to stress by remodeling and realigning (Silver, 1987). If stress is applied therapeutically in appropriate directions and planes, then realignment of fibers occurs and fascial dysfunction resolves. This helps to normalize structural and postural balance (Figure 8.4).

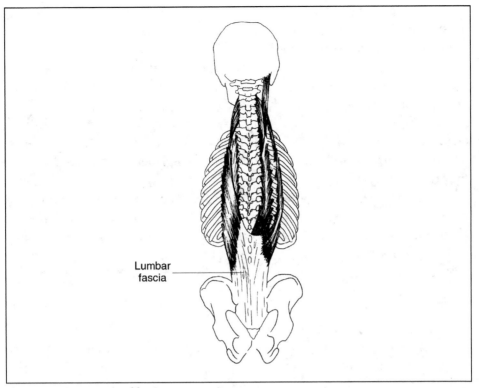

Figure 8.4. An example of fascia.
From *Anatomy of movement,* by B. Calais-Germain, p. 69. Copyright 1993. Eastland Press, PO Box 12689, Seattle, WA 98111. All rights reserved. Reprinted with permission.

Neurofascial Release

Neurofascial release (Davidson, 1992) is another fascial release technique. Whereas the focus of myofascial release is local, the focus of neurofascial release is global. After detecting a local area of stress for which range of motion is limited, the therapist palpates the body's fascial network to find the "key lesion." The key lesion is the area of fascial dysfunction, the fulcrum, around which the tissues have compensated. This fulcrum can be at a distance from the area of stress initially assessed because the fascia is continuous throughout the body. Ranges of motion are assessed before treatment and afterward to assess effectiveness.

A note of caution: There are other authors who have similarly named techniques, but these techniques differ in the way they treat the fascial tensions.

Visceral Manipulation

Visceral manipulation (Barral, 1989, 1991; Barral & Mercier, 1988) is a fascial release technique that focuses on the specialized fascia surrounding the organs of the cranial (brain), thoracic (e.g., the lungs and the heart), and abdominal (e.g., the pancreas and the liver) cavities. In simple terms, this fascia suspends the viscera within the skeletal framework. Visceral manipulation evaluates the movement or mobility of viscera in response to gross motor movement and also assesses the inherent motion of the organs themselves. Gross motor movement has an effect on and is affected by visceral mobility because all fascial sheaths of the body are interconnected. This reciprocal relationship exists because visceral fascia is attached to the bony skeleton (e.g., the pleura surrounding the lungs to the ribs) and directly or indirectly to the musculoskeletal system (e.g., suspensory ligament of the duodenum to the crus of the diaphragm to the anterior longitudinal ligament of the spine). In this arrangement, free mobility of the viscera accommodates bending and twisting of the skeleton, and free mobility of the skeleton accommodates the changes in size and shape of the visceral organs (e.g., the full stomach or bladder, or the pregnant uterus). Treatment entails applying small, gentle forces with the hands to improve mobility of the visceral fascia and thereby improve gross motor movement.

Craniosacral Therapy and Cranial Osteopathy

Progressing from treating biomechanical dysfunction (muscle energy) and muscle strain (strain and counterstrain) as muscle hypertonicity to treating fascial dysfunction (myofascial and neurofascial release, visceral manipulation), we arrive at central nervous system tissues and their role in structural dysfunction. Craniosacral therapy (Upledger, 1987, 1990; Upledger & Vredevoogd, 1983) and cranial osteopathy (Hruby, 1994, 1995) take advantage of the small but palpable, inherent, ongoing movement of and between the cranial and sacral bones. This movement, very broadly and loosely, characterizes the cranial rhythmic impulse also known as the craniosacral rhythm. The specialized fascia of the central nervous system, the dura mater (dural membrane) in particular, is attached to the cranial and sacral bones. Thus, if the normal pattern of movement of any of these bones is distorted, then normal tensions of the dura mater are disturbed. The dura mater is a part of the total body fascial network because it connects with the fascia outside the central nervous system by way of the spine at the intervertebral foramen. Therefore, abnormal tensions of the dura mater can affect fascial tensions in the rest of the body and ultimately distort structural/postural balance. This is a reciprocal relationship, whereby body fascia can translate tensions to the dural membrane. The assessment protocol evaluates, through palpation of the cranial (Figure 8.5a) and sacral (Figure 8.2a and b) bones, several parameters of the craniosacral rhythm, including

- Rate or cycles per minute (normal is 6–12),
- Rhythm or symmetry,
- Amplitude or range of motion, and
- Vitality or energy that describes the quality of the rhythm.

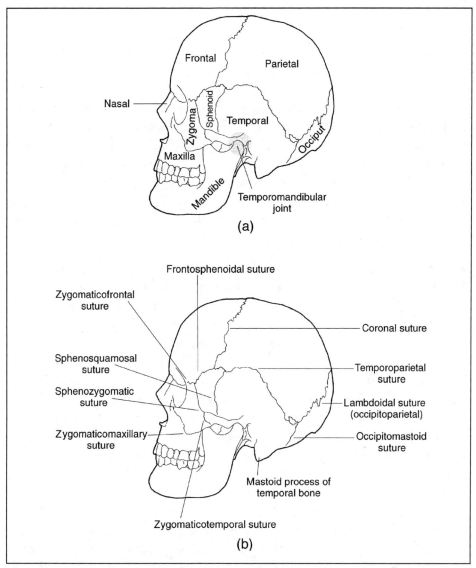

Figure 8.5. (a) External cranial and facial bones, and (b) some of their external articulations (sutures). These are components of the craniosacral system, which are evaluated to determine their mobility and their contribution to the symmetry, rate, and energy of the craniosacral rhythm. In addition, because of muscle and fascial attachments to these bones, and because of the nerves and vessels that pass through their foramina, their alignment and mobility contribute to head/neck movements, to oral-motor skills, and to visual and vestibular functions, to name a few. From *Craniosacral therapy,* by J. E. Upledger & J. D. Vredevoogd, p. 78. Copyright 1983. Eastland Press, PO Box 12689, Seattle, WA 98111. All rights reserved. Reprinted with permission.

Assessment scrutinizes the distorted movement to differentiate between sutural (bony) (Figure 8.5b) and membranous (dural membrane) restrictions. Also assessed is the mobility of the total body fascial network, with particular attention paid to the transverse diaphragms (the cranial base, the hyoid complex, the thoracic inlet, and the respiratory and pelvic diaphragms) that can impede fascial mobility.

Fascial and dural mobility may also be influenced by emotional stress (Upledger, 1990). Emotional stress, related to physical or emotional trauma, is internalized, and the area of the body affected becomes dysfunctional. Very broad analogies can be made to a headache or an ulcer that are the body's response to internalized emotional stress. During craniosacral therapy the areas of structural dysfunction triggered by the emotional stress may release. As the tissue tensions in the area normalize, the client may again experience the original emotional content of the trauma (MacDonald, 1992; Upledger & Vredevoogd, 1983). The release of this emotion is called *somatoemotional release* (SER) and is taught as a specialized treatment technique.

Craniosacral therapy and cranial osteopathy treatment techniques mobilize sutural, dural membrane, and fascial restrictions to normalize the cranial rhythmic impulse and structural balance in general.

Zero Balancing

Zero balancing (Smith, 1986) recognizes that structural dysfunction is often due to disruptive forces at the interface of energy and structure in the body. *Energy,* defined as movement or vibration, is a distinctive force in the body. The assessment protocol requires observation and evaluation of movement. This movement is of two types: gross motor and energy. When assessing gross motor movements one looks for distortions in movement patterns and any disruption in the flow of energy. When assessing energy movement one palpates for energy blocks at the level of the joint. The end point of motion of a joint (the end feel) is where the energetics of the joint can be assessed; this is bone energy that is the primary focus in zero balancing. Structural dysfunction may develop or persist because energetic knots interfere with structural/postural balance. A muscle spasm or an "idea" (mental content) is viewed as held energy in the context of zero balancing. Treatment focuses on releasing energy blocks to promote the health of both structure and energy flow and also to allow for a balanced relationship between the two at their interface.

Wide-Range, Systemic Effects of Manual Therapy

The structural approach as described in the following case histories provides (a) alleviation of dysfunctions (e.g., depression, head banging, and hyperactivity) and (b) improvement of functions (e.g., gross motor and visual regard). One may ask why focusing on one area or structure of the body has such a wide effect. The structural approach treats the neuromusculoskeletal system, and dysfunction in this system has the potential to disrupt function in other systems (Barral, 1989, 1991; Barral & Mercier, 1988; Davidson, 1987, 1992; Greenman, 1989; Korr, 1978; Mennell, 1992). When assessing structural symmetry, mobility and articular balance of the joints, elasticity/flexibility of fascia, and muscle tone, each are considered both individually and as they relate to each other (Greenman, 1989; Weiselfish & Kain, 1991, 1993) and to other physiological systems (Barral & Mercier, 1988; Davidson, 1987, 1992; Korr, 1978).

If you think of a system of "levers and pulleys," then you can envision that the binding of a joint, a muscle, or fascia has the potential to disrupt the function of distal as well as local structures. For example, because the fascia envelopes nerves, muscles, and organs and is continuous and interconnected throughout the body, then, if it is binding (reduction in flexibility), it can cause wide-ranging systemic effects.

Citing a second example, muscle dysfunction can also have a wide range of effects. Muscle spasms (a dysfunction) are considered examples of a "facilitated segment" (Korr, 1978; Upledger, 1987, 1990; Weiselfish, 1994; Weiselfish & Kain, 1993). A *facilitated segment* is a particular level of the spinal cord that, because of long-standing sensory input, becomes hyperresponsive to stimuli and leads to hyperactive motor output. The hyperactive motor output (a function of the central nervous system) will increase the responsiveness of the corresponding level of the sympathetic nervous system. The sympathetic nervous system will, in turn, affect specific visceral functions, peripheral functions, or both. For example, if the fourth thoracic level is facilitated due to protective muscle spasm of the intercostal muscles, then heart function, by way of the sympathetic nerves, may be altered. Thus, facilitated segments have the potential to affect target organs of the sympathetic nervous system. In this case, treatment of a muscle spasm can, therefore, also affect the circulatory system.

"Levers and Pulleys": Illustration of Wide-Range Effects

Now that we have addressed anatomically based examples of the wide-range effects of manual therapy, let us examine a therapy-based example that further illustrates these effects. Let us look at a behavioral problem, inattention to task, in which the focus of treatment will be the dropped head posture. One can develop a treatment plan based on an assessment of structure. The assessment may reveal

- Significant malalignment of four cervical vertebrae;
- Hypertonicity of the right sternocleidomastoid (Figure 8.6) and left scalene (Figure 8.7) muscles, thus maintaining the head in flexion and left rotation; and
- Restriction of the fascial sheaths at the thoracic inlet.

This assessment has now identified three structures—vertebrae, muscle, and connective tissue—that are responsible for the individual's dropped head posture. The structures identified as dysfunctional are viewed as singular links in a chain or web of interconnecting links (Barral & Mercier, 1988; Greenman, 1989; Upledger & Vredevoogd, 1983; Weiselfish & Kain 1991,

Figure 8.6. (a) Protective muscle spasm of the sternocleidomastoid muscles can affect the function of the shoulder girdle and the respiratory and craniosacral systems because of their attachments to the sternum and clavicles and to the temporal bones. (b) Contraction of the right sternocleidomastoid muscle produces right side-bending (not shown) and left rotation of the head when the thoracic cage is fixed. (c) Contraction of both the right and left muscles produces flexion of the head when the thoracic cage is fixed. These muscles contribute to dropped head posture if maintained in a shortened state, as in protective muscle spasm.

From *Anatomy of movement,* by B. Calais-Germain, p. 80. Copyright 1993. Eastland Press, PO Box 12689, Seattle, WA 98111. All rights reserved. Reprinted with permission.

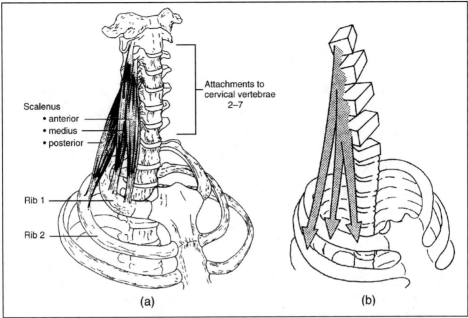

Figure 8.7. (a) Protective muscle spasm of the scalene muscles can affect the function of the respiratory system, thoracic inlet, and head and neck because of their attachments to the cervical vertebrae and ribs. (b) Contraction of the right scalene muscles produces right side-bending of the head when the ribs are fixed. These muscles contribute to dropped head posture if maintained in a shortened state, as in protective muscle spasm.

From *Anatomy of movement*, by B. Calais-Germain, pp. 77, 78. Copyright 1993. Eastland Press, PO Box 12689, Seattle WA 98111. All rights reserved. Reprinted with permission.

1993) that when dysfunctional, have the potential to set off a domino effect, resulting in dysfunction in other structures or systems. For instance, the hypertonic left scalene muscles that insert on the ribs may, over time, limit the expiratory mobility of the rib cage (Greenman, 1989). Eventually, this may interfere with breathing (respiratory system), endurance, or upright posture (musculoskeletal system), because the rib cage is now hypomobile on the left. In addition, the restriction of the fascia at the thoracic inlet may compromise the function of the vagus nerve (nervous system) to a point that the individual complains of gastric upsets (digestive system) (Barral, 1991). The attachment of the sternocleidomastoid muscle to the temporal bone (Figure 8.6) may affect its mobility and thus interfere with temporal bone function, resulting in identifiable visual-motor disturbance (sensorimotor systems) (Upledger & Vredevoogd, 1983). Through manual therapy treatment, needed structural changes can be achieved, and subsequently an individual's ability to function changes. These changes may affect motor, social, and perceptual behaviors as well as physical well-being. In our example—inattention to task—this would be, respectively, head/neck movements, visual regard, spatial orientation, and sensation (gastric pain or discomfort).

How Does Structurally Based Manual Therapy Differ From Traditional Sensorimotor and Other Functionally Based Therapies?

A goal of rehabilitation is to improve an individual's ability to function in some aspect of his or her life. There are several classical approaches in occupational therapy used with individuals with mental retardation and those with developmental disabilities that help to improve their capacity to function, including

- Exercise,
- Assistive technology,
- Environmental adaptation,
- Feldenkrais, and
- Sensory integration and sensorimotor therapies.

These approaches focus on functional aspects of rehabilitation (Weiselfish, 1994; Weiselfish & Kain, 1990). Then there is the structural approach (Greenman, 1989; Mennell, 1992; Mitchell et al., 1979; Upledger, 1987; Weiselfish & Kain, 1990), which does not immediately aim to augment one's ability to function but rather to unlock one's potential for function.

Traditionally, behavioral "symptoms" have been viewed and treated from two perspectives: behavioral and functional. Using the previous example of inattention to task in an individual with dropped head posture, the treatment by these two approaches is briefly elaborated and compared to structurally based therapy. The behaviorist will analyze the task and develop sequential steps of increasing difficulty and/or increased time on task to facilitate improved attention to task; he or she will also consider appropriate approaches to deal with any maladaptive behaviors. The health professional, who views this behavior from a sensorimotor or sensory integrative viewpoint, will notice the dropped head posture and may question the efficiency of righting reactions, vestibular function, and proprioception, recognizing their role in the ability to maintain focus. A practitioner using the structural approach, having noted the dropped head posture, will evaluate the structural integrity of the cervical and thoracic spines, the sacrum, and temporal bones, keeping in mind that dysfunction due to some or all of these will affect head/neck proprioception, vestibular function, and righting reactions. Clearly, all three viewpoints are productive; it is their interplay that expands the possibilities for the individual to achieve maximum functional performance.

Rationale for Using Manual Therapy With Adults With Mental Retardation

The structural integrity of an individual affects the potential for movement, socialization, perceptual acuity, and physiological health. Although functional approaches help to develop these potentials, to achieve maximum benefit from therapy—namely, to fulfill possibly untapped potentials—one needs to look first at structure and then at function.

To improve function in adults with mental retardation, I initially focused on sensorimotor and sensory integrative approaches. The clients' participation was difficult to engage because of sensory defensiveness, hyperactivity, intolerance for interaction, or visual inattention or because it was one more setting that placed demands of participation on them. The changes, although functional, were not easily transferred to other contexts (e.g., from the treatment environment to activities of daily living tasks). It seemed as if nothing was happening on a physiological level, from within the person, to facilitate meaningful change that would allow the individual to make choices during the execution of a variety of tasks. Persistent questions arose:

- How does the structural/postural framework affect movements, behaviors, and performance?
- Is there a biomechanical dysfunction due to joint or myofascial impairment?
- How could the individual's structural framework be influencing functional performance?

With these questions in mind, the idea developed to look at adults with mental retardation and other developmental disabilities not purely within the context of their medical/psychiatric diagnoses, but also as regards their structural makeup. Structural imbalance or asymmetry is often easy to observe: It includes dysfunctional gait, forward head posture, scoliosis, and facial distortions. In view of these departures from normal posture, the first thing to realize is that as "imbalances" they create stresses throughout the total structural framework. These stresses trigger compensatory responses both in the structural framework and in behaviors, as they would in any population. With structural imbalance, movement will be distorted and activity levels and tolerances will possibly be influenced, as will social and other behaviors (Simpson, 1996). For example, forward head posture may interfere with swallowing (Kraus, 1989; Mennell, 1992; Weiselfish & Kain, 1993) or may present as headaches (Mennell, 1992; Rocabado, Johnson, & Blakney, 1982–1983) or disturbances in equilibrium (Kraus, 1988). Thus, a key question presents itself: How can the structural framework be "normalized" to improve movement function and, possibly, behaviors in general?

To answer this question, a structural rehabilitative approach (Weiselfish & Kain, 1990, 1991, 1993) was decided on to influence essential and basic elements of function. The influence of structure on function has already been clearly documented (Barral, 1991; Greenman, 1978, 1989; Heinrich, 1991; Korr, 1978; Mennell, 1992; Upledger, 1987; Upledger & Vredevoogd, 1983). It is my contention that structural dysfunction can interfere with normal adaptive behaviors (Simpson, 1996) and, thereby, influence the potential of the adult with mental retardation to effectively respond to sensorimotor therapies. The structural approach affords new possibilities for facilitating change as well as a new way to view and better understand some behaviors.

Implementing Structurally Based Manual Therapy for Adults With Mental Retardation

Treatment Environment

The following case histories describe four male residents of state group homes that are established as intensive care facilities (ICF). Each home has six to seven residents, one is coed and the other all male, and both have 24-hour supervision. All residents participate in vocational day programs.

Because the homes are ICF residences for individuals with mental retardation, they are required by federal regulations (483.430{b}{1}) to provide those services that are deemed essential for the individual and to continue providing those services for as long as the health professional finds it appropriate and necessary. Each home has a multidisciplinary team of health professionals that includes a

- Pharmacologist,
- Psychologist/behaviorist,
- Occupational therapist,
- Physical therapist,
- Speech-language pathologist,
- Nurse,
- Social worker/case manager,
- Dental hygienist,
- Recreational therapist, and
- Program supervisor.

Quarterly and annual meetings are held for team members to share their particular professional perspectives on each client in order to develop a comprehensive picture of the individual and to evaluate progress toward team goals.

Occupational therapy treatment schedules are influenced by various factors. Clients are seen one to four times a month, as I am in each home once a week. On occasion it is necessary to increase the frequency of treatment to effect more rapid change in structural dysfunction for safety reasons. Most clients are receptive to a manual therapy approach in spite of the difficulty of staying in one place for a period of time or the difficulty of interacting; they always come and stay for therapy except during those times when illness, fatigue, or just "a bad day" defers therapy.

The treatment sessions are held either in the home's living room or in a bedroom. Sometimes if a client has roommates or if a common bathroom is in his or her bedroom, we opt to use another client's room with single occupancy. Visual and noise distractions are adapted to as needed. All residents have respected the common area used for therapy.

Treatment Session

Length of the Treatment Session
Treatment sessions range from 5 to 90 min. Shorter sessions may occur because the individual is not yet comfortable with the therapeutic process (the process of self-discovery and change) or with being treated and "touched." The initial process of developing trust between the client and the therapist may also initially preclude longer sessions.

Trust as Part of the Treatment Session
Trust plays a significant role in all evaluation and treatment sessions. The therapist must trust himself or herself, must trust the client, and must also have trust in the therapeutic process. Likewise, the client needs to trust himself or herself to change and the body to heal and needs to trust the therapist and the process. I consider myself a facilitator of change. The individual with whom I work needs to want change. He or she is the captain of the ship who directs the therapy; I am the navigator.

At this juncture, one should not become perplexed with the "mental retardation" condition of the client; wanting to change is not exclusively a deliberate decision. There are levels of functioning from which decisions are made that are not based on deliberate thought processes or cognitive function alone. These individuals seek me out for their sessions, and I see them come eagerly each week regardless of the discomfort of lying still, the discomfort of interacting with another person, or any discomfort experienced in the previous week's session. They keep coming. For me, this is a decision they have made, on some level. I must presume that they come because therapy feels good to them or because they recognize it as doing something good.

Implementation of Treatment Techniques
Once a detailed evaluation has been carried out (see "Evaluation Protocol" below), the manual therapy treatment approach has been decided, and the client is receptive, treatment can begin. Some treatment techniques (muscle energy, strain, and counterstrain) require the client to follow directions. This can be difficult because of lack of comprehension or because of muscle guarding that interferes with achieving specific positions. Other techniques (craniosacral therapy, fascial release techniques, zero balancing) require a relaxed supine position. Although this position is often a possibility, at times only moments are captured between motor restlessness or constant chatter. Neither of these situations is insurmountable. The initial implementation of a

technique might not be textbook style, but one can often apply the principles of a technique using some creativity. If you need someone to take a deep breath (very often not understood), ask him or her to blow and then catch him or her on the inhalation. If you need an isometric contraction, play a game of resistance. If you need quiet, work around the fidgetiness and catch those glimpses of quietude. There have been times when I have used an assistant for distraction or to implement multihand treatment. Instead of supine, use sitting. Often sitting, even while engaged in a task, is initially substituted for the relaxed supine position. Results from treatment obviously take longer to achieve, but the key is they can be achieved.

Sometimes gentle restraint—using the practitioner's arms, legs, or head—is necessary because of motor restlessness. Some situations are difficult to resolve. If you do not restrain, you cannot implement a particular treatment technique, and if you do restrain, muscle guarding occurs. This has been a persistent situation with Steve (see case histories below) when trying to release his occipitoatlantal joint. Frequently, the best way I have found to initially address these problems is to use treatment techniques that focus on the energetic component of a structural dysfunction, such as zero balancing, direction of energy or body unwinding (craniosacral therapy, cranial osteopathy), or therapeutic touch (Krieger, 1979). If fidgetiness is encountered during treatment, one needs to assess if this behavior is due to a discomfort of experiencing movement in an area in which previously there had been none (structural dysfunction), is due to pain, or is due to an emotional (Upledger, 1990) or energetic component (Smith, 1986) bound up in this area of the body. Finding an answer helps to make a decision as to which treatment technique is more appropriate.

Communication During the Treatment Session

Communication is an essential part of both the evaluation and treatment sessions. Treatment depends on a two-way relationship. It is important to learn to communicate with adults with mental retardation, to read their signs, including

- Body language,
- Changes in the quality of the voice,
- Changes in breathing pattern,
- Changes in tolerances,
- The quality of visual regard, and
- Changes in facial expression.

They often cannot verbally express the subtle or even the large changes occurring within themselves. Treatment cannot progress unless the therapist "hears" what is communicated and respects it. In addition, I talk to them, giving instructions ("Let this tissue soften"), telling them what I am doing, reassuring them, and telling them what they can do when experiencing changes in their body ("Trust yourself and your body to change" or "New movements may be scary"). This helps develop their trust in me and, I believe, they understand me, whether through language or touch. And remember: Many have receptive skills even if their expressive skills are negligible.

Adults with mental retardation, in addition to being receptive, are responsive to manual therapy. To see an individual with autism look up at you and smile while experiencing the release of fascial restrictions is heartening. More important, it is a confirmation of the benefit of the approach.

It is also important to communicate with group home staff and team members about the structural approach. Initially, it was surprising to experience others' relief at the possibility of finding a reason for maladaptive behavior other than finding fault with the patient's personality, which usually results in labeling the patient "uncooperative." Team members and staff will be more aware of what to look for in a person's behaviors and become better able to make referrals for therapy and to communicate their observations to you.

Ending the Treatment Session

Learning when to stop a treatment session is important so that one does not tax or overload neurophysiological systems (Breuer, 1989a, 1989b; Brown, 1993, 1994; Smith, 1986, 1996; Upledger & Vredevoogd, 1983) or exceed the client's tolerance. When working with Larry (see case histories), I would end the session when he covered his face—a signal of discomfort or possible forthcoming aggressive behavior. Eventually, I picked up on behavioral cues so sessions could end before his hand went to his face. It is preferable to end sessions on positive notes. One needs, however, to differentiate between discomfort experienced during tissue release, which is often part of the therapeutic healing process, and the discomfort of exceeding someone's tolerance for treatment. The latter may result in maladaptive behaviors.

Amount of Time It Takes for Change to Occur

Both structural and functional objectives are part of treatment plans; structural objectives are the building blocks for functional change. For example, improved biomechanics of the lumbosacral junction (structural) lead to improved sitting balance (functional). In my experience, the easily observable and tangible functional changes take 3 to 12 months to appear (treating once weekly). Large, observable improvements include changes in gait, chewing patterns, balance, and spatial awareness.

Subtler functional changes—such as increased smiling or more relaxed breathing—may appear earlier in treatment if they are the building blocks for larger ones, like improved social interaction, greater tolerance for sitting, or taking walks. However, subtler functional changes can take longer to occur if they are refinements of the larger ones, such as using more of the space around you by building on improved proprioceptive sense—itself resulting from improved pelvic girdle and spinal mechanics.

There are occasions when a structural dysfunction, which is a major component of a maladaptive behavior, is resolved, but the behavior does not change in all settings. In effect, the behavior, which over the years has become a learned behavior and is habitual, interferes with its own resolution. I have seen this with Brian (see case histories) when the chronic muscle spasms of the temporalis muscles resolved. At this point, all teeth grinding stopped during therapy sessions that were as long as 60 min. However, the teeth grinding continued outside the sessions. Final resolution of maladaptive behaviors is often accomplished by functional and behavioral programs developed by the team. Successful implementation of these programs requires group home staff to have higher expectations of the client.

Evaluation Protocol

All individuals are evaluated because of (a) observed deficiencies in the quality of their movements, such as hyperactivity, rigidity, or lack of movement, and/or (b) some obvious structural imbalance, such as structural malalignment (e.g., facial distortion, increased lumbar lordosis) and/or myofascial restrictions. Evaluation entails two steps. The first step is a general screening, followed by the second more formal and detailed assessment of structure.

In the first step, one screens for structural dysfunction by starting with observation. One looks at a broad range of behaviors to determine the presence of function versus dysfunction. These behaviors include

- Gross and fine motor skills
- Oral-motor skills
- Movement patterns (straight planes, rotation, fluidity)
- Gait (toe-walking, heel-toe)
- Transitions
- Perception (movement in space, body awareness, gravitational security)
- Visual regard
- Sensation (tactile, proprioception/kinesthesia)
- Concentration/attention to task
- Primitive developmental reflexes
- Maladaptive behaviors (aggression, irritability, depression, hyperactivity, self-injurious and pain behaviors)
- Physiological complaints (headaches, spastic colon).

When making these observations, one looks for structural imbalance (postural asymmetry, movement distortion, compensatory movements; Greenman, 1989; Mitchell et al., 1979; Weiselfish, 1994; Weiselfish & Kain, 1991, 1993) and maladaptive behaviors (Simpson, 1996). If there is dysfunction, the question needs to be raised, Is the dysfunction due, at least in part, to structural impairment?

As an occupational therapy practitioner, one already has some of the tools needed to consider the influence of structure (structural/postural strains) on function. Our sensorimotor background provides us with significant knowledge about movement and development: mobility developing from proximal stability and perceptual and cognitive functions developing from a sensorimotor foundation of exploration during infancy and childhood, to name just two. Importantly, this knowledge can be directly applied to a structural frame of reference because it provides a basic understanding of movement (dysfunction) that is the general focus of a structurally based manual therapy approach. By observing and assessing movement and function, one raises questions about sensory processing. Once sensorimotor and/or sensory integrative dysfunction is identified, one can begin to consider the influence of structural/postural imbalance on sensory processing before proceeding solely with a functional treatment approach. The idea is to take a different look at something familiar and explore additional reasons for it: Maybe the equilibrium system is impaired because there is impingement of neural tissue at the internal acoustic meatus; maybe the head droops because the cervical vertebrae are malaligned.

In the second step, one proceeds to identify specific structural dysfunction by more closely examining the components of structural integrity of the shoulder and pelvic girdles, spine, rib cage, head, and extremities. Because the various manual therapy treatment approaches address either different tissues (e.g., muscle or fascia) or different aspects of the same tissue (e.g., dural or visceral fascia), it is important to first decide if postural/structural integrity is impaired and then to decide which tissue(s) are involved.

First, static posture (Breuer, 1989a, 1989b; Greenman, 1989; Mitchell et al., 1979; Summerfelt, 1991; Weiselfish, 1994) is evaluated. It includes, but is not limited to, noting asymmetry of anatomical landmarks (eyes, shoulders, and iliac crests; Figures 7.2 and 7.3) and palpating soft tissue (muscle, fascia—inclusive of the dura mater) for texture, tone, and imbalance. Postural symmetry is evaluated in three planes to give a clear picture of three-dimensional structure and movement: coronal (a view from the front or back of a person), sagittal (a side view), and transverse (looking at anterior/posterior or rotational displacement). Effectively, the practitioner is assessing the height, depth, anterior/posterior displacement, and/or degree of rotation of bilateral bony landmarks. If these features are not equal or level, then structural dysfunction exists. Articular balance is also a part of the evaluation of static posture. Here, one assesses the degree of friction-free mobility of tissue interfaces. These interfaces may be bone to bone (glenohumeral joint), soft tissue to bone (cecum to ilium), or soft tissue to soft tissue (right kidney to duodenum).

Postural deviation in a static pose indicates the presence of structural dysfunction. It is also indicative of movement dysfunction (think "levers and pulleys")—most notably, hypomobility. Therefore, a dynamic postural evaluation (Breuer, 1989a, 1989b; Greenman, 1989; Mitchell et al., 1979; Summerfelt, 1991; Weiselfish, 1994) is carried out to include symmetry of movements, limitation of range of motion, functional strength, dissociation of movements, and compensatory or distorted movements. This dynamic evaluation represents the third part of structural integrity, namely, mobility; the other two parts, alignment and articular balance, have been addressed in the assessment of static posture (above).

The information gathered from the static evaluation is correlated with the limitation of movement(s) assessed in the dynamic postural evaluation. This helps to determine whether the movement dysfunction results from asymmetric muscle strength or pull (shortening, spasm), neurologic compromise (central or peripheral; Weiselfish, 1994; Weiselfish & Kain, 1993), articular imbalance, or fascial restriction.

At some point during assessment, sensory testing and reflex testing are also carried out. Finally, a differential diagnosis using the various treatment approaches is necessary. This determines which structure is contributing to the dysfunction: Is it muscle, fascia, or joint biomechanics that is impeding normal movement or interfering with adaptive behavior?

The above evaluation protocol is straightforward; however, it is not always as easy to implement with adults with developmental disabilities. By knowing what to look for and understanding the implications of postural asymmetry, even if you cannot completely and decisively carry out the postural evaluation, you can at least begin to visually, and sometimes manually through palpation, discern structural impairment. When this happens, it can be useful to prematurely begin cranial, energy, or fascial treatment approaches to initiate tissue releases while recognizing that evaluation is an ongoing process.

With the person with developmental disabilities there may be no complaint of pain, or the complaint of pain may be considered a "behavior." If there is a lack of postural symmetry, then there is structural dysfunction that is compromising that individual's level of performance and the efficiency with which he or she performs a task, possibly influencing adaptive behaviors. Is this dysfunction important if there is no obvious complaint of pain or discomfort? In my view, yes, because the dysfunction is now a "pathological" basis from which everything else is performed and a springboard for the development of more and more compensatory habits and maladaptive behaviors. When movement occurs, it is either from a well-balanced musculoskeletal foundation that allows for fluid and efficient movements or from one that is imbalanced and, therefore, pathological. The body automatically compensates to adapt to any imbalance. If the initial imbalance is chronic, then over time the compensation becomes part of the pathological foundation for movement. Compensation becomes one's "normal" way of moving. Eventually, the body's mechanisms of adaptation are depleted and movement becomes inefficient, energy consuming, impossible, and/or painful. Tolerances may be lowered to all types of environmental stresses. Therefore, the earlier structural dysfunction is alleviated, the easier it is to achieve well-being.

Treatment Protocol

Treatment is recommended based on the presence of structural dysfunction discovered during the evaluation. A treatment plan is developed to normalize function in areas of hypomobility. Hypomobility may be due to biomechanical stress, protective muscle spasm, inflexibility of connective tissue (fascia, visceral fascia, dura mater), or energetic restrictions. The treatment techniques used will depend on the practitioner's expertise and comfort with particular structurally based manual therapy techniques, but optimal results occur when the technique matches the dysfunction (e.g., craniosacral therapy for dural membrane restrictions).

Treatment plans have long- and short-term goals. The short-term goals focus on improving the structural dysfunction(s) assessed in the evaluation. The long-term goal is usually a functional/behavioral objective. The short-term structural goals are the building blocks that permit and support achievement of the functional goal. Once treatment is implemented, progress is monitored by reevaluating hypomobility, symmetry of anatomical landmarks, tissue texture, range of motion, quality of movement (resolution of compensatory movements), status of pain, quality of behaviors (more adaptive), and efficiency in performing activity of daily living tasks. Group home sensorimotor or structurally oriented programs are often developed to facilitate the integration of structural changes into functional performance and to augment direct therapy, respectively.

Development of a Treatment Protocol: An Example

I use the case history of Brian (see case histories) to focus on the relationship between structural dysfunction and "inadequate chewing" to demonstrate a structurally based manual therapy treatment plan, in this case for improving chewing skills. The static assessment revealed gross postural deviations of the

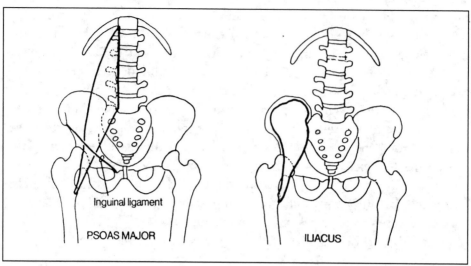

Figure 8.8. This figure illustrates an example of leg muscles with their attachments to the pelvic girdle and spine. Because of these attachments, any dysfunction of these leg muscles will not only affect normal movement of the leg but also that of the pelvis and spine.
From S. Goldberg, *Clinical Anatomy Made Ridiculously Simple,* MedMaster, 2004. Reprinted with permission.

spine, cranial structures, and shoulder and pelvic girdles. These postural strains correlated with limitations of movement (dynamic assessment) of the rib cage, spine, lower extremities, jaw, lips, and tongue. To improve oral-motor function, the gross postural strains had to be addressed first because proximal stability (axial structural integrity) is a prerequisite oral-motor skill (Alexander, 1988a, 1989b). Thus, the first structural dysfunctions to be treated were the pelvic and sacral imbalances, lumbar spine hypomobility, and lower extremity asymmetry (because pelvic dysfunction may be related to the abnormal pull of leg muscles on the pelvis) (Figure 8.8). Muscle energy was used to normalize muscle tone and length; a group home program of muscle strengthening and sensorimotor activity was established to integrate the ongoing structural changes into gains in functional performance. Further, treatment included craniosacral therapy that affects sacral and vertebral mobility by way of the dural membrane. The status of the membrane's structural integrity ultimately affects head/neck function (oral-motor skills). Myofascial dysfunction of the low back and of the thoracic spine and rib cage was then treated with myofascial release. At this point, improved postural alignment and lower body stability were providing Brian with a much more stable base of support from which to develop oral-motor function. Next, muscle energy, myofascial release, and craniosacral therapies were used to realign the shoulder girdle and cervical spine because of forward head posture. With the entire vertebral column realigned and the head and neck more appropriately situated over the trunk, stresses due to abnormal pull were lessened on the jaw and extrinsic tongue muscles, resulting in improved chewing skills.

In this example, three types of structural dysfunction that contributed to Brian's poor chewing skills were identified:

1. Biomechanical (pelvis, vertebrae, and hips)
2. Protective muscle spasm (legs, pelvis)
3. Soft-tissue inflexibility (fascia and dura mater).

Each of the structures identified as dysfunctional (pelvis, vertebral column, hips, and fascia) has the potential to produce an effect resulting in dysfunction in other structures or systems. In other words, structures and functions beyond the primary treatment objective can be affected. In Brian's case, while addressing oral-motor function (primary treatment objective), his breathing pattern (function) matured because structures associated with breathing (ribs, muscles) were directly affected by the structural changes occurring at the spine and at the pelvic and shoulder girdles.

Case Histories Using Structurally Based Manual Therapy

The following four case histories demonstrate the successful implementation of structurally based manual therapy with adults with mental retardation. There have been other individuals with whom I have had success, but there have also been those with whom I have had only limited success and some with whom I have been unsuccessful. The reasons are variable. A few individuals, themselves, did not want to change. One woman only wanted SER; every time I saw her, she would put my thumb way back on her hard palate and proceed to have an SER. There have been times when I could devise a step-by-step treatment plan but could not implement it. One man was so active and jolly that I could not find "glimpses of quietude" for treatment. And, there have been those with whom I just could not identify a specific structural problem. The following case histories should be read, keeping in mind that manual therapy is a new, important tool for treating adults with mental retardation and that it should be considered as one of several approaches for achieving improved function.

The following individuals, all residents of group homes designated as ICFs, have been receiving occupational therapy services, on average, for 6 years, with treatment occurring one to four times monthly.

Larry

Client Background

Larry is a 38-year-old man with a diagnosis of mental retardation with autistic features. Larry is nonverbal with good receptive language skills. He has been treated since June 1990 with a structurally based manual therapy approach; during a few preceding months he received sensorimotor treatment that was poorly tolerated. An assessment was requested because of rigid hand posture.

Brief Synopsis of Pretreatment Profile
Larry presented with robotlike movements, significant muscle guarding, and severe soft-tissue restrictions of the pelvic and pectoral girdles and along the spine. His gait pattern was a shuffle with toe-walking; he lacked balance reactions and held his fingers in hyperextension. Autistic behaviors interfered with social interaction, and little visual contact was made with people. Initially, treatment sessions were ended because of low tolerance for interaction; this was indicated by Larry putting his hand over his face. Larry did not initiate constructive activities.

Treatment Focus
The broad focus of treatment was to improve soft-tissue flexibility in order to facilitate improved motor function. Treatment techniques used were craniosacral therapy, myofascial release, neurofascial release, visceral manipulation, zero balancing, strain and counterstrain, and sensorimotor.

Major Structural Changes Resulting From Therapy
The primary structural changes that occurred from Larry's therapy were
- Greater elasticity of the fascial sheaths, including the dural membrane system.
- Significant resolution of muscle guarding.
- Alignment of the pelvic girdle.
- Greater mobility of the spine, pelvic, and shoulder girdles, especially the scapulothoracic and glenohumeral joints.
- Greater mobility of the sacroiliac joints (Figures 8.2a and 8.2b).
- Normal expansion of the rib cage.
- Release of restrictions at cranial sutures (Figure 8.5b) affording improved mobility of the occipitoatlantal joints (Figure 8.2b), sphenobasilar junction (Figure 8.9), and temporal and parietal bones (Figure 8.5a). The frontal bone (Figure 8.5a) has released (i.e., increased mobility), and decompression of the lateral cranial base is progressing.
- Improved function of the temporomandibular joints (Figure 8.5a).
- Improved mobility of the hyoid complex and of the hard palate (Figure 8.10). Proper functioning (alignment and mobility) of the hard palate (vomer, maxillae, and palatine bones) is important because of its relationship to breathing, oral-motor, and speech functions. This relationship between structure and function exists because of anatomic connections among the hard palate, facial, and cranial bones (Figure 8.5) and because of the relationships among the hard palate, tongue, and teeth.

Figure 8.9. (a) Inferior view of the base of the skull to picture the sphenobasilar junction. This is an articulation between the basilar part of the occipital bone and the body of the sphenoid. The dashed line indicates a midsagittal cut. Compression of this junction, along with compression of the occipitoatlantal and lumbosacral junctions, can cause clinical depression. Compression of the sphenobasilar junction may lead to the appearance of one sucking one's thumb, but one is actually pushing up on the hard palate in an effort to decompress the joint. Compression and lateral and vertical strains can cause myriad dysfunctions, including pain syndromes, personality disorders, and learning disabilities (Upledger & Vredevoogd, 1983). (b) This is a sagittal section through the cranium to view the sphenobasilar junction. Pictured is a vertical strain (a type of malalignment) of the articulation. If the articulating surfaces of each bone were brought into line, thus opposing each other, there would be normal alignment of the junction.
Fig 8.9 (a). From *Anatomy and physiology,* by R. R. Seeley, T. D. Stephens, and P. Tate, 1989, p. 164. Copyright Times Mirror/Mosby College Publishing. Reprinted with permission. Fig 8.9 (b). From *Craniosacral therapy*, by J. E. Upledger & J. D. Vredevoogd, p. 117. Copyright 1983. Eastland Press, PO Box 12689, Seattle, WA 98111. All rights reserved. Reprinted with permission.

In addition, following the implementation of the zero balancing protocol in 1995, Larry developed dorsiflexion of both feet, and for the first time there was fluidity of movement of the left hip and ankle; up to that time, muscle guarding at the ankles interfered with movement.

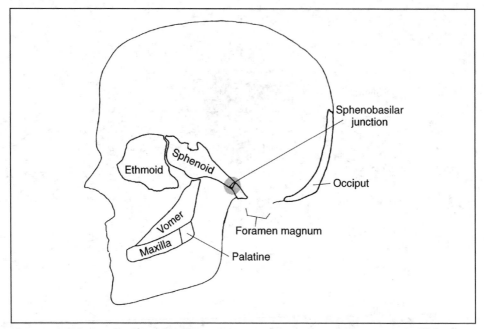

Figure 8.10. The bones of the hard palate are the maxillae and palatines bilaterally, and the vomer in the midline. Note the anatomic relationship to the sphenoid and, by extension, to the other cranial bones (see Figure 8.5, which shows the relationship the maxillae have to other facial bones). Proper functioning of the hard palate is important because of its relationship to breathing, oral-motor, and speech functions. (The ethmoid bone is identified to assist orientation.)
From *Craniosacral therapy*, by J. E. Upledger & J. D. Vredevoogd, p. 157. Copyright 1983. All rights reserved. Reprinted with permission. Eastland Press, PO Box 12689, Seattle, WA 98111.

Major Functional Changes Resulting From Structural Changes

Major motor changes. Dissociation of movements and rotation are now present and allow Larry to automatically make transitions through a series of positions (e.g., supine–kneeling–standing) rather than simply pushing up from supine to standing. Balance reactions have developed from a new ability to shift weight and dorsiflex his feet. During dressing activities he is able to sit on his bed in a relatively relaxed upright posture to put on his pants and socks in contrast to rigidly falling backward to perform the task. The upper extremities are now able to independently function in manipulatory tasks instead of supporting the lower body during movement or static positioning. Now, instead of using his arms to push himself up out of a chair, he is using his legs. Larry's gait pattern has changed to a normal heel-to-toe progression when walking. Spontaneous head/neck movements involving rotation and side-bending have appeared; the fingers are held in a normal, semiflexed position at rest; and depth of breathing is greater. At mealtime the lips and temporomandibular joints are functioning with larger and smoother movements. Since 1995, as ankle mobility improved, Larry has learned to hop and to kick a ball using appropriate stance and movements. During some sensorimotor activities Larry can now be described as "loose as a goose" because of improved spinal flexibility; his arms now reach above his head without any resistance due to muscle spasm or fascial tensions.

Major changes in other behaviors. Tolerance for interaction has changed dramatically, with eye contact now regularly made and with increased responsiveness to redirection and to prompts to engage in tasks. He tolerates being touched with no autistic behaviors and responds to interaction with a smile. He is more responsive to his morning routine without aggressive behaviors. We can now hold treatment sessions from 30 to 90 min. without his hand going to his face, and he often signs "more" when asked if we should stop. Larry now performs tasks using more of the space around him. In addition to seeking therapy, he has begun to seek other constructive activities. When his bedroom is being used to treat another resident, Larry comes in and spontaneously offers his pillow from his bed. He finds me and waits for therapy while I am treating another person.

Brian

Client Background
Brian is a 51-year-old man with the diagnoses of mental retardation, cerebral palsy, autism, rapid switch bipolar disorder, and seizure disorder. He has been stabilized on Tegretol and lithium since 1988. Brian uses language to tell a story but generally not to express needs unless cued. Previous therapeutic intervention consisted of guidelines for eating: the precutting of food and prompting to chew and swallow each mouthful. An assessment was requested to evaluate the appropriateness of his diet prescription. In late 1988, a structural approach to Brian's oral-motor dysfunction was implemented.

Brief Synopsis of Pretreatment Profile
Brian presented significant impairment of postural function: severe forward head posture (Figure 8.3b), flattened and flared rib cage (Figure 8.3b), retracted shoulders with arms maintained against the lateral chest wall, and increased lumbar lordosis (Figure 8.3b). Motorically there was poor dissociation of movements, especially of the lower extremities, and dragging of his right leg when walking; breathing was shallow and primarily diaphragmatic; and he had essentially no adaptive balance reactions. Oral-motor dysfunction presented as follows: poor lip, jaw, and tongue mobility; immature chewing pattern, that is, munching; temporomandibular joint dysfunction (Figure 8.5a), with the mouth opening only 13 mm (normal width is 35–40 mm); reverse swallow with fluids; and exaggerated swallow with solids. His craniosacral rhythm could be described as "stuck in the mud," because movement felt strained.

Brian had significant periods of hypomania and depression, screaming, hyperactivity, and euphoric moods. He also would grind his teeth.

Treatment Focus

A structural approach was implemented to establish more normal postural alignment to facilitate improved function of the oral-motor apparatus. Once this objective was attained, treatment focused on achieving greater articular balance to improve sensorimotor function, thereby increasing Brian's movement repertoire. Treatment techniques used included muscle energy, craniosacral therapy, cranial osteopathy, myofascial release, neurodevelopmental treatment, and other sensorimotor approaches.

Major Structural Changes Resulting From Therapy

The structural changes in Brian's postural profile were

- Improved alignment of the spinal curves with greater vertebral mobility
- Improved articular balance at the hip and pelvis with relaxation of shortened muscles and normalization of abdominal muscle tone
- Decrease in forward head posture (Figure 8.3b) with realignment of the shoulder girdle
- Improved mobility of the ribs, thus facilitating a mature thoracic-abdominal breathing pattern
- Release of the frontosphenoidal suture (Figure 8.5b), the sphenobasilar (Figure 8.9), and occipitoatlantal and lumbosacral junctions (Figure 8.2b)
- Release of the lateral cranial base
- Initiation of the rotary component of movement of the temporal bones (Figure 8.5a)
- Improved elasticity and flexibility of the dural membrane system
- Overall improvement in the craniosacral rhythm
- Improved alignment and mobility of the temporomandibular joint (Figure 8.5a), with the range of motion now 38 mm.

The following quotes are significant. At the time of the release of the frontosphenoidal suture, Brian spontaneously said, "I feel better," while appropriately pointing to his temples. With the release of the sphenobasilar junction, he announced, "I'm happy."

Major Functional Changes Resulting From Structural Changes

Major motor changes. Movement capabilities have improved in standing and sitting with the development of lateral weight shift and balance reactions. Function of the lower extremities has improved with greater dissociation between the hip and knee; dragging of the right foot during walking is essentially resolved. Physical stamina and endurance are improved dramatically such that Brian is now able to take walks of 1 to 2 miles and with reported greater stability.

The oral-motor functions that have developed with these structural and gross motor changes are

- Improved tongue mobility and maneuverability
- Normal swallow with fluids
- Active lip function
- A mature rotary chewing pattern
- Better respiratory and oral-motor functions for speech
- Better coordination of swallowing with breathing during mealtime.

These changes have allowed uncooked leafy vegetables to be reintroduced into his diet without the risk of choking.

Major changes in other behaviors. Brian's depressive mood swings have significantly decreased since mid-1991 with the release of the occipitoatlantal, sphenobasilar, and lumbosacral junctions (Upledger & Vredevoogd, 1983). Since these structural changes, Brian has had no resurgence of increased depressive periods during the past 5 years. Another change in behavior is a reduction in screaming, which coincided with the release of the temporal bones. For the 5 months before discontinuing therapy, teeth grinding was no longer occurring during therapy sessions. Eye contact with staff and clients has improved, focus on tasks has increased greatly, and Brian is more easily redirected when maladaptive behaviors do occur.

Occupational therapy services were discontinued in 1996. Sensorimotor skills, particularly of the lower quadrant and oral-motor apparatus, had improved significantly because of improved structural integrity. It was felt that Brian's needs could now be better met by regular engagement in gross motor activities to promote and to help maintain overall strength, biomechanical integrity, and overall well-being.

Steve

Client Background

Steve is a 29-year-old man with the diagnoses of mental retardation, attention deficit disorder with hyperactivity, and chronic sinus and ear infections. His medication regimen consists of Beconase and allergy shots, with Sudafed and Tylenol for congestion, headaches, and/or sinusitis. Steve is nonverbal with good receptive language skills. Prior to a manual therapy approach (December 1990), I attempted a developmental sensorimotor approach to facilitate fine motor skills, but because of severe attention deficit and hyperactivity, this was discontinued.

Brief Synopsis of Pretreatment Profile

Steve's hyperactivity consisted of perpetual and vigorous striding throughout the house and/or rocking on furniture, and attention to task was severely limited. He used only peripheral vision to regard objects or people. He indulged in self-abusive behaviors, most notably head banging. He held his thumb in his mouth up against the hard palate (he was not sucking his thumb). Steve was an individual with dysmorphic facies, severe lumbar lordosis (Figure 8.3b) with sacral hypomobility, and rigid neck posture. In supine he avoided flexed postures and often shot into rigid extension, especially when his feet were touched. His craniosacral rhythm was barely detectable.

Treatment Focus

The premise for implementing manual therapy was that structural abnormalities, especially of the cranium, were significantly contributing to a feeling of discomfort. In an attempt to rid himself of the discomfort, self-abusive behaviors ensued. It was felt that the head banging was not behavioral in origin, although it may have become learned behavior. To work toward improved structural integrity, the following treatment techniques were used: craniosacral therapy, zero balancing, and principles of visceral manipulation.

Major Structural Changes Resulting From Therapy

The structural changes that have occurred are numerous and include
- Unlocking of the occipitoatlantal joints (Figure 8.2b) and occipital condyles
- Release of the right lateral and vertical strains of the sphenobasilar junction (Figure 8.9)
- Decompression of the sphenobasilar junction
- Release of the frontal bone and associated sutures (Figures 8.5a and 8.5b)
- Release of the occipitomastoid suture (Figure 8.5b)
- Decreasing compression of the temporal bones (Figure 8.5a), with symmetrical rotation now present
- Release of the thoracic inlet (Figure 8.1)
- Developing mobility and decompression of the hard palate complex (Figure 8.10)
- Greatly improved elasticity of the intracranial membrane system
- Improved dural tube mobility
- Moderately good craniosacral rhythm in both range of motion and quality
- Overall improved fascial tensions throughout the body
- Pelvic realignment, with resolution of the exaggerated lumbar lordosis.

Facial contours have consequently changed. The bump on the right side of the forehead is gone; as a staff person exclaimed, "The egg is gone!" The furrows in the forehead are significantly shallower, eliminating the appearance of scowling, and his eyes do not appear as deeply set under the brow. The corneas went from a dull, yellowish color to white.

Since 1995, treatment has emphasized areas in which fascia (including the dural membrane and visceral fascia) and energy are binding. Subsequently, remarkable improvements in mobility have occurred in the following areas: oro- and nasopharynx, right occipitoatlantal joint, right temporal area, hard palate, and the area of the left ocular orbit. With the improved mobility, there has been a significant decrease in Steve targeting his left eye when head banging. Also, since the hard palate became more mobile there have been increased periods of calm both during and outside of the treatment session.

Major Functional Changes Resulting From Structural Changes

Major motor changes. There has been a significant decrease in hyperactive behaviors: (a) the frequency and intensity of running through the house has decreased; (b) when excited, Steve now rarely laughs loudly or waves his hands in front of his face; and (c) he is spending more time on tasks and is more focused, with greater attention to detail. From May 1991 through May 1994, Steve tolerated dental visits without the use of a papoose; the first of these visits immediately followed the release of the frontal bone. However, since 1995, circumstances of the visits have changed—including staff changes—and the papoose has again been used. Beginning in 1992, Steve has tolerated the wait in doctors' offices without head banging. With the implementation of the zero balancing protocol in 1996, Steve is tolerating the lifting of his feet and legs and does not push into an exaggerated extension posture. Muscle tension has normalized throughout his body, especially at the neck and low back; he now places his head down on the therapy table rather than holding it up.

Major changes in other behaviors. Steve now gives direct eye contact. Socially, his mother reports him as being a "happier person"; he smiles more frequently and is more affectionate. A staff person said, "It seemed he never had time before to be cuddled." Since the fall of 1996, Steve has been making uncharacteristic sounds, also reported by his mother. Some of these sounds seem to carry the intonation and rhythm of normal speech patterns. Laughter is more appropriate. The frequency with which he holds his thumb in his mouth has significantly reduced with release of sphenobasilar compression (Upledger & Vredevoogd, 1983) (Figure 8.9).

The frequency and intensity of head banging dropped dramatically following improved alignment and mobility of the occipitoatlantal and sphenobasilar junctions and of the temporal bones; this occurred between 8 and 12 weeks after the implementation of a manual therapy approach. Before this

Steve bucked like a bronco during sessions with arms flailing, but he always came and stayed for the session. Since these releases his motor behaviors have ranged from only twisting and turning to periods of complete calm lasting 5 to 25 min. Head banging decreased from a high of 9.7 incidences a month in the last two quarters of 1990 to somewhat over one incident a month in 1993 but has averaged about three incidences a month during the following 3 years.

Of particular note are changes in a range of behaviors in 1996 that accompanied release of tissue restrictions in the neck, face, and head. Steve is demonstrating increased expressiveness with appropriate grinning, smiling, and laughing. It seems that cognitive function has improved or been unlocked because eye contact is now very strong in response to verbal instructions during treatment, and behaviors are now interactive, such as being coy. In addition, he stops moving and twisting to listen when instructions are given or when I am communicating something about treatment.

In the fall of 1996, we were able to address the chronic restriction of the right occipitoatlantal joint in a more formal manner because of the increased periods of calm. During and following each of two sessions, Steve had dramatic treatment reactions. As noted previously, these reactions are SER (Upledger, 1990; Upledger & Vredevoogd, 1983) because accompanying the release of structural tensions is the release of emotion. For the first time Steve was expressing sadness and anger. Group home staff reported "he couldn't sit" and that he banged furniture hard when repositioning it. They reported he appeared very angry and uncooperative (uncharacteristic behaviors). Steve's work site reported he was pushing staff and stomping his feet. Both the group home and work site reported him crying uncontrollably (he has never been known to cry). He uncharacteristically hit/pushed others during transport from work—he has never previously shown any aggression. During therapy he repeatedly slammed his legs down on the therapy table. During the emotional releases he did not attempt to pull my hands off his body nor bang his eye. These behaviors continued for two to three weeks and then stopped. Steve's medical status was reviewed to identify any possible medical problem; none was found. As of this time, the only functional changes discernible following the SER episodes are significantly decreased motor restlessness during therapy and a calmer demeanor, which Steve now brings to therapy.

Henry

Client Background

Henry is a 33-year-old man with diagnoses of mental retardation, chronic undifferentiated schizophrenia, obsessive-compulsive disorder (diagnosed in 1994), and a history of seizures. He is presently on a regime of a decreasing dose of Mellaril while implementing a trial of Klonopin for the psychotic disorder, and he is taking Paxil for the obsessive-compulsive disorder. During the 7 years I have been working with Henry, psychotropic therapy has varied. The psychotropic drugs had no apparent effect on the quality of motor behavior, except when Mellaril was started in April 1992. At that time, motor restlessness subsided following a period of increased maladaptive behaviors. Before this, he had not been taking psychotropic drugs for 1 year. It has not been determined if the perioral movements and cogwheel-like rigidity, both inconsistent, have been signs of tardive dyskinesia and/or extrapyramidal signs. Henry is verbal.

Henry was participating in a time-on-task program when I started to work with him in late 1988. A review of the data showed him successfully meeting the objective of 20 min. on task many times, but this was inconsistent and dependent on mood; the program was discontinued. I subsequently developed a sensorimotor program to help integrate movements and decrease motor restlessness (King, 1974; Levy, 1974) to increase time on task. However, because of Henry's lack of involvement, this program was continued only as a group home program, and direct therapy began implementing a manual therapy approach in mid-1990.

Brief Synopsis of Pretreatment Profile

Henry demonstrated significant motor restlessness (i.e., pacing, rocking) that interfered with task focus and interaction. Movements were rigid, with extreme muscle guarding, and he moved as if from within a suit of armor. His gait was bouncy with hip-hiking and toe-walking. Even movement capabilities he possessed (like swinging his arms in a circle) he could not use because of poor body awareness. Spinal curves (Figure 8.3a) were flattened with severe loss of segmental mobility. He had frequent complaints of headaches and stomachaches. Henry exhibited a flat affect, a monotone voice, and minimal facial expression. Breathing was shallow.

Treatment Focus

The focus of treatment was to develop movement capabilities to decrease motor restlessness. The supposition was that with more coordinated and fluid movement, motor restlessness would decrease with a release of soft-tissue tensions. To address the structural dysfunction, craniosacral therapy, strain and counterstrain, myofascial release, and sensorimotor therapies were used.

Major Structural Changes Resulting From Therapy

The structural changes that affected improvement in Henry's behaviors and movement capacity include

- Greater and freer mobility of the entire spine
- Development of scapulothoracic mobility

- Improved mobility of the thoracic inlet (Figure 8.1) and respiratory diaphragms
- Decompression of the sphenobasilar junction with some resolution of a left lateral strain and an inferior vertical strain (Figure 8.9a)
- Decompression of the temporal bones (Figure 8.5a) with noted increased rotary motion
- Improved alignment of the temporomandibular joints (Figure 8.5a)
- Significant improvement in craniosacral function
- Improved elasticity and flexibility of the fascia and dural membrane
- Decreased hypertonicity of the anterior neck muscles (Figure 8.3b)
- Significant alleviation of chronic paravertebral muscle spasms along the thoracic and lumbar vertebrae (Figure 8.2b). The latter was due in great part to a group home program of strain and counterstrain that was implemented twice weekly and then as needed.

Major Functional Changes Resulting From Structural Changes

Major motor changes. Motor restlessness abated during the first year of a manual therapy approach with the initial release of the occipitoatlantal joints (Figure 8.2b), improved temporal bone (Figure 8.5a) function, and increased range of motion and vitality of the craniosacral rhythm. Pacing is essentially resolved; Henry even sits down to converse or have a soda. Rocking now tends to occur only with exacerbation of psychotic behaviors. Muscle guarding has essentially been eliminated from his profile, although high muscle tone remains. Dramatic changes are noted in his gait pattern: He is no longer hiking his hip or toe-walking, and arm swing has appeared. When rolling over he now uses segmental rolling patterns. Dissociation of movements between body parts (hip and knee, shoulder and pelvis) now occurs, allowing for greater and safer dynamic balance. During activity of daily living tasks arms are functioning with greater ease. Adaptive movements are more spontaneous in response to his environment, and the rotational component of movement has appeared. Along with improved head/neck function, swallowing is easier at mealtime, and thoracic–abdominal breathing has improved with greater expansion of the rib cage.

What stands out since 1995 is a tremendous leap in proprioceptive awareness, contributed to by the decrease in chronic back spasms and subsequent improved vertebral mobility and craniosacral function. Henry is gaining an awareness of movement such that, on request and after a hands-on demonstration, he can perform trunk rotation, head/neck movements, and shoulder movements. He can now balance on one foot. Fluidity of movement and ranges of active motion are greatly improved.

Major changes in other behaviors. By the end of the second year of a manual therapy approach, the team nurse reported that Henry was essentially without complaint of headaches, and consequently, the use of Tylenol dropped dramatically; also, complaints of stomachaches have subsided. Of note are Henry's comments during sessions: "I feel better." "My headache is gone." "Do more." In addition, his facial appearance is more expressive. Like Steve, despite motor restlessness, Henry stays for sessions, some as long as 90 min. Like Larry, when asked if therapy should continue or stop for the day, he says "more."

Perspective

The functional performance of the adult with mental retardation is clearly improved using a structurally based manual therapy approach. It can be concluded that at least some dysfunctional behaviors often displayed by these individuals—motor, social, self-injurious, perceptual—are due in part to structural imbalances rather than solely to mental deficiency. This therapeutic approach looks to treat structural causes as a basis of behaviors rather than treating the behaviors themselves, as other approaches generally do. The objective is to provide the individual with a healthier structural foundation rather than solely adapting the environment to his or her needs or adapting the behaviors to the environment. Improvement of structural integrity will provide the individual with more options to respond to internal and external stimuli because a healthy structural framework is more adaptive, providing the individual with new potential for response. Thus, manual therapy differs from other approaches in that it is able to uncover underlying potential to support future changes in function because it addresses the relationship between structure and function.

Even if one comes to accept this essential relationship between structure and function, one must still overcome traditional views about adults with mental retardation. These views, unfortunately, foster the sense that these adults, because of inherent limitations, have little ability to change. However, as demonstrated, these individuals do, indeed, have untapped potential, and acknowledgment of this can lead directly to therapeutic intervention.

These ingrained views about mental retardation often interfere with the natural establishment of trust and communication in the treatment environment. Even deftly skilled therapists, when faced with an adult with mental retardation, fall back into "conventional wisdom" and assume there is little or nothing therapy can do for these individuals or presume that adults with mental retardation cannot participate actively or even passively as we look to others to do. There is no expectation of comprehension. Yet, they come without bias or preconceived notions about therapy and readily perceive tissue movements and changes. They come because they develop trust in the therapist, and from there everything begins. I was lucky when I started learning manual therapy techniques, particularly craniosacral therapy, because I started with this population. I found in many of these clients that craniosacral rhythms were barely palpable. However, fresh from workshops, I applied these new skills and found that change is indeed possible, first structurally and then functionally. When I then started treating the "normal" population, I was clearly surprised because they already had "strong" craniosacral rhythms; they were just there. How could there be anything wrong? What I came to realize is the extreme nature of the dysfunctions with which I work. If I had started working with the "normal" population, I, too, may have palpated such gross dysfunction in the adult with mental retardation and mistakenly presumed that little could be done.

Stasis, however, is not an acceptable state for one's health, and because potential to change is inherent in all individuals, if we find structural dysfunction, then we always have somewhere to begin and a reason to prescribe therapeutic intervention. Potential need not leap out at you, but it may occur in small packets of change. Change is facilitated by the therapist and is dependent on the individual's ability to trust himself or herself to change.

Questions need to be shared and answers explored among the different professions to better understand the whole person and his or her needs. Traditionally, behavioral "symptoms" have been viewed and treated from behavioral and functional perspectives. Through a better understanding of the implications of structural imbalance, perhaps we can now facilitate more fundamental changes.

Some common areas of structural dysfunction that I have frequently observed in the adult with mental retardation are the sphenobasilar junction (Figure 8.9), occipitoatlantal joints, sacrum, temporal bones, and frontal bone (Figures 8.2 and 8.5a). Hard palate (Figure 8.10) and pharyngeal space restrictions also appear, as does muscle guarding. The thread that seems to connect all of these is the fascia. The clinical impression is that the normal, balanced elasticity of the fascia and dural membrane system is lacking and that this fascial inflexibility distorts postural, sensory, and proprioceptive functions. There is an apparent restriction or lack of internal mobility primarily of the fascial sheaths, the elastocollagenous complex (as proposed by Upledger & Vredevoogd, 1983) that supports locomotion and physiological health. It seems that function is not based solely on the integrity of joints and muscle but more on the integrity of the physical properties of soft tissue. Following the release of soft-tissue restrictions with manual therapy techniques there is a potentiating of the internal structural environment, which can lead to the (re)establishment of soft-tissue mobility. It is presumed that what then follows is an internalized awareness by the individuals of a newly established balance from within which internal tissue tensions resolve or dissipate. They all seem to have a new sense of orientation/groundedness and movement based on this new internal balance. This balance is the mobility of the fascia, inclusive of the dura mater, which is essential for externally produced gross and fine motor movements. Without this flexibility, there is a presumed discomfort with the physical body due to the soft-tissue restrictions; these, in and of themselves, may cause pain behaviors and lower tolerances and may result in distortions of responses to stimuli from the internal or external environment. Clinically, following treatment, proprioceptive sense seems heightened as it relates to body and self-awareness and to spatial awareness and relations.

It is important to consider that the dysfunctional behaviors may be signs and symptoms of structural dysfunction, placing the individual at a disadvantage to respond to and react to his or her environment. Manual therapy treatment techniques are able to normalize structural stresses, thereby unlocking latent potential for improved functional performance. This approach is of fundamental importance in the treatment of individuals with mental retardation and developmental disabilities in general.

Acknowledgments

I would give special thanks to Shirley Breuer, Charles Gilliam, and Marion Eagan for their time and comments on the chapter. And to Marion for her generosity in sharing with me her knowledge and skills through so many years. To Tracy Simpson—whose excitement with learning has inspired me to look behind the obvious—for his stream of thought-provoking questions and for his assistance beyond any and all reasonable expectation.

Some of the material presented in this chapter is based on data and interpretations originally presented by this author and published in *OT Practice, 1*, 40–45 (November 1996).

References

Alexander, R. (1988a, September). Oral-motor treatment programming for the infant and young child with neuromotor involvement [Course]. Marlborough, MA.

Alexander, R. (1988b, November). Rib cage: Focus on the rib cage for improvement in respiration/phonation, postural control and movement [Course]. Milwaukee, WI.

Banus, B. S. (1971). *The developmental therapist.* Thorofare, NJ: Slack.

Barral, J. P. (1989). *Visceral manipulation II.* Seattle, WA: Eastland Press.

Barral, J. P. (1991). *The thorax.* Seattle, WA: Eastland Press.

Barral, J. P., & Mercier, P. (1988). *Visceral manipulation.* Seattle, WA: Eastland Press.

Breuer, S. (1989a, October). Muscle energy for the lower quadrant [Course]. Hartford, CT.

Breuer, S. (1989b, November). Muscle energy for the upper quadrant [Course]. Hartford, CT.

Brown, R. (1993, April). Zero balancing I [Course]. Hartford, CT.

Brown, R. (1994, March). Zero balancing II [Course]. Hartford, CT.

Davidson, S. M. (1987). *Manual medicine: A primer.* Phoenix, AZ: Practical Publications.

Davidson, S. M. (1992). *Setting the fascia free.* Phoenix, AZ: Practical Publications.

Greenman, P. E. (1978). Manipulative therapy in relation to total health care. In I. M. Korr (Ed.), *The neurobiologic mechanisms in manipulative therapy* (pp. 43–52). New York: Plenum Press.

Greenman, P. E. (1989). *Principles of manual medicine*. Baltimore: Williams & Wilkins.

Heinrich, S. (1991). The role of physical therapy in craniofacial pain disorders: An adjunct to dental pain management. *Journal of Craniomandibular Practice*, 9(1), 71–75.

Hruby, R. J. (1994, November). Direct cranial osteopathy, craniosacral therapy— Level I [Course]. Hartford, CT.

Hruby, R. J. (1995, January). Direct cranial osteopathy, craniosacral therapy—Level II [Course]. Hartford, CT.

Jones, L. H. (1981). *Strain and counterstrain*. Indianapolis, IN: American Academy of Osteopathy.

Jones, L. H., Kusunose, R., & Goering, E. (1995). *Jones: Strain-counterstrain*. Boise, ID: Jones Strain-Counterstrain.

Jones, L. H., & Wendorff, R. (1994, April). Strain and counterstrain, level I [Course]. Sturbridge, MA.

Kain, J. (1996, March). Visceral manipulation Ia [Course]. Hartford, CT.

King, L. J. (1974). A sensory-integrative approach to schizophrenia. *American Journal of Occupational Therapy, 28*, 529–536.

Korr, I. M. (1978). Sustained sympathicotonia as a factor in disease. In I. M. Korr (Ed.). *The neurobiologic mechanisms in manipulative therapy* (pp. 229–268). New York: Plenum Press.

Kraus, S. L. (1988). Cervical spine influences on the craniomandibular region. In S. L. Kraus (Ed.), *TMJ disorders: Management of the craniomandibular complex* (pp. 367–404). New York: Churchill Livingstone.

Kraus, S. L. (1989). Influences of the cervical spine on the stomatognathic system. In R. Donatelli & M. J. Wooden (Eds.), *Orthopaedic physical therapy* (pp. 59–70). New York: Churchill Livingstone.

Krieger, D. (1979). *The therapeutic touch*. New York: Prentice Hall.

Levy, L. L. (1974). Movement therapy for psychiatric patients. *American Journal of Occupational Therapy, 28*, 354–357.

MacDonald, R. (1992, October). SER I [Course]. Hartford, CT.

Mennell, J. M. (1992). *The musculoskeletal system: Differential diagnosis from symptoms and physical signs*. Gaithersburg, MD: Aspen.

Mitchell, F. L., Jr., Moran, P. S., & Pruzzo, N. A. (1979). *An evaluation and treatment manual of osteopathic muscle energy procedures*. Valley Park, MO: Mitchell, Moran, & Pruzzo, Associates.

Ramirez, M. A., Haman, J., & Worth, L. (1989). Low back pain: Diagnosis by six newly discovered sacral tender points and treatment with counterstrain. *JAOA, 89*, 905–913.

Rocabado, M., Johnson, B. E., Jr., & Blakney, M. G. (1982–1983). Physical therapy and dentistry: An overview. *Journal of Craniomandibular Practice, 1*(1), 46–49.

Silver, F. H. (1987). *Biological materials: Structure, mechanical properties, and modeling of soft tissues*. New York: New York University Press.

Simpson, L. (1996). Seeing the forest for the trees: Treating adults with mental retardation through structurally based manual therapy. *OT Practice, 1*(11), 40–45.

Smith, F. (1986). *Inner bridges: A guide to energy movement and body structure*. Atlanta, GA: Humanics Limited.

Smith, F. (1996, November). Alchemy of touch [Course]. Hartford, CT.

Summerfelt, M. (1991, September). Manual therapy for the pediatric patient [Course]. Farmington, CT.

Tehan, P. F. (1980). Functional technique: A different perspective in manipulative therapy. In E. F. Glasgow, L. T. Twomey, E. R. Skull, & A. M. Kleynhans (Eds.),

Aspects of manipulative therapy (pp. 94–96). Melbourne, Australia: Churchill Livingstone.

Upledger, J. E. (1987). *Craniosacral therapy II: Beyond the dura.* Seattle, WA: Eastland Press.

Upledger, J. E. (1990). *Somatoemotional release and beyond.* Palm Beach Gardens, FL: UI Publishing.

Upledger, J. E., & Vredevoogd, J. D. (1983). *Craniosacral therapy.* Seattle, WA: Eastland Press.

Weiselfish, S. (1994). *Manual therapy with muscle energy technique for the pelvis, sacrum, cervical, thoracic, and lumbar spine.* West Hartford, CT: ANA Publishing.

Weiselfish, S. (1996, June). Visceral manipulation Ib [Course]. Waterbury, CT.

Weiselfish, S., & Kain, J. (1990). Introduction to developmental manual therapy: An integrated systems approach for structural and functional rehabilitation. *Physical Therapy Forum, 9*(6), 1, 3–5.

Weiselfish, S., & Kain, J. (1991, June). Myofascial release [Course]. Hartford, CT.

Weiselfish, S., & Kain, J. (1993, December). Manual therapy for craniocervical, craniofacial, and craniomandibular pain and dysfunction [Course]. Hartford, CT.

CHAPTER 9

A Five-Stage Model for Adults With Developmental Disabilities

Mildred Ross, OTR/L, FAOTA

Introduction

People in good health, who feel good about themselves, are able to take control, exercise choice, and know their feelings. It is another story for individuals whose energies are drained by the presence of a chronic disability and the lack of coping skills. For them, extra warmth, support, and structure need to be supplied, so that such individuals can succeed in learning these skills and retain their available energy. The Five-Stage Model serves as a basic group model for those people who require that extra portion of support and structure. The stages provide activities for

- Orientation and welcome,
- Movement and energizing,
- Perceptual tasks and sensorimotor skills,
- Cognition for expressing feelings and reflections, and
- Closure and preparing to take control (Ross, 1987, 1991, 1997; Ross & Burdick, 1981).

The Five-Stage Group is a systematic and sequential method for organizing the presentation of activities in a group format. It is developmental, as each stage is dependent on the stage before it to enhance its acceptance. It is hierarchical, in that each stage makes incremental demands on group members to respond to challenges as one stage flows into the next. Tasks chosen for each stage must be able to be graded up or down according to the functional and developmental level of group members. No two groups can ever be alike, as they take the group process from the "here-and-now" situation as that is presented by members during each session. Observations from peers and therapists are processed throughout the session, as a reflection of what is happening. Its greatest advantage, for those who do not learn particularly well from language, is that these observations relate more to the action and behavior displayed at the present moment by the participants, as they respond to a task and to others engaged in a task rather than to personal stories or the feelings expressed by participants.

Activities, used in the Five Stages, refer to all the physical actions and verbal exchanges that happen during the session. Therefore, the initial handshake, a bell that members ring and pass, exercises they follow, an anxious member exiting, any interruption occurring, a concern voiced, two items matched in a perceptual task, or the members describing what they are learning can be considered by the therapist as material to be processed or ignored within the group. When an event is processed, it becomes an activity.

Activity is used to organize behavior. Activities provide the means for eliciting the adaptive responses by doing, moving, shaping, and changing, so that a desired response is achieved and, "in addition to their active creation, adaptive responses are believed to have an internally organizing and integrative effect on the performance components or subsystems of the human as occupational being" (Wood, 1996, p. 631). It is this internal organizing, within the group session, that is expected to result eventually in behavioral and physical changes. When members become more calm and more alert, it is because the selected activity has organized them. The feeling of being organized helps members to be motivated for change.

Almost all techniques and activities known to occupational therapists can be adapted for use in the Five Stages. Therapists can use items that provide stimulating sensory qualities, such as sound, texture, color, special touch, joint mobilization, and exercise and movement, or introduce the cultural arts, relaxation techniques, and productive discussions. *How* and *when* these techniques and skills are introduced are the key principles of the Five Stages.

The goal of the Five-Stage Group with the adult population with developmental disabilities is to provide, in a structured framework, the means to practice good social interaction, to experience competencies, and to exercise choice. The Five-Stage Group accommodates people who may not speak and may be very cognitively limited but will accept sitting next to another person. It is the quintessential opportunity for peers to learn how to help and be helped by peers. It is a special boon to those people who like to be with others but are eliminated from the group experience by a flawed criteria that may insist on speech or some level of knowledge.

Description of the Five Stages

Stage I: Orientation

Purpose

The purpose of this stage is to recognize each member individually, to arouse each member as much as possible, and to review the purpose of the group (Ross, 1997). The therapist can review the purpose with a single statement that covers the intent of the session, such as "We meet together to work or share time and to learn from each other."

How an activity is introduced is most important. The following chapter describes how information is received by the central nervous system. It is relevant here. Discussions are inappropriate in the Orientation stage: Emotional issues, especially, are postponed for a later stage, when participants become more organized and focused, moving from self-absorption to greater awareness of others.

Content

Appropriate activities are any 1-minute activity, such as shaking hands; providing a backrub; saying names or hello in a foreign language; or passing a strong smell or lotion, a noisy or musical item, a fuzzy or rough item, or a weight or weighted object. These provide the opportunity to practice using items functionally; for example, using hand lotion mimics the way hands are washed, plucking a musical instrument promotes fine pinch, and handling a weight can correspond to holding a bottle of sauce and pouring it without dropping. People can respond to such small demands, and their interest is aroused.

Guidelines for Continuing on to the Next Stage

The allotted time for this stage may take 2 to 10 minutes. The therapist decides when to move on to the next stage. It is usually when most of the members become able to give some degree of attention.

Stage II: Movement

Purpose

The purpose of movement is to increase physical and cognitive readiness for the work of the group (Ross, 1997). Movement increases muscle tone, influences an automatic good postural alignment, and enhances body scheme through involving parts. Physiological changes can take place that will engender a response from the group member. Movement is the quickest way to obtain a response as therapists demonstrate an action, make a request, or require members to reach for objects being passed around.

This stage is not a substitute for individual movement therapy, but it can offer a brief one-on-one to facilitate a better way to move. Individual help is offered when it does not interrupt the group as a whole or distract the individual too much. In this case, movement is meant to energize and to be a way of expressing oneself, as well as interacting with others very naturally. Copying one another, as well as creatively moving to suggest a new way to move, is applauded. Movement generates an increased interest, a good mood, and a sense of self and relatedness to others, and this is verifiable on oneself.

Content
Appropriate movement protocols for cardiovascular improvement, warm-ups, and strengthening can be borrowed from low-impact aerobics, adding weights appropriately for strengthening, and using stretching exercises. Resources for ideas can come from libraries, adult courses, and local state health departments, as well as from the local department for the aging. The ROM Dance on audiotape and videotape is an excellent example of a protocol that mobilizes all joints creatively (Harlowe & Yu, 1981). Placing items in the hands of members promotes novel ways to move. These items can include cans of food, theraband strips, batons, canes, plates, cones, or scarves. Heavy or lightweight items provide different sensory inputs and may be combined in the same session. Movements used in functional outcomes, such as donning clothes, reaching into closets, or negotiating steps, can be practiced by imagining the action and recreating it with group participants. Each member can lead a movement, work with a partner, and join with others by holding hands or holding on to a large sheet, parachute, or rope (Ross, 1997). This is a good time to encourage laughter and other expressions of enjoyment.

Guidelines for Continuing on to the Next Stage
As members appear more alert, the therapist can inquire, after a period of time, perhaps 10 to 20 minutes, if they want to try another activity.

Stage III: Visual–Motor–Perceptual Activities

Purpose
This stage chooses activities that combine sensory motor and cognitive skills to enhance awareness of self and the environment, challenge interpretation of stimuli, and force an adaptive response (Ross, 1997).

In this stage greater demands, of an incremental nature, are placed on the group member. Group action has moved from passive reception to self-directed movement, and now the requirement is to develop a more constrained, directed, and planned response to the selected activities presented.

Content
In this stage, tasks can require less physical exertion but do require thoughtful action, such as identifying, organizing, and interpreting sensory data and making a more precise, meaningful response. Tasks are selected that will

Figure 9.1. Problem solving: "Whatever shall we do with these envelopes?"

bring successful outcomes for most members within two to four attempts. Therefore, grading activities (making them more or less difficult to perform) is an important concept in presentation. Tone of voice, pace of presentation, and deciding whether to show a complete example or one step at a time are also ways to grade an activity.

Appropriate occupations can range from learning functional tasks such as how to open and close a tie or plastic bag, how to use a tool like a reacher to pick up a variety of objects, or how to manipulate any item like a top or Jacob's Ladder that requires starting the action and letting go. Almost all activities carry a message or a lesson, and conveying that message through performance can be powerful. Manipulating an item successfully leads to "Wow, I can do that, although I did not believe I could at first!" A group endeavor can demonstrate how the members work well together as each one, in turn, joins one link to another to make a single design or necklace. Other activities have been found successful:

- Identifying tools in a bag
- Identifying sounds, smells, or weights
- Discriminating between shapes
- Judging distances and force by throwing bean bags, aiming golf balls into electric putters, or knocking down plastic bowling pins with a plastic ball.

Sequencing a story from a series of pictures or showing each member's favorite time of the day on a clock with movable hands invites interest and can be discussed more fully in the next stage.

Figure 9.2. Decision: "Let's see how fast we can fill them up." (This activity was not competitive; each person was improving on his or her own past performance.)

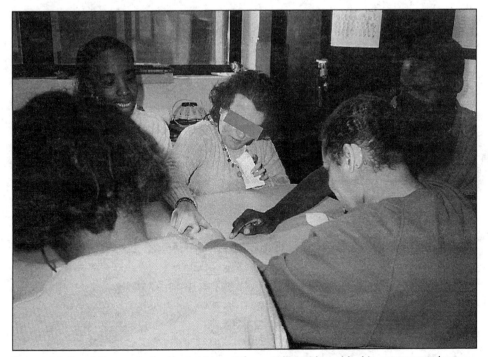

Figure 9.3. Carefully spotting and reaching out for supplies without blocking someone else.

Relaxation techniques may be introduced here. Guided imagery can be started with the suggestion of a boat floating in water under a blue sky; each member can then be asked to add to this image. Alternately, the therapist can guide the group with a simple relaxation message, allowing those who want to close their eyes. A member can illustrate a special dance, music, meditation, or the way to massage one's own limbs.

The therapist may pass around heavy items that provide proprioceptive input to joints and can induce calm when members need extra assistance to focus. For example, group members can be asked to hold a weighted mirror and then to select a favorite facial feature on themselves. In the cognition stage this can be used as a memory activity: Each group member is required to remember what others have said was their favorite feature.

Guidelines for Continuing on to the Next Stage

This stage can take up most of the time of the group if it is a group where world or local current events are discussed, something is being taught like a dance or a game, or members have stories to share. As suggested, Stage III may merge into Stage IV as members begin to express feelings and closure to the activity.

However, when the activity presented is quickly accomplished by group members, they can be asked if they want to go on to another one, and this becomes Stage IV.

Stage IV: Cognition

Purpose

This stage crowns all that has gone before, as group members have the opportunity to demonstrate organized thought and behavior in their performance and in relating to each other (Ross, 1997). This is the time to remember any issue that was postponed for discussion at the beginning of the group. Emotions are less intense, focused attention is at its height, and resolution of problems appears to happen more easily. Often the group directs itself, and members will assume roles of leadership, even if temporary. Therapists promote and support these outward signs of civility and inner security by not interfering.

Content

This stage need not be verbal. Music can be played and clapping to the rhythm encouraged. Questions can be asked and responded to with a recognizable "yes" or "no" from members. Items used in the group can be displayed and each member invited to go and pick up his or her favorite one and use it again. A discussion can be initiated; if one or two members are able to verbalize, members can guess how others may answer, and that can be verified with the member. The therapist can call attention to an item in a picture and ask the others to point out other features. An activity such as catch, holding hands, or moving some object around the room like a marionette can be used to further reinforce the feeling that the time spent has "connected us all" together.

When verbal communication can proceed, invite discussion of a previous activity, such as a description, how it felt to perform, and what could be learned or changed in the performance. Therapists can model answers as well.

There can be the introduction of poetry, storytelling, reminiscences, pictures, and birthday or other cards that play a tune as they are opened. The sequence of activities in the group session may be reviewed. Members may introduce the subject of holidays, birthdays, boyfriends, or other situations they want to share. A short slide presentation can be presented, with each group member participating by taking a turn in moving slides forward.

However, as closure approaches, too much novelty, alarming news, or the creation of intense feelings should be avoided.

Guidelines for Continuing on to the Next Stage

The therapist gauges when it is the opportune time to remind the group that it is nearing the time to close the group.

Stage V: Closure

Purpose

The purpose of this stage is to provide the use of familiar activities that signal the closing of the session on a positive, affirmative note (Ross, 1997).

Content

In this stage, brief activities are used so that group members experience the benefits of accomplishment and an inner sense of balance. A repeat of the same activity presented in Stage I can be used. A review or summation of what has occurred in the session and each individual's contribution or performance is provided (Cole, 1993).

The therapist may decide whether the group members require a closure that contains additional arousal or maintains prevailing mood or whether members require additional calming.

- *Arousal:* Some fast routine, clapping to a song, or providing a cold beverage.
- *Even flow:* Hold hands, repeat some affirmations, or have members express themselves in some way.
- *Additional calming:* Members hold hands with closed eyes or may tell the group what they plan to do when the session is over. Some may linger after the session.

Stage V is never omitted.

Anticipated Outcome

Members feel relaxed, and this can be expressed in their facial features, by their postures, or by a statement. They are alert and calm, starting or appearing to have experienced some pleasure or satisfaction.

Special Opportunities

Suggested Procedures for Specific Problems

The following needs or problems of adults with developmental disabilities may be addressed in an occupational therapy group by introducing the subject for discussion, creating graded activities to practice correction, and reviewing the progress.

Sensorimotor Features

Sensory and Perceptual Processing

Clients bump into each other. A client blocks another's view or gets too close while passing.

> It always is a group function for the therapist to emphasize spatial distances that permit safe exercise and seating where no one's view is blocked. This function can promote distances that are appropriate for sitting near one another, talking to one another, or walking around with greater awareness. This has occurred with good success, at least during group sessions.

Figure 9.4. Stage V: First, we held hands; then some could reach for elbows, and others made it to the shoulders.

Clients do not look in all directions and do not scan on either side so that work or other objects, if not placed in front of them, are not seen and not used.

> Passing objects around often and turning one's head to watch what is happening can be a frequent activity in the group.

Clients find sorting and matching shapes and objects difficult. They do not recognize mistakes in performing tasks or take steps to correct.

> In the frequent handling of objects being passed around, clients have opportunities to use these objects in special ways. Sometimes several trials may be necessary to achieve results. Members build the experience of knowing success while getting to recognize the process of achieving it. Items like two-piece puzzles that make a picture, or something to squeeze or pump for action, are suitable at the very lowest level. Success may be limited, but the activity allows peers to help each other when it is done in a group format. Frequently, members are asked gently during a group activity, "Did you do that right?" Adults appear to enjoy it when they either guess or know they did something right.

Clients find it hard to locate their own elbows, the calf of their legs, or the middle of the back, even with demonstration. Clients do not appear to be familiar with all parts of themselves, as clothes are torn, bunched up, or twisted. They may not recognize where their discomfort is located on their bodies.

> Items in movement, such as batons or plates, can be used to touch body parts. Learning to massage arms and legs and pulling sleeves up and down can be done, as well as pantomiming gestures, like sleeping and so forth. Although full success may not be achieved, some surprising results are possible.

Clients have excessive needs for touch stimulation or to avoid many forms of touch as in handling textures or being touched.

> Use of the vibrator has been seen to neutralize this behavior. Putting a hand-held vibrator into the hand of a group member to use as desired is one option, and offering it on the back, moving slowly, is another. Very rarely is this rejected, but it should never be used to surprise. (Ross, 1997, Appendix)

Neuromusculoskeletal

Clients sit slumped in chairs. Clients are unaware of how to choose good chairs in which to sit. Clients complain of backache or pain in the legs, neck, and shoulder; they may fall out of the chair.

> When group members must look around, attend, and participate, their heads are up, their shoulders braced, and their trunks are stabilized with feet flat on the floor. This feeling is a good one that

they can get often during group sessions. Rarely are people slumped in a group session.

Clients lack strength in holding a 3-pound beanbag and lack endurance standing and moving in a group for 30 minutes.

Use beanbag activities regularly to build endurance. Just passing a beanbag around is a proprioceptive activity that influences relax-ation. The beanbag can be placed in a stretchy cloth parachute, held, and waved up and down by all members together. It should never be used to throw, as gauging how members will throw is too unpredictable.

While standing, clients cannot shift weight or maintain good standing balance.

Clients can hold one another's hands or wrists while moving all together. Place a two-by-four in front of each client for him or her to step onto and over. Some may need help, but this activity is a very good one for people who lack the experience. However, where poor balance is due to neurological conditions, extreme caution and watchfulness must be used to ensure sufficient support is pro-vided. Additionally, poor balance may be due to visual problems, and this factor needs to be ruled out.

Figure 9.5. Learning to squat, to take care of the back, and to coordinate desired movement.

When ambulant, clients demonstrate poor balance; tripping; falling; or bumping into walls, furniture, or each other.

Clients can stand behind and hold onto chairs to practice balance while moving and swinging legs in different directions. Precautions should be taken that sufficient distance exists between group members doing this exercise. This is another way to teach awareness of others. Neglect of either side can be observed and followed up with help. (Author's note: I refer here to unilateral neglect, which means that an individual ignores using one or the other side of the body.)

Bilateral Motor Coordination

Coordinating the carrying of objects with foot movement, alternating limbs in movement, and passing an item from one hand to another hand can be difficult for members in a group. The adult needs to be reminded to use both hands in a task. Members also do not know how to handle many familiar objects and explore their use, such as stretching a rubber band around an object, winding up a gadget, cutting off tape from a dispenser, or pouring from a pitcher.

Use Stages II and III as the time to practice these skills. Exercise can

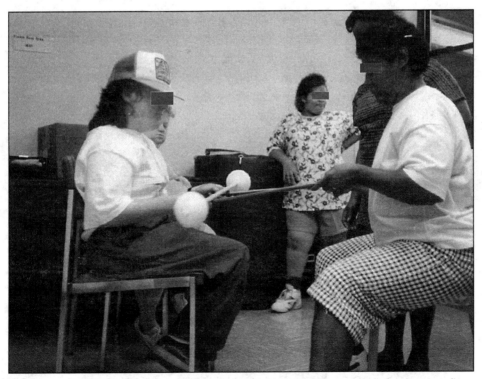

Figure 9.6. Working together as partners is important while learning control of movement, direction with coordination, and focus. Even the helpers learn to attend with consideration.

be devised with just these movements in mind as well. (Ross, 1997, Chapters 2–3)

Clients find it hard to grade muscle tension and movement direction. Clients initially find it hard to handle paper without wrinkling or tearing it or to not break objects by pushing, pressing, or pulling too hard. Grasping, holding, and placing are developmental skills that need much practice. Improvement can be achieved only by doing many similar kinds of activities repetitively, consistently, and with good humor. Improvements have been observed over 3 to 6 years, with very few exceptions.

Use musical instruments to pluck, strum, press, and strike, for example. Carefully undoing sugar-free candies has been useful. Bounce a light wad of paper on a plate, or throw and catch a soft ball.

Cognitive Integration and Cognitive Skills

Clients cannot attend to a task without some degree of verbal or physical prompts, or both. They never know when it is their turn.

Ask other group members to remind them. Provide group games where this skill can be practiced often. Recognize that an occasional success may be what can be achieved and praise it. (Ross, 1997, Chapters 3–4)

Clients display confusion in understanding environmental cues, such as where to sit in a room; who to watch; how to use and pass an object; and how to use cues such as pathways, aisles, and other guides.

Clients do not ask for help. Clients do not help one another, may hurt one another physically, or may give away their property. Responsibilities of ownership and rights are not understood.

All issues may never be resolved, but finding activities that incorporate these skills can help. (Ross, 1997, Chapters 4–5)

Two adults find it hard to wait their turn or mistreat each other.

Adults are required to work this out between themselves, immediately. This activity has met with success.

Group members demonstrate no comprehension of winning a game, being competitive, or improving their own performance. Alternately, members cannot bear to lose a game or a turn.

Group membership provides these experiences over and over. Regular participation in a group gives these clients a chance to know one another and experience these difficulties in familiar surroundings with familiar people. The experience of group membership can help to lessen these difficulties.

Adults cannot remember the sequence of a task and, if some part of a task is learned, the memory of how it is done suddenly is forgotten. What was learned one day may be forgotten by the following day.

> Other members are encouraged to wait before helping or to help with only one step at a time. Learning how to help others can be important for peers who are able to grow in this understanding.

Psychosocial Skills

It is observed that clients can increase their ability to perform motor and perceptual tasks when given the opportunities to practice them. However, it is in the world of feeling that they live, and that influences their social behaviors. The interactive skills appear to be the hardest to acquire and depend greatly on internalizing new attitudes through encountering new experiences in the group.

Psychological

Adults may demonstrate unrealistic attitudes developed through the years, such as "all work is exhausting" and "extending themselves in work is benefiting others rather than themselves." They may believe either that fun is all they should expect or that fun is childish and must be disguised when participated in singly or collectively. Many other examples of lack of establishing one's own values, interests, and self-concepts exist.

> Sharing, awareness of the needs of others, and awareness of the differences that exist in each individual must become a part of the client's engagement in all activities.

Social

Adults display such self-absorption that a balanced view of their place in the order of things is skewed. For example, discrimination between great wrongs and small ones cannot be made, emotional flare-ups are too frequent, and the efforts of others are not appreciated. This self-absorption impairs role performance, social conduct, interpersonal skills, and self-expression.

> A more balanced view can be learned by many adults if consistently worked on in the group. Role models do emerge in a group setting. Therapists need to praise every good action observed and briefly draw its implication for the group.

Self-Management

Concepts that can be reviewed include
- Being on time,
- Allowing sufficient time,

- Planning and making the preparations ahead of time, and
- Assuming responsibility for mistakes and fixing them.

Summary

The Five-Stage Group sessions have had accomplishments. At the very low-est level, crying and uncontrolled bladder behaviors have become controlled. At the more moderate levels, outbursts both physical and verbal have become better monitored by almost everyone with these problems. At the highest level, these adults have been able to demonstrate leadership behaviors, such as taking charge of a stage in the group. They are able to open the group using the welcoming steps and to lead the movement stage. These adults can be assigned to supervise and assist others with more physical or cognitive problems, setting up their lunch so independent eating is possible, assisting them during the day in removing and donning outer clothes, and keeping an eye out for the needs of those who may not know how to ask for help.

Occupation is defined as "chunks of culturally and personally meaning-ful activity in which humans engage" (Clark et al., 1991). By attending the group, members are thus involved in an occupational act, and anyone who wishes to come (or who simply follows other members as they come to the group) is initiating engagement in an intended personally meaningful activi-ty. Within this major category of occupation fall the myriad tasks or activi-ties selected for use in the Five Stages. These are different from the kinds of general activities used in other groups and may differ in the way they are pre-sented. This concept is important to understand and is why a variety of activ-ities are suggested as examples under each stage description. Throughout the session, the selected activities involve every member separately in a 1-or 2-minute task. Alternatively, all the members are involved at the same time in an interactive game, discussion, or collective project that can take about 10 to 20 minutes. Each member gets a turn—a chance to be singled out, but only briefly—each time it is his or her turn. Activities need to be adapted to fit within that time period. Everyone in the group is working to some degree on the goals of relaxing, experiencing, and connecting with one another. Activi-ties are chosen that can be completed successfully within three attempted tri-als whether or not these trials require another demonstration, a verbal cue, a physical assist, or a hand-over-hand help from the therapist or from another member.

Advocacy

With the recent advent of managed care and cost containment in areas of chronic care, funding has become less available. As institutions close and class action suits are initiated, new arenas emerge for serving a population

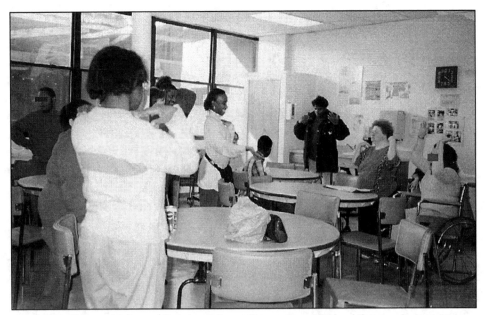

Figure 9.7. Alternately, the two female adults on the extreme right lead the exercises.

Figure 9.8. Alternately, the two female adults on the extreme right lead the exercises.

that is disabled: for instance, group homes, supervised apartment living, and day care programs. Even the structure of how the day is to be spent undergoes changes. Whatever those changes, individuals with developmental disabilities continue to need ongoing preventive care services in addition to medical and management care. The Five Stages Model is one of the means whereby behavioral issues can be addressed, social stimulation needs met, and hidden skills tapped in a cost-effective manner. Advocating for a nonintrusive means for instructing this population in stress reduction methods is now also in the mainstream of prevention. Using a group approach from which the individual's life narrative and needs emerge has historical precedence for other populations with disabilities. In referring to the need to preserve such methods as narrative and life history in the present climate, Burke and Kern wrote,

> The challenge for our profession is to fit these methods into the lexicon of functional and physically measurable change. Hence, each therapist must accept the responsibility for ensuring that methods such as narrative and life history are preserved regardless of the environments they find themselves in and that the data gathered from using these methods are talked about and documented in useful, outcomes-driven, consumer-oriented packages. (Burke & Kern, 1996, p. 392)

Group outcomes for the population with developmental disabilities can affect peers learning to help each other and management costs by requiring fewer controls as behaviors improve. The message here is that retaining a group approach also can be the challenge for our profession to fit "into the lexicon of functional and physically measurable change" (Burke & Kern, 1996, p. 392).

The group may not be a panacea for the ills that the adult with developmental disabilities acquires. However, there is great advantage to these adults when they know that they belong to a special association of persons who are interested in them beyond the need to feed them and keep them clean. Occupational therapists understand that their most impressive asset is advocacy. People who are involved in health care, managed care, politics, and insurance want results, but results that include a sense of satisfaction on the part of the consumer. Despite "bottom-line" arguments, consumer satisfaction will shape the way new services are delivered. When therapists believe in the efficacy of groups for treatment, then groups will be done.

References

Burke, J. P., & Kern, S. B. (1996). The Issue Is—Is the use of life history and narrative in clinical practice reimbursable? Is it occupational therapy? *American Journal of Occupational Therapy, 50,* 389–392.

Clark, F. A., Parham, D., Carlson, M. E., Gelya, F., Jackson, J., Pierce, D., et al. (1991). Occupational science: Academic innovation in the service of occupational therapy's future. *American Journal of Occupational Therapy, 45,* 300–310.

Cole, M. B. (1993). *Group dynamics in occupational therapy: The theoretical basis and practice application of group treatment.* Thorofare, NJ: Slack.

Harlowe, D., & Yu, P. (1981). *The ROM Dance Network.* (Available from P.O. Box 3332, Madison, WI 53704-0332)

Joe, B. E. (1997). Managed care: Does it measure up? *OT Week, 11,* 14–16.

Ross, M. (1987). *Group process.* Thorofare, NJ: Slack.

Ross, M. (1991). *Integrative group therapy* (2nd ed.). Thorofare, NJ: Slack.

Ross, M. (1997). *Integrative group therapy: Mobilizing coping abilities with the Five Stage Group.* Bethesda, MD: American Occupational Therapy Association.

Ross, M., & Burdick, D. (1981). *Sensory integration: A training manual for therapists and teachers for regressed, psychiatric, and geriatric patient groups.* Thorofare, NJ: Slack.

Wood, W. (1996). Legitimizing occupational therapy's knowledge. *American Journal of Occupational Therapy, 50,* 626–634.

Additional Reading

Vohs, J. R. (1996). Jumping tracks. *Developmental Disabilities Special Interest Section Newsletter, 19,* 1–3.

Writing about her 23-year-old daughter, born with cerebral palsy and cognitive difficulties, the author of this excellent article described how using a vocabulary of "slots, facilities, placements, coverage, 'day hab,' functional skills, acquisition, resident, consumer" brought limited and frustrating results for her and her daughter throughout many years. When the author began to use a contrasting vocabulary for goals for her daughter consisting of "home, neighborhood and community, friends, job contribution, citizenship, lifelong learning and education, and adventure," her daughter's needs began to represent the needs all people have. This freed up approaches and promoted the achievement of many of her daughter's dreams. We can do the same and reduce the separation between "normal" populations and populations born with disabilities. Set goals for the population with developmental disabilities using an effective language of "lifelong learning, education, and adventure," so that they will achieve social integration, continue skill learning, and realize some dreams.

CHAPTER 10

Groups Are Physical, Social, and Emotional Therapy— "A Chance to Tell My Story"

Mildred Ross, OTR/L, FAOTA

> When I talk to you and you listen to me, not only do we see and hear one another, but, insofar as either of us remembers the occasion, it is because we produce long-term changes in the function and structure of the nerve cells in each other's brains.
> *Eric Kandel, Professor, Columbia University (1992, p. 31)*

The purpose of this chapter is to demonstrate how group treatment can be used for the management and delivery of service to adults with developmental disabilities. Getting these adults to sit together and meet as a group is an important intervention, and changes for a better lifestyle may be possible. The benefits and results of such intervention for this population are discussed. The kinds of groups used, the various aspects of the role of the therapist, and the application of physiological and psychological features that influence success are described. The immense diversity existing in this population, the variety of topics and activities to offer to groups, and the similarity in the needs of this population compared with all other populations are detailed.

Group Membership Enables and Enriches Social Development

Feeling comfortable in a variety of group settings is an acquired skill for most people and a very important one. To assume that those who cannot talk, are slow in thinking, or are limited in verbal expression cannot benefit from a group experience is simply wrong. A person must be in a group to learn how to be in one. Social skills, like other human skills, are acquired chiefly through engagement and practice. Social skills must be experienced with other peers who can offer a challenge not too great yet not too comfortable so that learning occurs. No one should be excluded. Some memberships even have life-saving properties.

An Individual Needs to Belong to Many Kinds of Groups

In general, group experiences in addition to family are presented naturally as one encounters diverse peer gatherings in school and joins social, religious, athletic, or other kinds of groups. Such associations provide the advantages of learning how to play, to struggle, to share with others, to be praised, to express hurt, to find redress, to help others, and to accept help until, finally, the person develops a good identity and rewarding relationships. Through these memorable events, the necessary shaping of advantageous long-term changes in the personality occurs (Kandel, 1992).

These different kinds of group opportunities are not accessed readily by the individual born with a disability or by the individual who becomes disabled, traumatized, or diseased early in life and who may have been institutionalized for long periods. Disability often creates so many demands that even within the family the need for normal socialization can be overlooked and never achieved. When attention is turned to these needs, therapeutic groups are a proven benefit.

We Learn Through Our Nervous System

There is a persisting perception that groups are purely psychological events, perhaps because "feelings" are so much discussed. However, it is simultaneously a physiological event owing to the chemical exchange that accompanies the action that takes place in the group (Kandel, 1992). This chemical exchange is the communication code that is transmitted from neuron to neuron throughout the nervous system. The motor and behavioral responses are put together from the summation of the interpretation of the communication message. Among the cortical structures involved, the limbic system (the limbic lobe is considered the emotional brain) especially registers the event. The amygdala collects and processes the responses from other lobes, coordinating emotion with memory association, and reports via chemical discharge to the hypothalamus, which regulates the autonomic nervous system. The autonomic nervous system influences brain stem regulation of the internal organs. The immune system via the hypothalamus and pituitary gland is informed and responds by supplying stress hormones appropriately. The relatively new field of psychoneuroimmunology informs us "that the immune system is not an autonomous agency of defense, but part of an integrated network of regulatory mechanisms serving homeostatic functions" (Ader, 1992). "Recent research demonstrates that there are bidirectional communication pathways between the immune system and central nervous system . . . with each providing important regulatory control over the other" (Maier, Watkins, & Fleshner, 1994, p. 1004).

When members demonstrate the ability to concentrate and participate during a group session, it can be assumed that therapists, discussions, activities, and myriad other factors are influencing the immune and central nervous systems of members. Internal balance (homeostasis) is the result of the satisfying stimulation provided in the group session. When members seen in the group setting are unable to participate and override their symptoms, therapists then have elements to evaluate for their behaviors. Therapists can assess the acuteness of the person's illness or lack of readiness for the particular group, the depletion of the person's immune system, or the flawed stimulation presented in the session (Ross, 1997).

Depending on the intensity of the input of the event to each person, cardiovascular, respiratory, sensory, and motor behaviors will be critically affected. Pupils may widen, and respiration and heart rate slow in a learning mode. There will be observed outward changes to information heard or to conflict seen. The group members will smile or laugh, relax visibly, and straighten up in their postures. Some participants will stand up and pace, move vigorously or even ominously, in some way. Anxiety, envy, fear, and other negative feelings can be expressed by a rush of words, loss of attention, sweaty palms, yawns, sleepiness, or a flushed face. If you introduce the subject of a forest fire or the suicide death of a person, the changes in body behavior may become very evident. As they receive and process sensation, each person exhibits a seamless melding of their total physical, emotional, mental, and spiritual self all at once. Josephine C. Moore said, "We are our nervous system. It's our behavior: It's who we are. You cannot separate neuroscience from behavior" (as cited in Royeen, 1990, p. 10).

Application of Nervous System Learning and Meaningful Stimulation to Occupational Therapy Groups

When conducting a group of people with chronic disabilities, this writer suggests two guiding principles. The first principle is to consider when and how the planned activities are to be introduced. The knowledge of how different kinds of stimulation affect the nervous system is a crucial tool in the acquisition of skill that must be acquired to conduct groups of adults with developmental disabilities. The skilled therapist must learn—through knowledge of neuroscience, through careful observation, and through experimentation—how and when to change activities.

Some operational principles may be stated simply:
- Whatever is novel, alerts.
- Whatever is fast, excites.
- Whatever is routine or familiar, soothes and composes.
- Whatever is slow, relaxes.

The second principle builds on the first, namely, that a moderate approach to arousal achieves longer lasting results. Group events should not become too exciting or too dull. Consider that if you use novelty too soon or too much with anxious group members, you will lose their attention because too much stimulation is disorganizing. Overfiring of one system can make it difficult for the complementary system to recover, such as keeping the sympathetic and parasympathetic systems in balance. Relaxation may not be easy to achieve as quickly as it may be required (Lutz & Ramsey, n.d.; Noback, Strominger, & Demarest, 1991). Furthermore, there is the chance that the event may be canceled out as individuals in the group do not relate the excitement to a realistic plan for follow-up. In a therapeutic group the goal is to obtain a sense of inner control, calm, and balance, and flooding the system requires a lot of coping skill and self-management to regroup.

Information-processing deficits exist with mental retardation. Can these be reversed, considering the deficits with which such a nervous system begins? Reduced density of synapses, those important sites over which chemical and electrical communication cross, is reported in fetuses and infants with Down syndrome (Neistadt, 1994). This means there is less opportunity for available information to permeate the system. Observed deficits in memory, abstract thinking, learning strategies, and attention spans exist. The question is, Can these be improved substantially? Reviewing the physical, biochemical, and electrical properties of the information-processing system that underlies all human learning, the validity of plasticity assumptions for learning following brain injury after birth is very good in its promise (Moore, 1990; Neistadt, 1994). It is not clear how information processing in a brain that begins with prebirth injury or deficiency can be improved. Reason and observation show that exposure to meaningful stimuli, practice within a context, repetition, innate motivation, and an inner state of satisfaction can bring about learning in the individual with developmental disabilities.

General Benefits of Groups

When individuals become uncomfortable and inappropriate with others, they need a setting where appropriate behaviors and attitudes can be practiced safely. In such a setting, people with extreme and immoderate behaviors that interfere with the safety and rights of others learn to curb those behaviors. Such a setting is also a way for those who are withdrawn to test the waters: There is the opportunity for learning from peers about what to say or do in a group while preserving a sense of safety and privacy. Skilled facilitators encourage the group to distill both general wisdom and individual skills. Good groups provide consistent feedback, so that members can be stimulated and nurtured to change behaviors and acquire hope. Adults who cannot

or do not use language to express themselves, or those with poor comprehension, dementia, or cognitive disturbance, especially benefit from group
membership as they continue to learn at their pace and make themselves better understood. In a well-conducted group, each member consistently gets a
sense of being respected by and connected to others: Participants feel more
comfortable about changing their behavior. Here, at least, tension and conflict are able to be voiced, not met with punishment or demeaning coddling.
For example,

> Kevin is a man who was discharged from a state facility for men-
> tal retardation to a group home. From there he was referred to a
> work service program. Here he attended my Five-Stage Group. For
> about 5 years he displayed minimal independent function and was
> nonverbal. Then at one session, Kevin and the others were holding
> onto a stretchy parachute. A sandbag had been placed in the cloth
> to make it heavier to lift. The weight fell out of the raised stretchy
> cloth and landed near Kevin. In a very unusual gesture for him,
> Kevin bent down, picked it up, hesitated, and then placed it back
> onto the cloth. This was the first time he had initiated an act of
> involvement with the group. This act made him a part of what was
> going on and, for the first time, he did something to stay a part of
> it. He continued with more acts of involvement and fewer isolating
> mannerisms. Kevin's behavior in the workshop gradually changed
> too, requiring fewer prompts to stay on task.

> Another young adult, Sam, frequently stayed out all night in
> bad neighborhoods and would not accept individual counseling.
> However, he agreed to attend my occupational therapy group and
> participated in sharing his issues for about 4 years. In this group,
> he began to report his unsafe behaviors and eventually heard the
> message of the group members, so that the extreme nature and fre-
> quency of his unsafe actions were greatly reduced. Eventually, Sam
> began to respect and trust his peers sufficiently to be able to eval-
> uate many of his situations with them.

> A middle-aged adult, Dolores, presented with unpredictable
> temper tantrums that interfered with her work. She chiefly attend-
> ed groups that taught relaxation techniques, such as using tapes,
> guided imagery, and exercise. This appeared to reduce her defen-
> siveness better than a direct confrontation about her escalating
> behaviors. When Dolores joined our verbal-sharing group, she
> willingly shared those experiences that were either pleasant or
> aggravating to her but quickly displayed irritation by groaning or
> withdrawing from the group when others were describing theirs.
> Dolores demonstrated that not everyone wants to talk things over;

exercising, engaging in group activities, and learning to share in this way are preferred by some more than others. Dolores joined group sessions that were structured to include less verbal sharing and more movement and relaxation activities, and she was able to redirect her inappropriate behavior. She now continues on a job with a job coach.

Another participant, Louise, has mental retardation with serious neurological deficits in perception and tactile sensation but good verbal skills. Although she displays limitations in understanding world events, she shows good ability to profit from her extensive life experiences. She can reflect on these personal, concrete, and meaningful events and learn from them with the help of others and her own willingness to do so. She benefits greatly from expressing herself in groups that she had attended for more than 10 years. As a member of an occupational therapy group, Louise is able to empathize and to relate how, by self-control, listening, and self-evaluation, she took on similar problems shared by group members of fighting, willfulness, and disrespect to others. That ability has greatly influenced, directed, and benefited the group members. Louise told how she threw plates and had to clean up the mess and how she lost privileges when she screamed. Louise shared how she began to recognize that certain family members disturbed her, that people taunting her in the street made her feel ashamed, or that a pain or sore so frightened her that it triggered her uncontrolled behavior. She explained how describing these feelings to people who listened was helpful to her. Louise could say, "You have to admit when you are wrong," and she got the message across to members by articulating the steps to take to achieve goals. Louise realizes that, despite her ongoing struggles, she is seen as a role model, and she expresses her pride in this. There is no better learning than that received from peers who can share.

Therapeutic Groups at Goodwill Industries

Therapeutic groups usually consist of five to nine adults. In my groups the members usually chose to be with others of similar abilities, and therefore, much of the time group membership could be homogeneous. I facilitated three different groups. One group consisted of adults of all ages whose cognitive functioning fell below 45 IQ or in the low–moderate to severely impaired ranges. These people could not use language for a number of different reasons or were limited verbally to a word or phrase with difficulties in articulation. The second group consisted of individuals with moderate cognitive impairment between 45 IQ and 65 IQ, also displaying very limited verbal skills. The third group consisted of people who possessed verbal skills with varying abilities and degrees of comprehension. These adults were considered in the high range of moderate to mild cognitive impairment, approximately 65 IQ and above. In addition, individuals with average or better cognition and diagnosed with traumatic brain injury, autism, or other psychiatric diagnosis were referred to this group and chose to attend. In this group, participants chiefly wanted to verbalize and share their experiences. There were some individuals who could float between two and even three of the groups because of their interest and their ability to learn from different kinds of experiences. The Five-Stage format (Ross, 1997) was used consistently with the first two groups, and principles from the Five Stages were incorporated as much as possible into the third group. Usually, this latter group had two coleaders, but in the last year of its existence (1997), only one facilitator was present. All examples of verbal responses described in this chapter came from this third group, which met once a week. Descriptions of the changes in physical behaviors that occurred are illustrations from all the groups. More information on the structure of the Five-Stage format is provided in Chapter 9.

Examples of Therapeutic Group Experiences

Members Learn to Realize That They Need Their Peers

During their life most group members experience the extremely transient contact with people who are hired and who move in and out of their life. The peers they meet may be their most enduring contacts, like acquiring an extended family. Group members say this in one way or another. There are so few ways to meet formally and feel a sense of relatedness to each other. For example, in a special sharing session one member brought pictures of his family. He insisted that the facilitator must see them first. It made him feel important to bequeath this special honor, but it sent the wrong message to group members about their value. The facilitator reminded him that because all members had the same interest, she would wait her turn. He still could feel important about what he had to show to the group as members responded with good interest and he, again, saw how they cared for him.

Member Has Her Moment to Receive Attention

Once, when members were asked to give their reasons for coming to the group session, Mary answered that it was "a chance to tell my story." She recites the same scenario over and over many times, but it is a grand way to say that we all need to relieve the burden on ourselves by reciting our chores, our grievances, our unnoticed victories, all of which make us feel recognized and acknowledged. This population is at risk for the stifling of this very human need.

Members Learn to Listen to Others and Gain Various Advantages

One member reported that she learned about giving and getting "respect" when she began to listen to others without interrupting them before they were finished speaking and, conversely, could assert her right to be listened to in this way. Another person demonstrated that in listening to and learning from each other, different solutions can be gathered to solve a problem. This phenomenon occurred when one member related her frustration and difficulty at being required to pack up all her winter clothes and take them to another area for storage. How to do this and how to carry it all loomed as an immense obstacle for her to overcome. The group members attended to this concern with numerous practical suggestions. The discussion diminished her need to be dependent and helped her to learn to do for herself.

Attending to Group Process

Between and among groups of people there are walls, such as developmental disabilities, that separate one from the other. These walls need to be breached and weakened. A lack of experience and information, an inability to read and pursue continuing education, and inequality in relationships with members from other populations exist. Group process in the hands of a skilled practitioner can facilitate communication among members to ameliorate these serious deficiencies. As group members experience the rules regarding attacking, shaming, or blaming others, as in any other group, they begin to examine issues, learn more factual information, and see where they can take responsibility for their actions and consequences.

> Group member Mary, describing her discomfort with a vaginal rash, attempted to better clarify her situation by beginning to expose herself. A broad range of social know-how existed in the group, and several members registered distress. The facilitator seized on this occasion to teach members to notice how others are listening to them. Rarely are issues of such sensitivity explained, developed, reinforced, and rewarded with this population.
>
> The therapist interrupted Mary and requested that she look at the faces around her. Most of these faces were expressing some degree of discomfort. One young man was halfway out of his seat about to leave but sat back down when Mary was interrupted. Mary, however, could not interpret what the expressions meant, and another member who could explain it did so very simply. One member was very contemptuous of Mary. However, her contempt presented the opportunity to discuss the difference between private and public self-touching. This issue illustrated exactly the kind of help members can give to each other. The member who showed

contempt relented in her strong feelings, as she saw the incident worthwhile through the eyes of the therapist. Others also learned their right to express their discomfort instead of rolling their eyes and trying to leave when "touchy" subjects arise. In addition, members learned how to get help. In this instance, a nurse was able to help Mary. The members learned that they can go to different people and places to get help with their problems and that a variety of outcomes are available from many sources. They began to understand what subjects can be discussed in groups and when to protect their privacy.

Many adults with developmental disabilities have no experience with group membership. Therefore, the evolution of the group through the usual stages of development in which members struggle for control or leadership may not happen. Role development—such as of leader, arbiter, or role model—even when it occurs is tenuous and depends greatly on the facilitator to help it flourish. Just the hint of an energizing connectedness among members may be all that happens for a long time.

During an activity group with seven young adults with moderate to severe cognitive impairment, the time "to talk" had arrived. They were asked to talk about something good or kind that had recently happened to them. In this group about half of the members could not produce sound. It sometimes required another member to volunteer to speak for a member, sometimes a member had to explain the request in "code" words to the other member, or sometimes the group members would make guesses. This is how it worked. When it was Vivian's turn, she thrust her hands forward to show she understood. Although considered to have very low cognition and to be deaf and without speech, she persisted until the group understood she was proud of her newly painted fingernails. Vivian then began to untie her shoes. This was a puzzle at first but, when asked if her toenails had been painted as well, she nodded affirmatively and stopped untying her shoes. It took time, but she was able to reveal that her mother was responsible. All this time group cohesion was building, and it was intense as members enveloped her. They could be happy for her—with maybe a tinge of envy—which made this occurrence so human.

Good reasons exist for creating groups with a mixture of different diagnoses so the advantages each population brings can be shared. At times, individuals with traumatic brain injury or psychiatric problems have joined the group of adults with developmental disabilities. These individuals with other diagnoses bring the capacity to verbalize and generalize, which may be lacking in people with developmental disabilities. This ability promoted greater understanding as everyone contributed to explanations from different levels; everyone grew by helping or being helped.

Ben, a young man with a history of autism and psychiatric problems who demonstrated good intelligence, attended the group for 2 years. Ben joined because he "felt so empty inside." At one session, near the end of his stay, he turned to Jenifer, an adult with developmental disabilities, who was venting her aggravation at taking a bus to work that carried noisy teenagers, and said, "You are not alone. I feel that way too on that bus!" With the help of Jenifer, Ben was able to recognize and connect with his feelings. The facilitators knew he had graduated. He, in turn, provided a model for Jenifer of how she might offer a meaningful response when she connected with others.

Content and Conduct of the Group

Therapists can introduce a rhythm to the group to maintain a sense of balance or to promote the return to homeostasis that is the desired goal. This rhythm consists of increasing or decreasing the degree of excitement by using selected activity and discussion to achieve a balance, so that the members' available energy will be sustained throughout group.

When conducting the group, a welcoming smile, a pleasant environment, comfortable seating, and a very brief activity such as a handshake or passing an object will start any kind of group momentarily. Experience showed that when the therapist attended to each individual member very briefly, general focus was achieved. However, an activity must follow quickly to maintain the attention.

Movement or some novel theme creates additional motivation. To maintain this focus, the next step is to create more energy and interest. To do this, novelty in subject matter or movement that is fast paced can excite and alert.

Consider how touch tracts and their pathways to certain structures like the cerebellum can be effective. Stimulating these pathways initially with an alerting kind of touch, followed up with more moderate-pressure touch, helps to reduce emotion and invites an interest to learn (Ross, 1987). Providing items to handle or introducing different kinds of movement can also accomplish this. Examples are provided in the previous chapter, "A Five-Stage Model for Adults With Developmental Disabilities." Even if a group member does not know the date or cannot articulate many words, the person can relate very naturally on a sensorimotor level and follow simple movements and good touch (Ross, 1997).

Having the group aroused by the movement activity and successfully interested in what is happening provides the optimal time for performing a perceptual task or having a meaningful discussion:

Novelty should be introduced judiciously with an entertaining or exciting question or observation to continue the interest. As a moderate amount of interest is sustained, the group becomes able to evaluate the experience or to concentrate on one person's problem or exert more patience while waiting for a response from a slower member.

Nearing the end of a session, any immoderate behavior like a buildup of enthusiasm or even the realization of hurt and pain can cause the emotional flooding of the whole nervous system. This situation is not conducive to calm deliberations of the activities of daily life after the group session is over for the day. Therefore, every group needs a cooling down such as closure activities:

> Focusing again on each member individually, stating plans to meet again, and some formal touch that is beneficial for the group are some ways to signal the nervous system that events have remained safe, the familiar is back in focus, and there is incentive to move on.

Role of Therapists as Group Leaders

Therapists need to call on members and ask, "What did Mary just say?" When what Mary said cannot be repeated, it might mean that its significance is not understood. The facilitator cues to encourage Mary's continuing contribution. The leader seeks clarification when the adult who is explaining uses the same words over and over again. John may offer an interpretation that is still unintelligible. At this time another member can be asked, "What did you hear John say, Susan?" Susan may be familiar with the code that one word may symbolize, can help interpret John's message, and then get his verification. Mary can be asked again "If we are all talking about the same thing" she introduced. The leader is in charge of following the ping pong ball of this communication as it flies back and forth and keeps the discussion focused.

All explanations must be very brief. Two or three sentences that are descriptively concrete are all that is necessary from the facilitator. The group members can do a lot of the work. The leader steers the group members to teach. To a young adult man who insisted that his age of 30 years entitled him to make his own rules about curfews, the group members provided examples about establishing trust, demonstrating responsibility, and simply stating what one expects from others. The young man was convinced eventually to change his actions. The facilitator started this discussion by stating that "behavior, not age, makes people believe in someone." Attention spans are not experienced sufficiently to stay too long on any one person or topic and need constant spurts of brief redirecting remarks. Memories seem to disappear at times. However, repetition, practice, and the human desire to learn lurk in all populations. The opportunity to be listened to strikes a responsive chord.

With other populations, facilitators might use more neutral comments. However, with this population, frequent and extravagant (but sincere) praise supplies, supports, and maintains interest. This reinforces members' growth and good decisions.

The ease with which issues of control can be aroused in therapists working with adults with developmental disabilities has to be recognized. Control issues can be a pitfall. In a group of adults of very low function, everyone was requested to bring his or her own chair to make the usual circle. Some needed to have help initiating the action, but all completed it alone. When the chairs were placed, a picture was taken, followed shortly by a second picture. On viewing the pictures later, the facilitator was amazed. In comparing the first picture of the group (with members completing the circle on their own) with the next picture of the group as it began, the scene was very altered. The first picture showed an uneven and more oval space between members. In the second picture, group members were evenly spaced in a precise circle. Obviously, in the second picture the need "to control" by rearrangement could not be resisted by the therapist. Therapists need to be very mindful of allowing flexibility, extending patience, and continuing to grow in understanding.

Leadership is ever alert to "fading out" whenever the group demonstrates that it is finding its own voice: Leadership can never consider itself as purely directive. The leader serves as a facilitator, keeping members focused and dropping the reins when it is possible. Groups demonstrate they have found their own voice when members make suggestions and these are followed up. All members are called on for answers, definitions, and reactions, even if they are unwilling to contribute at a particular time and refusal is accepted. As stated previously, a more active facilitator may be required with some populations than with others, but as soon as possible all learned dependent behavior is deflected using the same group dynamic skills regulating all groups.

A sense of superficiality may appear to exist at times; therapists may also feel discouraged about the direction a session may take. However, it is the accumulation of group sessions that yields results, and a quick fix cannot be expected. Under any circumstances, these cannot be short-term groups: The usual short-term verbal group is not effective with this population.

The group format is very applicable to the issues that concern adults with developmental disabilities, like self-respect and conflict resolution. Gaining self-respect can be guided by helping this population use more assertive interactions. Learning rights and expressing them assertively, however, must be done in stages. To this population, assertiveness can be construed as showing a range of behavior from bad manners to civil disobedience for which there will be reprisals. Fear of reprisal from caregivers can be very real and confounds the learning process.

As in any group management, conflict occurs and needs to be addressed. Addressing conflict allows the group leader to guide the group toward the practice of assertive behavior and appropriately expressing what one wants.

Conflicts between members are handled at the moment of occurrence and in a direct and clear manner. Many sessions are required to recognize rights and learn appropriate requests. Once these skills are mastered, the therapist can then introduce a variety of ways to reduce frustration, anger, and rage before these feelings escalate. Gradually, it becomes possible to teach members to use relaxation techniques to reduce their quick emotional responses and increase more reasonable behavior. Learning mantras or using mental pictures, tapes, and music can build inner strength to reinforce the new practice of meeting needs with more effective behaviors.

Some adult members tell of the restraints that belittling caregivers may offer when they see them using relaxation techniques, and these are very real obstacles to address with everyone. Some quickly learn how to hide their new growth and understanding when they perceive it to be threatened. For example, Jeanie, a member with Down syndrome, described how she made sure her bedroom door was locked when she retired to do the meditation she was taught in the group. She knew her parents would laugh at her because they would not understand. She had had no success in keeping them from checking out her tied boxes in her dresser drawers. Jeanie also could describe her improved relationships with her stepfather as a result of sharing her issues in the group. She began to understand over several years' attendance in the group that she had a right to privacy, that she had a right to do what was required in the context of her situation, and that there was a difference between being "fresh" and being assertive. Therapists learn to proceed at a slower pace to achieve new learning and explore with the group members a variety of means to arrive at desired goals.

When it is appropriate that a decision be based on majority agreement, all members are helped to understand what this means and that it must be respected. Group members can be blunt with another member. For example, Betty, a member with dual diagnoses, often would not talk about herself but referred repeatedly to vague and off-topic issues like "the meaning of boundless" or "belief in heaven or in hell." Group members told her they did not understand what she was talking about and that such words reminded them of death and dying or made them sad. The facilitator would reinforce the group's wishes by reminding Betty that she should not refer to the unwanted topics even though the members were inconsistent in their attempts to do this. With a more able group, peers are expected to take care of their needs, and such protection is not rendered by the leader. With this initial support from the leader, Betty's group was able eventually to take responsibility for enforcing its majority decision that each person talk about himself or herself and for deterring Betty from acting on her obsessive thoughts. When necessary, one or another member headed off any "forgetfulness" on Betty's part. This helped Betty, and when she was asked to describe the group to a new member she stated, "We talk about ourselves." The facilitator took advantage of this by asking quickly, "Can you give an example?" Caught by surprise, Betty answered, "I pick out my own clothes." Betty was very pleased with the group's approval. Another time she was asked what she liked about the group, and she stated it was the "good conversation." She appeared to have more difficulty than anyone in conforming appropriately, but she was committed now to change. For many years she had required a special "management program" in the workshop to control inappropriate behaviors. Now with the group experience, Betty has successfully appealed to have this behavioral program dropped. She never misses a group session.

There is a receptivity in this population that some may see as a learned compliance or as their inability to think quickly enough to combat a statement. The receptivity also can be a natural tendency to wish to live peaceably, to live in the moment, to accept limits, and to avoid being hurt or hurting others. The adult usually recognizes with an honest poignancy that he or she needs consistent support to do his or her best.

Group Language

In all cultures, special words are marked for use that may be understood more readily by the majority of members. In this subculture group, members have to help the facilitator learn their special language. Additionally, this population gets very little opportunity to have words defined for them, so it cannot be taken for granted that the meanings of even familiar words are understood. Frequently synonyms for words cannot be offered adequately by group members. Some words appear to carry great weight even when members cannot define them.

Respect

The use of "respect" appears to be very well understood by every member. It may be that society in general uses this word so often that everyone "overlearns" it. This word may convey all that needs to be said about anyone's behavior to another or to oneself. It has become the most effective word to be used in the group to bring about instant attention. "Respect her space," "respect his need not to tell us," "respect her point of view," "respect his right to make that choice," "we do not feel respect from you," and so forth all appear to promote understanding.

Control

On the other hand, it was seen in one group that, when members were exhorted to "control" a robot to keep it from falling off the table, the meaning was not understood until the request was changed to "let's play with it." To a population that rarely experiences "control" but appreciates "play," the latter word is understood better.

Game

However, calling an activity a "game" may discourage some group members from participating because their respective families have told them not "to act like a baby," which they associate with "game." Calling a game an "activity" may be more acceptable for some members. Therapists must learn each group's sensitivity to certain words because there are no hard and fast rules. At certain levels of higher function, avoiding the word "play" may be necessary, whereas at lower levels the word is helpful.

Angry

Words like "hurt," "upset," or "aggravated" may be more acceptable than "angry" or "mad" because most members have been told it is bad or wrong to be angry or mad. It is hard for some to separate the feeling from an action. "Angry" may carry with it the intent to do violence, and some cannot unlearn this interpretation easily.

Advocate

An example of an often-used word requiring definition arose when group members learned of congressional action being taken to reduce Medicaid at the federal and then the state level. The word "advocate" was heard and required clarification. One person described it as "the person who takes you places." Others went further, stating, "they speak for you," "like you," "stand up for you," and, concluded one member with one word, they are your "backup." Members then saw that a sister, a friend, or a state worker acted in this capacity. The group discussion continued as the facilitator inquired, "Can you be your own advocate?" This question led to a very lively discussion and indicated how each member was at a different stage in accepting and using this concept.

Kinds of Groups

The adult population with developmental disabilities benefits from groups that meet to
- Cook,
- Reduce stress,
- Exercise,
- Enhance community involvement (Edgerton & Gaston, 1991),
- Improve work concepts,
- Teach arts and crafts,
- Dance,
- Advance the understanding of sexuality (Ludwig, 1995), and
- Promote healthy relationships.

All of these groups can enhance self-esteem and self-expression as well as require problem solving and choice making. When people choose their own groups and goals, it is more likely that they will show greater initiative in carrying on what they have learned (Neistadt, 1995). Only lack of available facilitators; lack of transportation; and lack of money to purchase services, supplies, or admission tickets limits the kinds of groups that can be developed for all levels of functioning (Schleien, Meyer, Heyne, & Brandt, 1995).

This population demonstrates the broadest, most diverse range of individual aptitudes and levels of understanding within any one group of same-age people. In a group of young men and women, one man exhibits timidity on the subject of romance, denying any interest. Another man has a special friend but is vehement about his lack of readiness for more than that. One woman likes having her boyfriend but also wants to play the field without him knowing this because she is sure her mother will never let her marry. Another accepts attention from one but confides that she really loves another to whom she has never spoken. Yet another woman wants to concentrate on her boyfriend, taking the relationship seriously and expecting it to offer more physically to her when she feels ready. She hopes that eventually she will marry. In the same group, stages of readiness, maturity, degree of dependence, and comprehension differ when another kind of subject matter is introduced. This diversity makes it possible for peers with more wisdom in one area to help and share and then on another occasion receive enlightenment from others.

The many changes taking place in the approaches toward long-term support for the population with developmental disabilities assist in the exploration of preventive means, the development of new attitudes such as that reflected in the Special Olympics, and the realization that there are universal natural needs. Deinstitutionalization, community involvement, work experience, and the use of purposeful groups will push progress further. In the Midwest, statewide Associations for Retarded Citizens (ARCs) have very vocal members among the adults with developmental disabilities and provide programming that promotes the integration of adults into existing groups in the community (Johnson & Olsen, 1982). The ARC is a grassroots organization, as opposed to a professionally created organization, that was started by families of people with developmental disabilities and that is an important resource for advocacy. The Association on Aging with Developmental Disabilities describes a retirement support group in its newsletter (Association on Aging with Developmental Disabilities, 1995).

Observations After Providing Groups for 10 Years to Many of the Same Clients

- Ninety percent of the consumers like the group. They come as soon as it is announced. Those who are verbal will repeatedly ask for the group if a group is disbanded.

- Clients who act out with hostility on many occasions do not do this on the day they attend the occupational therapy group. Once or twice a year there may be an exception, but adaptive behavior for that day is the norm.

- Improved motor behavior is seen over a period of 3 to 5 years by participants in the Five-Stage Group. With the exception of a very few participants, this change occurred with people who had been institutionalized for most of their lives. Those starting with a more kindly, individualized environment can expect a faster rate of change in their abilities. For example, everyone improves from her or his initial performance in the ability to follow visual demonstration or verbal directions. These are important gains because the improved agility affects physical safety and behavior. People who cannot bend with stability to pick up or place an item on the floor learn to maintain their balance. Then they are not knocked over so easily when someone brushes against them. Clients who cannot grasp and release, such as when throwing a ball, grading hand movements while filling a bag without ripping it, or crushing paper inserts to put in a box, all improve. The success is first seen in the group and then observed in the workshop, and because both have an impact on the client, it may be that both workshop and group activity have to coexist.

- In the activity group that consists of activities and verbal processing, there are gains in social behavior. During group sessions, members exhibit greater awareness with respect to each other's space. They consciously consent to sharing attention and items with each other as they begin and continue to watch each other more consistently. How this may generalize into actions outside the group meeting has not been established. Yet, if it is the case that poor behaviors are learned for general use, then healthier behaviors also can be learned for general use. One hundred abstracts (PsycLIT, Journal Articles 1/90–6/95) were reviewed on research outcomes for this population using groups as a means of accomplishing change in undesirable behaviors presented by individuals. However, no groups were reported being used for preventive measures or for teaching methods for change. Single-case studies were used frequently to report on individual behavioral programs that never included any group attendance. All of the latter studies were concerned with challenging behaviors. Introducing choices of various activities in recreation and meals "produced significant decreases in frequency and severity of challenging behaviors" (Ip & Szymanski, 1994). A good group provides multiple choices in activities and themes for discussion and can be cost-effective. Documenting measurable outcomes "of challenging behaviors" as a result of group membership can be a good subject for research.

- A clear outcome of the use of activity and discussion/sharing groups with adults with developmental disabilities is that each person improves in verbal and nonverbal self-expression when offered the opportunity. Nowhere else is the adult listened to or attended to with the consistent patience shown by the group with a supportive facilitator. Under other circumstances, the adult is often talked to rather than listened to because it is easy to do this. Solutions appear simple. However, there can be a depth of reasoning for which the adult is not credited or helped to explore fully. To illustrate, a woman was assigned the job of breaking down boxes in the workshop. She had severe dyspraxia, and she was accustomed to experiencing a long waiting time between job assignments. When her hands became bruised in the handling of the boxes and she saw another worker's canvas gloves lying around, she donned them and continued working. She was accused of taking something that did not belong to her. No one allowed her time to explain that she usually had to wait too long for others to solve her problems, that she was only borrowing the gloves, and that she was tired of sitting around waiting for a job assignment if she would be taken off this job. In the group she was guaranteed a chance to explain all of this and took the time to do so. Because the matter already had been resolved, the opportunity in the group to express all of her feelings provided closure for her.

- Self-confidence grows as group members first acquire the ability to articulate, then to expand on their verbalization, and finally to take action. As an illustration, a young woman named Sally said that she came to the group to learn more about herself and others. However, she remained unable to apply the new assertive language that she rehearsed in the group to the conditions she experienced in her group home. After attending sessions for about 5 years, she was asked what single lesson she had learned in the group. She responded, "Other people's problems are not my responsibility." Indeed, she constantly worried about what she was expected to do when things went wrong around her. Sally described that her roommate, who worked in the same workshop, was getting up to give kisses to the man sitting next to Sally. She thought this was poor manners, and the bosses would not like it. When asked what she would do about it, Sally responded, "Nothing, it's not my responsibility. But it isn't right." Sally demonstrated that she could relate what she learned from the group as she acted on that rationale.

Others show stronger attempts but still slip back too easily into their old passive behaviors if not constantly supported by group meetings to maintain newly acquired learning. It may be expected that outcomes evolve naturally from talking to taking action. This only reinforces the need for using groups with this population.

Members of the population considered developmentally disabled often are patronized. The nervous system records it even when the person cannot articulate it. The fight-or-flight mechanism is triggered frequently in many people in this population. Usually the fight idea is stifled in favor of withdrawal and emotional blocking. This frequent stimulus of being kept in one's place can create ongoing, chronic, and unpredictable stress (Moore, 1990). Physically and emotionally, endurance is reduced. Eventually, when enough toxins are released within the system, the body can shut down completely. A good group can transcend the need for participants to choose fight or flight and become the one place where members are able to relax from their tensions. Groups can do this when respect and caring prevail; dialogues are fair, honest, and clear; and activities teach something that is useful. Then the group becomes an occasion to remember and increases the possibility for needed changes to occur (Kandel, 1992).

Acknowledgments

Deep gratitude is expressed to scholarly friends who reviewed this manuscript for tidy and explicit expression and clarity of thought. Great appreciation is extended to Susan Bachner, MA, OTR/L, FAOTA; Marilyn B. Cole, MS, OTR/L; and Valnere McLean, MS, OTR/L, FAOTA. Warm recognition is extended to my cotherapist, Laurie Donovan O'Brien, BS, who is a sensitive and dedicated advocate for people with developmental disabilities and with whom I have enjoyed many pleasurable years of work and discussion.

References

Ader, R. (1992). On the clinical relevance of psychoneuroimmunology. *Clinical Immunology and Immunopathology, 64*(1), 6–8.

Association on Aging with Developmental Disabilities. (1995). *Newsletter, 1*(1). St. Louis, MO: Author.

Edgerton, R. B., & Gaston, M. A. (Eds.). (1991). *I've seen it all! Lives of older persons with mental retardation in the community.* Baltimore: Brookes.

Ip, S., & Szymanski, E. (1994). Effects of staff implementation of a choice program on challenging behaviors in persons with developmental disabilities. *Rehabilitation Counseling Bulletin, 37,* 347–357.

Johnson, V. M., & Olsen, L. M. (1982). *A guide to alternative programming for older mentally retarded–developmentally disabled adults.* St. Louis, MO: St. Louis Association for Retarded Citizens.

Kandel, E. (1992). *The biology of mind.* New York: Columbia University.

Ludwig, S. (1995). *Sexuality: A curriculum for individuals who have difficulty with traditional learning methods.* Unionville, Ontario: York Region Public Health Department Healthy Sexuality Program.

Lutz, F. W., & Ramsey, M. A. (n.d.). *Complex organizations: The voodoo killer in modern society.* State College: Pennsylvania State University. [Copies of this report may be obtained by requesting it from M. Ross.]

Maier, S. F., Watkins, L. R., & Fleshner, M. (1994). Psychoneuroimmunology. *American Psychologist, 49*(12), 1004–1017.

Moore, J. C. (1990, April 23). Current concepts in the neurosciences. *American Occupational Therapy Foundation Mini-Course in the Neurosciences.* Rockville, MD: American Occupational Therapy Association.

Neistadt, M. E. (1994). The neurobiology of learning: Implications for treatment of adults with brain injury. *American Journal of Occupational Therapy, 48,* 421–430.

Neistadt, M. E. (1995). Methods of assessing clients' priorities: A survey of adult physical dysfunction settings. *American Journal of Occupational Therapy, 49,* 428–436.

Noback, C. R., Strominger, N. L., & Demarest, R. J. (1991). *The human nervous system* (4th ed.). Philadelphia: Lea & Febiger.

PsycLIT Journal Articles 1/90–6/95, SilverPlatter 3.11 PsycLIT Database, American Psychological Association.

Ross, M. (1987). *Group process: Using therapeutic activities in chronic care.* Thorofare, NJ: Slack.

Ross, M. (1997). *Integrative group therapy: Mobilizing coping abilities with the five-stage group.* Bethesda, MD: American Occupational Therapy Association.

Royeen, C. B. (Ed.). (1990). Neuroscience foundations of human performance. *American Occupational Therapy Association self-study series.* Bethesda, MD: American Occupational Therapy Association.

Schleien, S. J., Meyer, L. H., Heyne, L. A., & Brandt, B. B. (1995). *Lifelong leisure skills and lifestyles for persons with developmental disabilities.* Baltimore: Brookes.

Additional Reading

Kielhofner, G., & Miyake, S. (1981). The therapeutic use of games with mentally retarded adults. *American Journal of Occupational Therapy 35,* 375–382.

Toglia, J. P. (1985). Use of games in cognitive retraining. *Physical Disabilities. Special Interest Section Newsletter, 8,* 3–8.

Other Resources

Association on Aging with Developmental Disabilities, 1816 Lachland Hill Parkway, Suite 200, St. Louis, MO 63146.

Missouri Centralized Information and Referral Center for Older Persons with Developmental Disabilities, University of Missouri at Kansas City, 800-444-0821.

The ROM Dance Network, P.O. Box 3332, Madison, WI 53704-0332.

St. Louis Association for Retarded Citizens, 1816 Lachland Hill Parkway, Suite 200, St. Louis, MO 63146.

PART 4

Full
Participation

Work *Is* Occupation: What Can I Do as an Occupational Therapy Practitioner?

David J. Wysocki, MS, OTR/L, ATP
Ann T. Neulicht, PhD, CRC

Introduction

The field of occupational therapy has long recognized work as a significant area of human occupation and performance. Paid employment produces pragmatic and psychosocial outcomes. Work offers a means by which people can meet their daily needs, but it also sustains the larger social structure for meeting an array of social values and needs (Crist & Stoffel, 1992; Mitchell, 1985). Within the context of personal development, work can offer a sense of mastery over the environment and feelings of accomplishment and competence that lead to heightened self-esteem.

Occupational therapy practitioners who serve adults with developmental disabilities often express frustration at working in what seems an underrepresented field. That opinion is substantiated by the scarcity of current occupational therapy resources, especially in the area of developmental disabilities and work. As we prepared to write the chapter for the first edition, our literature search revealed a minimal number of current occupational therapy references. Again, while writing for this revised edition, a literature search of the *American Journal of Occupational Therapy* from 1999 to the present revealed a single article that directly addressed work-related intervention in developmental disabilities; its focus was on school-based practice (Spencer, Emery, & Schneck, 2003). Despite those limited resources, occupational therapists acknowledge that the field *is* rewarding and that it offers a boundless array of interesting practice experiences ("Adults With Developmental Disabilities," 1995). The field of developmental disabilities and work is not new to occupational therapy (Abbott, Franciscus, & Weeks, 1988;

Kirkland & Robertson, 1985). One result of the deinstitutionalization movement that began in the 1970s and that continues in this decade as the reform of the system of mental health services delivery has been that adults who traditionally were served in institutions now live in the community. They have left many of their conventional occupational therapy services behind. Today, the opportunities for increased community-based involvement (Spencer, 1990), coupled with the diversity of the population, offer a challenging and rewarding opportunity for the occupational therapy practitioner who works within an interdisciplinary team.

This chapter offers an overview of work as a practice area with adults who have developmental disabilities. Work is intrinsic to human life, and life without the choice of work, for any person, is incomplete. The scope of developmental disabilities presented in this chapter includes the cognitive and neuromotor issues associated with mental retardation, cerebral palsy, autism, and traumatic brain injury. For those who are new to developmental disabilities, or for readers who are more familiar with work primarily as a practice in industrial rehabilitation and work hardening, the chapter offers a comprehensive outline of the field, its history, and prevalent practices. For occupational therapists who have more experience in the field of developmental disabilities, it can serve as a common framework for a practice that is underrepresented in the current literature. For all readers, it can be a resource of contemporary information within the field and a report on the progressive changes of vocational perspectives in developmental disabilities, including some exciting examples of how those changes are manifesting. The chapter includes

- An overview of developmental disabilities issues as they apply to work,
- A background briefing on work and vocational programs for people with developmental disabilities,
- A description of service and work settings for adults with developmental disabilities,
- A summary of the types and areas of practice for the occupational therapist,
- A view on preparing adults with developmental disabilities for work in the information age, and
- A listing of resources in the field.

Scope of Issues for Adults With Developmental Disabilities

Developmental disabilities encompass a wide range of etiologies, diagnoses, issues, and severity (Reed, 1991). This is important because of the far-reaching effect developmental disabilities can have on functional performance. The specific disabilities—their severity and their depth—can have a significant and distinctive influence on the targeted programs, goals, and outcomes of any work-based intervention. It is essential, as with any type of occupational therapy, to perform appropriate assessments in developing individual treatment plans. Because of the lifelong nature of developmental disabilities, an occupational therapy practitioner can expect to establish long-term working relationships with clients. Familiarity with the population and a sense of the effect a particular disability can have on work performance will guide the experienced developmental disabilities therapist in targeting areas for assessment. A comprehensive occupational profile and vocational program will consider individual needs and strengths in all applicable areas and the interactive relationships among those areas.

The *Occupational Therapy Practice Framework* recognizes *work* as one of seven areas of occupation (American Occupational Therapy Association [AOTA], 2002). Under *social participation,* AOTA recognizes work as a component of the community. Extending this would allow one to recognize peers and friends (under social participation) as frequent components of one's work environment. From an occupational therapy perspective, most working people must also be successful in activities of daily living, instrumental activities of daily living, and education to be successful at work. This places the responsibility on the occupational therapist to address performance in at least five of the seven areas of occupation.

When one examines the interactive matrix of performance skills and performance patterns and the contexts, activity demands, and client factors as detailed in the *Framework*—and as required for successful employment—the breadth of potential interventions begins to be revealed. It is with this perspective that this chapter is written—that successful work outcomes are evidenced in addressing a comprehensive and integrated milieu of consumer interests, performance abilities, and environmental interactions.

Jerry: A Case to Follow

Jerry's story is a three-part case vignette to help illustrate the areas covered in this and following sections. His story progresses with the chapter as we address increasingly complex aspects of work intervention. It will be revisited at the end of the section on areas and types of occupational therapy practice in developmental disabilities and work and after the section covering modern employment options for people with developmental disabilities.

Jerry, a man in his early 30s, recently moved into a community group home from a residential facility for people with mental retardation and developmental disabilities. He was diagnosed with moderate mental retardation and mildly spastic quadriplegia. Jerry had worked at the institution shredding paper and assembling tool packets for a local electronics company. His new living situation allowed him to accept a job in the community, at a footwear distribution warehouse. His duties include assembling and sorting boxes by picture, number, and color. The boxes are used for bulk footwear that is sorted and packed before shipping to retail stores.

Jerry's new employer was not completely happy with Jerry's job performance. After almost 2 months on the job, Jerry had proved himself reliable and punctual. But the boxes were not always assembled and sorted correctly, and some of Jerry's co-workers had complained of hygiene issues. The incorrectly assembled and sorted boxes caused other problems down the line, where bar codes on the boxes are scanned before packing.

Jerry was scheduled for a comprehensive occupational therapy evaluation with the move to his new home. During the evaluation, Jerry demonstrated problems with visual perception, especially with form constancy and spatial relations. He also exhibited a mild nystagmus and difficulty in ocular motor tracking and accommodation. He was eager to perform well during the evaluation, but the heightened stress of the assessment revealed a significant increase in upper-extremity muscle tone that interfered with gross and fine motor control. The added stress also appeared to increase Jerry's salivation and drooling, which led him to repeatedly wipe his chin and mouth with his hands and shirtsleeves. Jerry's hypertonal spasticity was primarily in his extremities, and he exhibited hypotonicity in his trunk. This affected his endurance, especially under the stress of performing the assessment tasks. Jerry demonstrated excellent attention to task, applicable problem-solving skills, and functional memory. However, he also had a history of difficulties when changing jobs or environments, revealing a potential difficulty with immediately generalizing learned skills from one setting to another.

Overview: Services and Settings for Adults With Developmental Disabilities

Controversy over the care of people with developmental disabilities and mental retardation has existed for more than 130 years (President's Committee on Mental Retardation, 1977). In the 19th century, training schools were established by enlightened individuals who believed retardation could be "cured" by education and training. By the early 20th century, the view had changed: Little could be done to help most people with developmental delays. Confinement in an institution for life usually was considered the kindest solution for the individual, the family, and the community.

By the 1960s, much more had been learned about the abilities of people with retardation. Some parents and other advocates sought alternatives to over-crowded and dehumanizing institutions and began to organize community-based programs. As staff members and planners at institutions began to see that many residents of institutions could make greater progress living in the community, the use of schools and sheltered workshops increased.

Sheltered Work or Supported Employment

The sheltered workshop (now commonly called a "community rehabilitation facility") was intended as a long-term but transitional placement for people with disabilities. Program goals included skill training and work adjustment to prepare individuals for paid work in the community. A service continuum of vocational evaluation, pre-employment training, work adjustment, job placement, and time-limited employment services was developed to facilitate independent paid employment. Work generally involved labor-intensive bench work, assembly, packaging, and collating—tasks that are routine and repetitive and require little skill. Pay for this work typically is below mini-mum wage, and there can be a lot of down time in the workweek. Work gen-erally is supplemented with other rehabilitative services, such as compen-satory education.

The meaning of "long term" was intended to be "for as long as neces-sary," and program participants were to remain in a workshop only for as long as it took to become ready for competitive employment (Olshansky, 1971). The workshops have been severely criticized, however, because they segregated employees who had little hope of long-term success in competitive employment (Parent, Hill, & Wehman, 1989). A report published in the mid-1980s stated that 12% of sheltered workshop participants would be expect-ed to make the transition to competitive employment each year, and only 3% of that group were still in the workforce after 2 years (Bellamy, Rhodes, Bourbeau, & Mank, 1986).

Because of the low numbers of successful transitions from sheltered set-tings, current trends in the field emphasize inclusion and integration for peo-ple with developmental disabilities. Supported employment is an alternative vocational option that can accommodate the individual needs of people with severe disabilities. The *Federal Register* (1984, p. 17509) defined *supported employment* as

> paid work in a variety of settings, particularly regular work sites, especially designed for handicapped individuals (i) for whom com-petitive employment at or above the minimum wage is unlikely; and (ii) who, because of their disability, need intensive, on-going support to perform in a work setting.

Supported employment was intended to provide services for as long as some-one needed assistance and to provide flexibility in employment alternatives. The supported-employment model does not require that an individual be "job ready" before placement can occur. Often the necessary work and social skills are taught at work using a train–place–train–follow-up (Lagomarcino, 1986) or a place–train-follow-up (Wehman, 1986) model.

There are several current approaches to supported employment:

- **Individual placement** places the client in an integrated competitive employment setting with one-on-one support from a job coach. The support continues for as long as the worker is employed. Individual placement is also described as a *supported competitive employment model.*

- **Enclave** employment places a full-time supervisor with a group of no more than eight persons with severe disabilities. The place of employment is an industry or corporation where work is per-formed in an integrated setting. The supervisor and supported employees can be employed by the industry itself or by an employ-ment service program. Enclaves also are sometimes called *work-stations in industry.*

- **Mobile work crews** have full-time supervisors with groups of as many as eight workers who travel together to work sites in the com-munity. They engage in contracted work.

- **Entrepreneurial businesses** have private enterprises that operate as subcontractors or prime manufacturers. The businesses employ groups, no more than eight of whom are supported employees. Inte-gration is provided by including individuals without disabilities as coworkers and through regular contact with the general public.

- **Transitional employment** is paid work performed in integrated busi-ness and industry settings at assignments that typically last 3 to 9 months. The supported employees work part-time while they con-tinue their involvement in other services or support activities.

- **Supported jobs** integrate employees into a job site, although wages are below minimum. Pay scales are based on productivity, and sup-ported employees receive continuous training and advocacy from a job coach (Hill, Hill, Wehman, Revell, Dickerson, & Noble, 1987; North Carolina Vocational Alternatives Task Force, 1992).

Support involves activities that help the employee to acquire, strengthen, and maintain the physical, intellectual, emotional, and social skills needed to per-form the specific job tasks, work routine, and personal life activities that are critical to employment success. Support is not time limited and can involve years of service that will ebb and flow with work and life changes. Interven-tion involves identifying and analyzing jobs in the community, completing

functional consumer assessments, writing task analyses, matching job requirements with skills, identifying therapeutic needs (such as seating or positioning, mobility, vision, or spasticity management), using behavioral training
strategies, developing environmental or job modifications, and negotiating
for additional community support when needed.

Job carving might be necessary to define one or more components of a
job for someone who could be unable to perform all essential tasks. The person responsible for providing employment training typically is called a *job
coach*. A job coach actively assists a worker in learning a job and meeting
employer expectations. The coach provides advocacy, including the fostering
of workplace relationships and natural supports. The coach also monitors the
worker's progress and employer satisfaction.

There are several critical features of the success of a supported-employment model: job opportunities in an integrated setting, decent pay for meaningful work, community-based training that reflects labor market needs,
knowledge of vocational alternatives, and vocational choice (Wehman &
Moon, 1987). Community-based facilities and school-to-work transition
programs that provide supported employment services have undergone an
organizational change in converting services from segregated, center-based
approaches to community-based services that are integrated within the community. This conversion has required changes in goal definition, program
implementation, funding, staff training, and attitudes. The beliefs of consumers, parents, staff members, and employers that individuals with severe disabilities are not capable of integrated competitive work are being challenged.

Much like contracted work in sheltered settings, supported employment
typically is characterized by labor-intensive bench work, assembly, and distribution or by employment in food service or building and ground maintenance. Employees generally work part-time, there is little or no opportunity
for upward mobility or promotion, and fringe benefits are minimal or nonexistent (Kiernan, McGaughey, & Schalock, 1988). Unfortunately, the implementation of supported employment is incomplete, as evidenced by low
wages, lack of career choices, poor employment retention, and little real
opportunity for social integration (Dwyre & Trach, 1996; Wehman &
Kregel, n.d.). Expanding consumer choice, allowing more self-determination,
and promoting meaningful employment outcomes beyond initial entry-level
jobs must be considered as we face the challenges of employment for people
with disabilities.

School-to-Work Transition

The school system has a unique set of issues as a service agency offering
work programs for people with developmental disabilities. One concern of
the school system is the transition of emerging adults (14–21 years of age)

with developmental disabilities from school services into the community. During this transition, the clients and their families must negotiate the shift from a federally mandated system to a less regulated environment. This occurs simultaneously with a change in role expectancy for a client who is moving from childhood to young adulthood. Recent studies show that this transition into the community and into the role of worker does not go as smoothly for people with disabilities as it does for nondisabled people (Barber, McInerny, & Struck, 1993; Ward, 1996). Although in recent years the unemployment rate for the general population has ranged from 5% to 9%, the rate for young people with disabilities has been between 44% and 64%. That percentage increases dramatically, to 85%, for emerging adults with multiple disabilities, which can be contrasted with the 38% unemployment rate for emerging adults in the general population.

The federal government has responded to the need to incorporate school-to-community transition services into public education. In 1984, school-to-work transition was prioritized nationally by the Office of Special Education and Rehabilitation Services in the U.S. Department of Education, which stated that the goal of education and transition was sustained employment (Adelstein, 1992). In 1990, Congress amended the Education for All Handicapped Children Act to require that transition services be included in individual education plans for students over 15 years of age (and from 14 years of age on, when appropriate) (Costello, 1992). A 1997 change required that transition services begin by 14 years of age (Individuals With Disabilities Education Act Reauthorization of 1997, P.L. 105–17, 20 U.S.C. §1400 et seq.).

There is growing recognition in schools of the need for systematic transition planning that involves occupational therapy starting as early as possible in the student's life. According to a variety of researchers (Brollier, Shepherd, & Markley, 1994; Carrasco, 1993; Costello, 1992; Mitchell, Rourk, & Schwarz, 1989; Spencer et al., 2003; Ward, 1996), a best-practice, comprehensive school-to-community transition program should include the following:

- An interdisciplinary–interagency service delivery system consisting of individual vocationally based assessments, program planning, and implementation
- Direct occupational therapy involvement with job assessments, assistive technology, modification of the task environment, and development of an individual training plan
- Client involvement
- Parent involvement
- Business community involvement
- Prevocational programming, including independent-living and social skills training, beginning before high school

- Vocational training, started by 16 years of age, including job-sampling experience with job analysis, accommodation, and matching services
- Successful, paid, supported-employment placements that begin before a student leaves the school system
- Follow-up of former students to evaluate the effectiveness of the transition program.

Several model programs have been implemented around the country that have successfully included elements of these key factors into their services. They include the Little People's School and the Gaebler Children's Center in Massachusetts, the Career Training Workshop in North Carolina, Project STRIVE in the Boston public school system, and a community-health–based program for adolescents called the Life/Work Planning Group (Adelstein, 1992; Brollier et al., 1994; Carrasco, 1993; Costello, 1992; Mitchell et al., 1989; Ward, 1996). Such programs offer examples of how more intensive and systematic responses to transition issues can make a difference in the lives of clients and their communities.

Residential or Institutional Settings

Despite deinstitutionalization and the movement to more integrated and normalized employment opportunities, large residential centers for people with mental retardation or developmental disabilities still operate in most states (Prouty & Lakin, 1996). The centers mostly serve people who have multiple disabilities or disabilities that are characterized as severe, some with significant medical or behavioral components. The centers face added challenges in helping their clients make the transition to community settings. Limited funding, community constraints, and the concomitant scarcity of openings in group homes in many states have restricted the number of possible community placements. In 1960, 342 large state facilities were in operation to serve people with mental retardation and developmental disabilities. By 1995, 119 had closed, with peak closure occurring in the years after 1988. On average, 10 facilities closed each year. From 1995 to the present, however, an average of 4.4 facilities were slated to close each year (Sandlin, Prouty, & Lakin, 1996). That brings the closure trend back nearly to the 1970s rate.

Many of the extant large centers provide work and work-related opportunities through sheltered workshops, campus employment, and supported employment. The issues faced by people with developmental disabilities in those programs in some cases can be addressed by occupational therapy. The need for occupation-based intervention becomes more important for people with severe or multiple disabilities. It is sometimes possible to use a successful work experience to help someone who has spent most of a lifetime in a large residential center make the transition to community life.

Areas and Types of Practice

Each setting—whether it is a community-based facility, school system, or residential institution—will have a unique service protocol and expectations for occupational therapy involvement. Regulatory and payer mandates, facility culture and philosophy, history with occupational therapy services, and the amount of occupational therapy marketing and education performed locally and statewide affect practice. The amount and type of services expected of the occupational therapist also are influenced by the occupational therapist's employment status. Therapists work as direct employees; indirectly, on contract; or as self-employed, private-practice providers.

In general, occupational therapists provide evaluations and treatments directly to clients, work with interdisciplinary teams, and offer consultative services for the interventions provided to the client by people in other disciplines. The provided services can be directly involved with the client's work program as *work-based* interventions (performing a job analysis or implementing environmental accommodations), or they can be *supplemental* to the work program (seating–positioning, vision, neuromotor, or ADL [activities of daily living] assessments). A literature review can show the variety of ways the occupational therapy practitioner can serve people with developmental disabilities. Occupational therapy is a broad-based profession, and each practicing occupational therapist offers a unique background and set of competencies. If a therapist is proficient in an appropriate occupational therapy service that is meaningful to the client, that service should be considered for inclusion within the client's interdisciplinary service matrix.

Settings and Occupational Therapy

Federally funded settings must offer interdisciplinary team services that include occupational therapy. For adults in community-based and large residential-based services, the client programs are developed by teams and monitored and maintained as individual program plans (IPPs). The IPP includes long- and short-term goals and assessments, and it provides recommendations for health care, education, and vocational development. Occupational therapy services can fit into any of these program areas.

The community-based plan, often called the "person-centered plan," will tend to have a greater orientation to independent-living skills and vocational programming than will the IPP, which generally offers more emphasis on health care. The school team's individual education plan (IEP) is used to meet the client's entitlement to a free and appropriate education. Since 1990, the federal government has required a school-to-community transition plan—an individual transition plan (ITP)—in addition to the IEP. The ITP must address the student's vocational preparedness. Although occupational therapists have been oriented toward earlier intervention in the schools, they could fill an important role in school transition vocational services as well (Brollier et al., 1994; Ward, 1996).

Vocational Teams

A treatment *team* is an integral part of providing effective vocational or work intervention. The makeup of the team varies from one setting to another, and it can include a few to many service providers. The primary member of the team is the client. Family members and other people significantly involved in support also should be added to the team—with the client's consent. The team can include vocational professionals (rehabilitation counselor, job analyst, vocational evaluator, job developer, job coach), educators, community-oriented professionals (social worker, case manager), psychologists, rehabilitation engineers, physical therapists (as needed, primarily for functional mobility, seating, orthopedic conditions), and other health care providers. The occupational therapist's role will depend on the service delivery agencies involved. The occupational therapist should identify how best to complement the team on the basis of client needs, team composition, and the occupational therapist's knowledge.

Types of Practice

Work-Based Intervention

A variety of work-based interventions can be performed by an occupational therapist:
- Prevocational assessment and training
- Vocational assessment and intervention
- Functional capacity evaluation
- Job analysis
- Environmental assessment and modification
- Assistive technology or work jigs.

Many work-based interventions require a degree of specific experience or training and are often done in partnership with vocational professionals. The occupational therapist's contribution to the team-based assessment can lead to direct occupational therapy treatment, or it can be used to inform the assessments provided by the team to establish goals and provide the services by which the client can attain those goals.

Prevocational Assessment and Training

Prevocational intervention is often used for, but should not be limited to, clients who have not yet entered the workforce. It can be especially effective as part of a school, community, or job transition plan, and it should be implemented as early as possible, before the expected transition. As part of a comprehensive vocational plan, prevocational services examine a client's *vocational readiness*. Vocational readiness is "the process of assessing and treating deficits in performance components that interfere with the individual's ability to participate in productive occupations throughout the life span" (Kirkland & Robertson, 1985, p. 2).

Prevocational intervention addresses job and career preferences, the skills involved with getting and keeping a job, social- and community-living competencies, personal care, and leisure activities (Brollier et al., 1994; Reynolds-Lynch, 1985; Ward, 1996). All of these performance areas are dynamically integrated and should be considered together with the effective performance components and contexts as found in the *Occupational Therapy Practice Framework* (AOTA, 2002).

Vocational Assessment and Intervention

Vocational intervention also addresses vocational readiness, but usually as it applies to clients who are already in or about to enter the workforce. A vocational evaluation should be as inclusive as the prevocational assessment but oriented to a client's immediate, functional relationship with his or her job situation. If prevocational intervention has occurred, there should be less emphasis on work objectives and preferences and more focus on work performance.

For a client who is preparing to start work, this also can include simulated work, work sampling, supervised job experiences, internships, or monitored volunteer work. Unpaid work, however, can tend to place the client in an inferior position as a viable employee and lock him or her into a career of uncompensated employment. For the client about to enter the workforce, or for someone who has already begun working, the vocational assessment can be geared to issues more specific to the prospective work situation. The vocational intervention should include a functional capacity evaluation (FCE) (also called a "physical or work capacity evaluation"). In industrial rehabilitation, the FCE is geared primarily to physical issues, including functional strength and endurance (sitting, standing, lifting, carrying, pushing, bending, repetitive use, grasping). Naturally, this is important to the client with developmental disabilities too, but the design of the FCE should integrate the physical and cognitive issues relevant to the client's disability status and prospective work. It is important to examine current functional ability and the potential for improvement.

The occupational therapist's contribution to the vocational assessment (ADL and work performance areas; sensorimotor, cognitive, and psychosocial components; temporal and environmental contexts) should be integrated into recommendations for remedial and compensatory treatment and lead to a client's improved ability to work (Kornblau, 1996). (Note: The *Occupational*

Therapy Practice Framework [AOTA, 2002] offers a comprehensive review of all applicable areas for occupational therapy assessment.)

A job analysis also is part of a comprehensive vocational plan that is critical to matching prospective workers with appropriate employment. The objectives of a job analysis are as follows:

- Identify the elements of a job, including essential and nonessential functions, tasks, and duties
- List the skills required to perform the job
- Explore the compatibility and adaptability of the job for the client.

The job analysis assesses the job's physical and cognitive demands, aptitudes required, educational or training requirements, stress factors, objectives or outcomes, required tasks, equipment used, environmental conditions, and safety issues (Blackwell, Conrad, & Weed, 1992; Havranek, 1992; Jacobs & Wyrick, 1989; U.S. Department of Labor, 1991a).

The environmental assessment is an integral part of a comprehensive job analysis. Environmental factors can have a substantial effect on the success of a person with disabilities entering the workforce (Kielhofner, 1992; Velozo, 1992). The sense of mastery of one's environment, elicited through the physical, cognitive, and psychosocial accessibility of the workplace, can greatly influence the meaningfulness of and fulfillment offered by the work experience (Kielhofner, 1992). An environmental assessment should examine the facility as a whole and not be limited to the immediate task surroundings. For example, the physical, cognitive, and psychosocial accessibility of coworkers, supervisors, personnel representatives, front door, restrooms, lunch and break rooms, snack machines, emergency exits, safety equipment, and reference material, in addition to the job itself, take on significant importance for people with developmental disabilities. The assessment should consider all of the environmental contexts of the setting, including the physical, social, and cultural contexts.

Sometimes it is necessary for an occupational therapist to facilitate a change in the worker's environment to improve conditions that adversely affect performance. Environmental modifications can occur within any context, and they are compensatory interventions that can be considered concurrently with remedial client intervention. Physical modifications could include increasing accessibility to a restroom, changing the quality of lighting in the work area, adjusting the position of a computer monitor to reduce glare, or using assistive technology to improve the use of a workstation. Social modifications could include changing the proximity of a coworker to the client, improving coworkers' disability awareness, or facilitating natural supports. Cultural modifications could include management education about accessibility regulations and mandates, leading to employer-directed changes in the environment. Employer-directed change could encompass physical or nonphysical changes, such as adjustments to work schedules.

Assistive Technology

In *Assistive Technologies: Principles and Practice,* Cook and Hussey (1995) define *assistive technology* (AT) as including "a broad range of devices, services, strategies, and practices that are conceived and applied to ameliorate the problems faced by individuals who have disabilities" (p. 5). AT devices are simple or sophisticated; they can be custom designed, off-the-shelf, or modified; and they can include products designed specifically for people with disabilities or standard consumer products used in an assistive manner. AT can be general and applied to a variety of environments or a more specific modification to the workplace or job.

One type of AT frequently referred to in work environments for people with developmental disabilities is a *jig*—a device often custom-made for a particular job or task—that increases a worker's cognitive or physical ability to perform a task. Examples include paper folders, templates, or work holders. Computer key guards, expanded keyboards, and switch-adapted trackballs are all jigs, even though they are not commonly viewed as such.

AT services include team-based assessment, identification, recommendation, procurement, delivery, training, and follow-up. An AT team should consist of the client, a supportive peer or family member, direct service providers, case manager or leader, therapists, and the appropriate technology practitioners. If off-the-shelf AT is being considered, the team also could include an AT supplier. A rehabilitation engineer is another team member who can provide an array of technical support for vocational intervention (Gordon & Kozol, 1984). For vocational AT services, the team also should include vocational service providers and can include the employer.

AT is a broad, dynamic, and increasingly interdisciplinary field. The Rehabilitation Engineering and Assistive Technology Society of North America (RESNA) has developed ethics and standards for AT practice and a credentialing program for AT practitioners and AT suppliers (Minkel, 1995, 1996). The RESNA AT certification is a value-added supplement for rehabilitation professionals, including occupational therapists, who are already in practice.

Because of the extensive and dynamic nature of the field, most AT specialists concentrate in one or two practice areas (computer access, seating and positioning, environmental controls, work modifications). Other than possibly the rehabilitation engineer, the AT practitioner is more likely than any other practitioner to work both as a regular member of the vocational intervention team (as an occupational therapist, educator, vocational professional) and in AT practice. If the client has multiple AT needs, the team could include more than one AT consultant. For example, the team could have an occupational therapist who specializes in workplace modifications or computer access and another with expertise in seating, positioning, and mobility. In coordination with occupational therapists who have specific AT training, occupational therapists who have a general awareness of AT can contribute greatly to the work of a team (Angelo & Gross, 1994). For example, an occupational therapist with extensive experience in developmental disabilities assessment and intervention can collaborate with another who specializes in general computer access to offer a more complete and effective service to the client.

Occupational Therapy Practice: Supplemental to Work

In addition to work-specific intervention, occupational therapy can contribute globally to the vocational success of a person with developmental disabilities. As a team contributor to the client-centered plan, an occupational therapist can perform a comprehensive occupational therapy evaluation. The information garnered can be applied to specific program goals, including vocational planning and treatment. An occupational therapist can help the team to identify areas that interfere with the client's success at work and make recommendations for strategies and services that respond to those issues. For example, an occupational therapist can analyze ADL performance issues for grooming, hygiene, or mobility. The occupational therapist can then assess the client's environment for factors that affect those issues. The client's cognitive, sensory, perceptual, or motor performance could be involved, or there could be something in the environment that is affecting the client's ability to perform. With that information, the team can better address the client's needs as they relate to current and potential skills and abilities. An occupational therapist can be a key team member in helping the team to identify any potential inhibitors to work performance and help guide the team to the best ways to address those issues.

Other Elements Affecting Vocational Services

Other programs exist that can directly or indirectly influence vocational programs for people with developmental disabilities and the provision of occupational therapy services. They include technology-related assistance grants, state vocational rehabilitation services, and the Americans With Disabilities Act (ADA; P.L. 101–336, 42 U.S.C. §12101) (Crist & Stoffel, 1992; Metzler, 1995; Shelly, Sample, & Spencer, 1992). The Technology-Related Assistance for Individuals With Disabilities Act of 1988 (amended in 1994), P.L. 100–407 and P.L. 103–218, often is called the Tech Act. Its purpose is to increase access to and awareness of AT. Most states have received federal funds, matched by state money, to establish projects that promote systems change and increase interagency coordination in the provision of AT services.

Occupational therapists who are interested in AT can contribute to the development and applications of state Tech Act programs, which may include services for people with developmental disabilities and work issues. State vocational rehabilitation (VR) services generally are funded through the Rehabilitation Act of 1973, P.L. 93–112, 29 U.S.C. §701 *et seq.* (amended in 1998). State VR services fund community-based vocational services to enhance employability and independent living for people with disabilities, including severe developmental disabilities. Among the services are the following:

- Vocational evaluation
- VR planning
- Access to rehabilitation facilities and support services, including occupational therapy, physical therapy, rehabilitation engineering, and AT services
- Education and training assistance
- School-to-work transition planning, work adjustment, supported employment, job placement assistance, and follow-up.

Another avenue for consumer job opportunities is ADA, the far-reaching civil rights law promoting *full* participation in community-based life, including work, for people with disabilities. ADA includes comprehensive sections on public access, employment, transportation, and telecommunications. Under ADA, employers with more than 15 employees are prohibited from discriminating against qualified people with disabilities in hiring, firing, advancement, compensation, training, and other employment-related areas. ADA mandates *reasonable accommodations* that allow qualified individuals with disabilities to work. Reasonable accommodations include on-site modifications to job tasks, environments, or work schedules. The services of occupational therapists can be useful in the process of identifying the essential job functions, environmental or job modifications, and any appropriate AT to enable people with disabilities to work (AOTA, 1992).

Jerry: A Case Revisited

As a result of Jerry's occupational therapy evaluation (see "Jerry: A Case to Follow" above), the team agreed to several additional interventions to help improve Jerry's work performance at the footwear distributor:

- Jerry was referred to a developmental vision clinic for more extensive vision assessments and recommendations for vision intervention.
- Staff members at Jerry's group home were contacted by his occupational therapist and asked to help Jerry learn socially acceptable and improved ways to manage his drooling.

- A team consisting of Jerry's occupational therapist, rehabilitation counselor, and job coach performed a job analysis, including an environmental assessment, at Jerry's work site. The group also performed an adapted FCE for Jerry.

The vision assessments showed that Jerry had potentially treatable deficits in visual perception and identified exercises that could help him improve his visual accommodation and perception. Jerry's nystagmus was very mild and consistent with his increased spasticity under stress.

The environmental assessment and job analysis revealed several areas in need of further intervention. Jerry had broken new ground as the company's first employee with a developmental disability. Jerry's employer cared about him and wanted to employ more people with developmental disabilities. However, a general lack of disability awareness existed at the site.

The assembly and sorting problems with Jerry's work included incorrectly sorted boxes, which were to be sorted primarily by number, and boxes that were assembled with bar codes partially covered. The numbers used for sorting were difficult to locate because they were part of a longer system of numbering. Jerry also had no workstation. Instead, he stood over the pallets of unassembled boxes, using the unformed boxes as a makeshift worktable on which to perform the assembly. The pallets were located in the back stacks of the warehouse, near a drafty freight door and where the lighting was poor. Jerry's FCE had revealed a problem with endurance, especially because the job required that he stand for long periods and bend constantly.

The team made several recommendations, based on the updated information:

- Create a company disability awareness program, directed by Jerry's employer, based on standard information modules supplied by the team.
- Open a pathway to have the box pallets transported to an area with better lighting and climate control and in better view of the other employees for inclusion.
- Set up a workstation with a height-adjustable worktable and chair that also has a back that gives lateral support; the workstation should give Jerry adequate visual access to easy-to-follow patterns for assembling the boxes.
- Set up clearly marked sorting bins on wheels, positioned for easiest access, for assembled boxes; the wheeled bins allow for easier transport to the packing area by the other employees.

- Develop a work jig for Jerry to use with assembled boxes that covers nonidentifying numbers, so he can sort the boxes more easily and accurately.
- Design another jig to help Jerry with the folding and holding tasks on the smaller boxes.
- Assign Jerry a job coach during his transition period for supported learning of the new job skills and to help him develop natural supports with the other employees.
- Implement a schedule change for Jerry to balance the more physically demanding periods with less demanding times.

Preparing Adults With Developmental Disabilities for the Information Age

What *More* Can I Do as an Occupational Therapy Practitioner?

The increased use of technology has changed the way societal transactions are conducted by creating a constant demand for quick access to and analysis of information. This directly affects the knowledge, skills, and abilities required of producers and consumers of goods and services.

Modernizing Work Options for People With Developmental Disabilities

As the first edition of this book was being prepared, it was projected that by 2000, labor-intensive work would represent only 15% of what was done in the American workplace and that the unskilled person would be structurally unemployable (Daggett, 1995). Recent studies and projections indicate similar concerns (Hecker, 2001; U.S. Department of Labor, 2002; U.S. Department of Labor, Bureau of Labor Statistics, 2001). The November 2001 issue of *Monthly Labor Review* projects that "occupations requiring a post-secondary vocational award or academic degree, which accounted for 29 percent of all jobs in 2000, will account for 42 percent of total job growth from 2000 to 2010" (Hecker, 2001, p. 57). Jobs that require less training and more labor will not be major contributors to overall job growth. The Bureau of Labor Statistics reports that *production occupations* (as found in most sheltered workshops) constituted only 9% of total employment and that by 2010 people in those jobs will account for just 8.2% of the workforce (U.S. Department of Labor, Bureau of Labor Statistics, 2001). Although some routine, labor-intensive jobs will always exist, they will require the ability to track employee time, maintain schedules, and document production electronically. Most workers will no longer manipulate machines or perform routine tasks at specific workstations. The work world will be characterized by increased automation and robotics; flexible production schedules will require frequent resetting of assembly lines; and there will be greater use of information technology, computer interfaces, and computer-mediated processes. Workers will be required to exhibit multiple skills; multidimensional knowledge of products, processes, and procedures; and higher-order language and thinking skills to work with computers. The workforce will shift from production, craft, assembly, and task-oriented work to work based on knowledge, service, and process outcomes (Ryan, 1995).

The information-age workplace will challenge workers to demonstrate the following abilities:

- Interface with multiple platforms in a constantly changing environment
- Adapt to job demands that are assignment specific rather than task specific
- Periodically relearn and retool
- Interpret symbolic, written, oral, and visual representations
- Independently execute tasks that require problem-solving and decision-making skill
- Fund and train personnel to provide multiple interventions and long-term follow-up.

Although the new array of technology will present challenges to workers with disabilities, the application of computers and technology also creates opportunities:

- Ways to perform complex, multidexterous tasks using standard user-to-computer interfaces or access
- Accommodations for physical, sensory, perceptual, cognitive, and performance limitations
- Reduction of multiple-step tasks to a single action, through the use of buttons, symbols, or icons
- Consistency in format and content of various activities
- Analogous operating concepts for similar tasks across different platforms.

Historically, employment opportunities for people with developmental disabilities have been limited to jobs that we would now expect to become obsolete (Kiernan, McGaughey, & Schalock, 1988; U.S. Department of Labor, 1995, 2002). Education and skill training for that population generally has been task specific, with little or no integration of learning for a functional purpose. People with disabilities often are unable to develop along career paths or meet the needs of new work environments because they are not given the opportunity to develop employability or transferable skills. Often, people with developmental disabilities who can be placed in specific jobs are not employable in a changing environment.

To increase employability for information-based and automated work environments, training strategies must integrate critical thinking, decision making, and problem solving with social and job-related skills. The use of computers can offer such an opportunity. In recent years, teachers, therapists, and researchers have discovered the power of computer technology as a tool for circumventing learning difficulties associated with disabilities. Computers are a motivating medium that can enable individuals with disabilities to experience the information world in a mainstream fashion. Computers can be used to help people improve language skills and enhance their ability to read, comprehend, and communicate. Computers also can provide meaningful opportunities for reading and writing and offer options for the understanding and execution of instructions, mastery of decision-making and problem-solving abilities, and internalization of cause and effect. Independent use of cognitive skills (learning, decision making, problem solving) is inherent in the successful execution of computer tasks. When computer training can be integrated into programs that address other critical vocational education for job-seeking skills and for social, community, and personal-living competencies (Krantz, 1971), options for employment and employability are enhanced.

The computer is an integral part of modern business, including the business that occurs in rehabilitation settings (Burkhead & Sampson, 1985; Sampson, McMahon, & Burkhead, 1985; Schmitt & Growick, 1985). Office, communication, clerical, and administrative support tasks are now done by or with the help of computers and microprocessors. Computers have created entrepreneurial opportunities as well as options for job sharing and work in home offices (Murray & Kenny, 1990). The use of computers and AT has expanded access to new work environments by people who have been traditionally excluded—those with severe physical or cognitive disabilities. Computers also are evident in many non-technology-based jobs. The ability to use a keypad or keyboard is necessary even in low-skill, labor-intensive positions where employees must clock time, enter employee or job numbers, and access benefits. Leisure, ADLs, and access to routine services such as banking, customer service, libraries, and even snack machines often require the ability to key in information to obtain services or products.

Pioneering Efforts to Expand Available Work Options

Results of computer skills training programs for people with developmental disabilities indicate that such training can improve clients' communication skills, concentration, memory, perceptual skills, reading skills, dexterity, cognition, independent functioning, vocational development and exploration, self-esteem, and socialization (Armstrong & Rennie, 1986; Fiedorowicz, 1986; Links & Frydenberg, 1988; Wood, 1986). Among the successful computer training efforts and providers are Careers in Automation for Persons with Severe Physical Disabilities (Lash & Licenziato, 1995); Project COMPETE (Mann & Svorai, 1994); Goodwill Industries, Hartford, Connecticut (Ross, 1991); and the Hawaii State Planning Council on Developmental Disabilities Computer Training Project (Peet, Saka, & Nakasone, 1985).

Several North Carolina programs have provided computer and technology training and jobs to people with physical and cognitive limitations. Adaptive Technology Centers, Inc., has served some 280 clients with severe disabilities since 1988. More than 75% of those trained have secured work as office, data entry, and mail clerks and in shipping, handling, and order-processing positions (S. Primlani, personal communication, January 8, 1997). Copymatic Document Solutions, a company started in 1988 by United Cerebral Palsy (UCP) of North Carolina, uses an entrepreneurial business model (Ranii, 1994; S. Collura, director, Copymatic Document Solutions, personal communication, February 14, 1997). Through Easter Seals UCP North Carolina, the company has grown to provide digital printing; copying; computer graphics; database management; bulk-mailing services; and documentation, storage, and inventory management. The nonprofit company employs adults with severe to moderate disabilities in an integrated setting with nondisabled employees. The company employs workers with disabilities in all aspects of the business in four North Carolina cities.

Project COMPUTE (Computer Utilization Training for Employment) was a 2-year project in North Carolina designed to use computer skills training to encourage changes in service delivery and vocational outcomes for people with developmental disabilities (Neulicht, Primlani, & Chewning, 1995). The project's grant activities also included a study tour of existing training programs, a labor market analysis, a multidisciplinary assessment, a program guide, and a videotape. Project COMPUTE involved 12 clients between 21 and 42 years of age, most with multiple impairments that included mild mental retardation, autism, cerebral palsy, severe visual impairment, and psychosis. The only criterion for program entry was a desire to learn to use a computer to improve vocational options. Three clients were not literate, and the remaining eight had minimal reading and writing skills. Ten of the clients had been working in a traditional workshop, performing assembly and production tasks. The average training time to develop general and job-specific skills was 350 hours. The program provided 16 hours of training each week over a 12-month period to two groups of six clients each. The staff-to-student ratio generally was 1:6 but varied by activity. One-to-one instruction was used to teach clerical skills and for literacy instruction. Clients who were trained through Project COMPUTE demonstrated a marked increase in the ability to access and use computers. They also demonstrated significantly increased self-esteem, self-confidence, and work-appropriate behaviors.

Project TechWork started as a grant-funded project to help people with severe developmental disabilities obtain gainful technology-based employment through the use of computers and AT. The grant portion of TechWork was a multiple-agency collaborative effort led by the Murdoch Center, a state residential facility for people with mental retardation and developmental disabilities. TechWork involved clients from the Murdoch Center; from INCO, a community rehabilitation facility and supported-employment contractor; and from the Granville County Schools Transitional Program. More than 120 referrals were screened, and a training program began at each of the three sites.

TechWork's clients have moderate to severe mental retardation and mild to severe physical and mental disabilities. Other state agency collaborators have been the North Carolina Division of Vocational Rehabilitation (DVR), the regional community college, the North Carolina Assistive Technology Program, and the University of North Carolina at Chapel Hill. A three-part screening tool is used to assess, identify, and prioritize candidates for vocational technology services. A computer-based access evaluation also is used to identify job access issues, AT recommendations, and client training needs. Adaptive software modifies existing business-based data management systems to the cognitive and physical needs of clients. The software is used to augment computer skills training and for mailing-list jobs. A four-unit, 150-page basic curriculum guide was developed for clients who might have minimal reading proficiency, delayed learning rates, visual deficits, attention deficits, learning disorders, or various physical challenges (Plachcinski, 2000). The guide is now reproduced by TechWork employees and published for sale.

Some TechWork clients work for bulk mailers, updating customer lists and printing labels (a value-added service to the already-existing job of folding mailers). Others scan documents for digital archiving and retrieval (back-file conversion) and for resident artist publishing, reproducing works for a variety of retail graphic art products. Graduates of the community-based TechWork programs have attended regular community college introductory computer classes, and several other TechWork clients have participated in a partnership program of UCP North Carolina and the state's DVR to continue development of paid community-based jobs for people with multiple barriers to employment.

For many people, the long-term result of contending with multiple, complicating issues in developmental disabilities is having virtually no community-based work opportunities. The partnership program of UCP North Carolina and the state's DVR was established as a joint effort between public and private agencies to increase participation of people with multiple physical and developmental disabilities in supported employment in the state. The program has recognized that, nationally, people with multiple physical and developmental disabilities are among the least served in supported employment; that group makes up only 1.3%–3.0% of the total supported-employment population. Issues associated with systemic barriers, internal or psychological barriers, and the inability of any single conventional service to successfully address the complex list of obstacles combine to result in historically low outcomes. Thus, the program's objectives include the following:

- Remove systemic barriers to clients' successes
- Effectively respond to internal barriers
- Generate innovative solutions for individual job carving, job creation, and small business development
- Develop methods that facilitate coordination of services by several agencies that serve this population
- Develop best-practice methods for job coach training and management.

In the process of implementing the objectives, the program's operators recognized the need to include community-based occupational therapy services as an integral component of both the team and the methodology. Occupational therapy services, as part of the program, have addressed a range of issues. For example, the program's clients have had little or no history with successful community-based work. Because of this, common issues typically surface in such fundamental areas as efficient ADL performance at home and work, safe transfer methodology, seating and positioning, functional vision, functional mobility, expanded communication needs, neuromotor performance issues, and spasticity management.

Results for the first 3 years of the partnership program have included the following:

- Development of a reliable quality service team (QST) process whose team members include
  - clients, their peers, and family members;
  - DVR offices and counselors;
  - independent-living centers and counselors;
  - community-based allied health professionals;
  - UCP job coaches and managers;
  - mental health, developmental disabilities, and Community Alternatives Program case managers;
  - AT specialists; and
  - VR engineers.
- Establishment of seven service regions across the state with a different QST in each region
- Provision of service to more than 70 clients, with job placements in data entry, medical billing, office assistance, child care, greenhouse work, product stocking, and pizza box assembly.

Although the job outcomes have included information-based and labor-intensive work, the program has established the clients' presence in the workforce, many of them for the first time in their lives. This offers continued employment possibilities across a range of job types. As an example, some clients whose first jobs were assembling pizza boxes have gone on to jobs that include computer-based order handling.

Modern Job Market Areas for People With Developmental Disabilities

The job analyses and industry interviews conducted through Project COMPUTE and TechWork confirmed that the work world is information based. To be used effectively, information must be generated, updated, stored, and distributed. The computer is the most prevalent tool used in the coordination of these tasks.

Work involving computer-based technologies involves user input to operate equipment or to manage data. The data can range from simple, discrete units of information to complex continuous text and graphics. Similarly, the operating procedures can range from simple to complex. Computer tasks can be categorized as command and control, discrete data entry, document processing, graphics, and systems integration, including programming. The focus of Project COMPUTE's and TechWork's labor market research was on jobs involving production, maintenance, and distribution of information.

Of most promise for people with severe disabilities are command-and-control tasks. Those tasks often require the operator to make routine selections from data sets or to use a computer interface to operate the equipment. Examples include touch-screen interfaces to operate high-volume copiers, mail-handling equipment, and communication equipment such as fax machines. Automated copiers perform a range of collating, binding, and stapling tasks to produce a variety of bound and loose-leaf documents, thus reducing the physical demands of mail room or copy center positions. Digital document scanning and storage (backfile conversion) offers a range of physical and computer-based tasks that ties in with the growing need for document-based information archiving and retrieval. Discrete data-entry tasks, such as entering or updating a database, are included in jobs that involve order processing, payment or remittance processing, inventory, or data entry. Potential document-processing tasks include paginating and formatting, cutting and pasting, cutting and archiving, assembly of boilerplate paragraphs, and merging and printing of form letters. Another potential market is in the online transcription of messages for telephone paging companies. Even though it is production work, messages can be abbreviated, lending themselves to standardized message formats and reducing the number of keystrokes required.

Office automation itself can be considered an accommodation with positive vocational outcomes for people with severe disabilities. For example, the industry trend is to simplify decision making and provide for standard operating procedures: using bar codes for data entry, icons or symbols to represent tasks, and scanning to reduce keystrokes. Conveyor belts, hydraulic lifts, and spring-loaded carts and trays can reduce material handling and physically demanding lifting and carrying tasks. The manufacturing sector also relies on many machines that are operated by computerized touch pads.

Other mainstream workplace advances offer accommodations, such as hand-held microcomputers with keypads and bar code scanners, which are designed to accommodate all types of users; some devices are even voice activated. Those tools help manage inventory in stores and in distribution centers, and the warehouse clerk, micrographics technician, or order processor need understand only the codes for location and item before entering the number of units requested. Manual tasks that require shelving or removing of items, for example, have literacy demands that are relatively low.

Program Planning in a New Work Age: Staff, Equipment, Support, Consumer Assessment, Job Marketing, Training, and Job Procurement

Before starting a computer skills training program, one must consider staff and equipment resources. Instructors, including job coaches and job development specialists, must be computer literate to train employees and market services to the business community. Equipment must be in good working order and able to support all desired software and AT applications. As with any new service, the attitudes of and acceptance by staff members, clients' families, and employers might be guarded at first. Active community involvement through a business advisory council or an employment advisory board is necessary to develop jobs. Funding through private, community, state, and federal grants should be solicited to begin the effort, or a fee-for-service agreement through the state division of vocational rehabilitation should be sought to maintain and expand training and placement.

A profile of the client issues and strengths is important for modern job matching. Some common issues become especially important to consider in preparing clients for contemporary work. For example, literacy remediation is likely to be an issue for people with developmental disabilities and must be included in an integrated program rather than treated as an "add-on" service. Visual-processing difficulties involving ocular motor control, visual–motor integration, field deficits, visual acuity, visual accommodation, and visual perception are critical for people who will use computers (Cook & Hussey, 1995, pp. 87–92). Numerous studies among participants with developmental disabilities and acquired brain injury reveal dramatically high incidences of ocular motor dysfunction, significant refractive errors, strabismus, accommodation deficiencies, visual field deficits, visual perception issues, and glaucoma (Ciner, Macks, & Schanel-Klitsch, 1991; Scheiman, 1990; Suchoff, Kapoor, Waxman, & Ference, 1999). Often, those conditions remain hidden unless the client is specifically evaluated for them or until the more demanding functional requirements of information access come into play.

If vision deficits remain unidentified, the client is often described as having other physical, cognitive, or behavioral difficulties. Among the professionals who provide services for people with developmental disabilities, occupational therapists typically are alone in having a background in vision function and assessment. However, despite the high numbers of clients with visual deficits seen by occupational therapists, there seems to be no systematic consideration of visual profiles (Scheiman, 2002). "Because vision is dynamically interwoven within functional task performance, ignoring visual deficits is likely to result in invalid assessment, faulty clinical reasoning, and, ultimately, ineffective treatment" (Scheiman, 2002, p. 2).

Because of the high visual performance demands in most work settings, and especially those that involve computer-based tasks, it is essential that occupational therapists accurately assess for any visual deficits and refer clients for qualified intervention. Other critical sensory areas to consider are hearing, as used for auditory computer feedback, and tactile and proprioceptive ability for computer input, especially when adapted computer input is used and visual and auditory cues are not immediately available.

A client-centered, comprehensive vocational plan is essential to placing people with developmental disabilities in the modern workplace. The inclusive vocational plan, coupled with an awareness of the particular issues related to modern jobs, will greatly increase the client's chances for success. For their part, programs must make a commitment to critically but creatively analyze the job market, develop a profile of client skills, and create a job match that goes beyond traditional food service and janitorial positions so that people with developmental disabilities will be employable in the modern job market.

Case Examples

The following case examples illustrate individual progress (personal and professional) as a result of computer skills training.

Jake

Jake is a 22-year-old man with Down syndrome who earned a high school diploma through participation in a self-contained educable mentally handicapped (EMH) program. Jake functioned in the moderate range of mental retardation and was not literate. A baseline evaluation revealed that he was unfamiliar with basic punctuation marks and rules for capitalization; his verbal skills were limited to simple phrases. Before training, his computer experience was limited to playing games on an Apple IIG; he used non-rhythmic random keyboarding.

During training, Jake required both oral instruction and demonstration because he had difficulty with written instructions. He also demonstrated social immaturity with mildly inappropriate social behaviors and hygiene issues. A word prediction program was used to enhance generative writing and improve language. His ITP goals included a focus on reading and following instructions, maintaining and following a schedule, and increasing social and vocational maturity by learning job expectations and behaviors.

At the conclusion of about 500 hours of training over a 4-year period (200 hours in a 2-year, school-based model), Jake was independent in his use of the keyboard and mouse. He demonstrated functional use of a standard computer operating system, including drop-down menus and keyboard commands. His typing speed using the complete keyboard was 12 words per minute (wpm), he could use a keypad at 15 wpm, and his rate of data entry was 1,600–1,800 keystrokes per hour (kph). He learned to recognize and interpret standard icons and symbols, use basic commands to independently operate a standard word-processing program, transcribe text, copy simple letters and memos, and generate simple sentences. He also learned to perform data entry and searching and correcting from source material, including alphanumeric and coded information. He learned to sort alphabetically and numerically using a sorter and became independent with most clerical and bulk-mailing tasks.

Jake has been competitively employed full-time as an office clerk. He rides public transportation, unassisted, to work. His duties include using a computer to enter weekly time sheets for all employees at a temporary agency, sorting incoming mail, metering and preparing outgoing mail, and operating a copier and document shredder. He is independent in his tasks and follows a general routine with occasional variation. Jake has become aware of his personal appearance and behavior (he has decided to change his eating habits so as to avoid burping in public; for Valentine's Day, he bought candy for his coworkers). He has moved from a self-contained EMH class with job expectations in food service or janitorial work to competitive employment in an office setting using technology, computers, and natural supports.

Michelle

Michelle is a 24-year-old woman with cerebral palsy and moderate mental retardation who uses a wheelchair for mobility. Activities using fine finger dexterity, grip, and grasp were difficult for her. She exhibited motor control and planning difficulty and problems with visual tracking and accommodation. She had difficulty sequencing, categorizing, and comprehending multiple-step oral instructions. Michelle was a nonreader who had a limited sight-word vocabulary and who used minimal decoding strategies. Michelle's strengths included excellent interpersonal skills and good communication and conversational skills. She was highly motivated to learn and perform new tasks well.

Michelle had no exposure to computers or keyboards before she entered. During the initial evaluation, she entered text without spacing or knowledge of punctuation and capitalization. She required frequent repetition of oral and modeled instructions and needed affirmation for each keystroke. Her ITP goals included increasing sight-word (work) vocabulary; executing single-word, stepped written instructions; maintaining a schedule; and increasing self-confidence.

At the conclusion of 320 hours of training over a 6-month period, Michelle was typing, using a nonrhythmic 10-finger method at 8 wpm; she used a keypad at 8 wpm; and her data entry rate was 980 kph. She was functional with simple list menus and had learned keyboard commands. She could enter text with spaces between words and some punctuation, and she had learned to enter alphanumeric data into a single screen. Her decision-making ability and self-confidence had improved to the extent that she was able to tell professionals at a national conference to give people like her a chance "because we can do it."

Michelle became employed full-time, with natural supports, in a competitive position as a greeter. She maintains a flexible schedule and has received compliments from her employer regarding her learning ability. Michelle has made the transition from performing below competitive standards in a workshop setting to competitive employment with natural supports. She has since married and has moved into her own apartment.

Jerry: What the Future Could Hold

Let's look back in on Jerry, after his successful transition to community-based work, and predict what the future could bring.

Jerry improved significantly on his job at the footwear distributor after his team-based vocational intervention. He was able to improve his visual and perceptual skills well enough that, together with the compensatory environmental and job modifications, his job performance improved to nearly competitive standards over time. He also received a pay raise, reflecting his improved performance. Moving Jerry into proximity with other warehouse workers and designing job modifications that helped everyone increased coworker interaction and significantly opened favorable relations between Jerry and the other employees. Jerry's subsequent improvement in social awareness and his improved hygiene skills, coupled with the increased awareness and involvement of his coworkers, had created a positive working environment.

Because of his positive experience, Jerry was interested in further vocational advancement, and he had expressed an interest in gaining new job skills. The rehabilitation counselor worked with Jerry to identify some interest areas. His employer and vocational rehabilitation services were contacted regarding Jerry's aspirations. One of his interests was to work in distribution and with the computer. (During his time at the footwear distributor, the shipping department had become more automated and now used a computer-based system.) Jerry's employer was interested in keeping him as an employee, and Jerry had expressed his satisfaction with the workplace. A computer access evaluation was performed by an occupational therapy assistive-technology practitioner (ATP) with a background in computer applications. The ATP teamed up with a vocational counselor and evaluator. The results showed that Jerry could benefit from basic computer and literacy training. It was recommended that his computer access could be improved by using a switch-adapted trackball in place of the standard mouse and a key guard to reduce the incidence of errant keystrokes caused by his difficulties with spasticity and motor control.

The distribution station also would require some minor access modifications and installation of an adjustable worktable. Because the automated distribution system uses bar codes for inventory identification and shipping lists, it was recommended that Jerry begin by spending part of his day performing some of those tasks. His employer agreed and initiated the natural supports to begin training Jerry on the new tasks. Based on a commitment from Jerry's employer, VR services implemented a training program that included an adapted computer class and literacy training. After some discussion concerning who was financially responsible for the recommended job accommodations, an agreement was made. Jerry would be lent his AT by the state's Tech Act program during his training classes. After training, Jerry's employer would take advantage of ADA tax adjustments and implement all necessary job modifications at the company's cost. With support over time and with the appropriate intervention, it appears that Jerry could be on his way to permanent employment in his community.

Conclusion

Work is essential to our development, social contribution, and livelihood. It is a means by which we provide for our daily needs, and it sustains a shared context for meeting an array of social necessities. Work offers us a sense of mastery over our environment as well as an awareness of accomplishment and competence, leading to a heightened sense of self-esteem. All too often, opportunities to experience these same qualities of life are thwarted for people with developmental disabilities. However, with appropriate and comprehensive vocational-related services, people with developmental disabilities have been able to contribute more to their quality of life and to their community.

Occupational therapy practitioners can play a pivotal role in providing the team-based services that foster significant work and community outcomes for this population. Vocational services for adults with developmental disabilities have gone through notable changes since the beginning of the 20th century. The shift in approach to services since the 1970s has opened new opportunities for more meaningful community-based living, bringing about an array of increased challenges for people with developmental disabilities and their service providers. Because of the range of developmental disabilities and their effects on work, those opportunities and challenges vary among individuals and their service delivery environments. An awareness of the issues is critical to providing appropriate and effective vocational services for people with developmental disabilities.

Because of the increasing shift toward providing community-based services, effective occupational therapy intervention is needed more now in the community than in institutional settings. This need adds to the required knowledge base for occupational therapists who practice in the area of work and developmental disabilities. Occupational therapists can contribute to the vocational intervention team with specific work-based practices or with more general occupational therapy services. Generally, an occupational therapist's role, as part of the team, is to help identify potential and actual inhibitors to a client's work performance. The occupational therapist can make the recommendations necessary to help remediate and compensate for the identified issues, often leading to improved work performance by the client.

AT is becoming an increasingly applicable tool to facilitate successful work outcomes for people with disabilities that should be an expected part of occupational therapy service provision. Occupational therapists can now provide AT services as RESNA-certified AT practitioners and suppliers, or they can bring awareness of AT to bear on their work with the team to provide appropriate referrals to AT service providers.

The workplace continues to become less labor-intensive and more based on technology. People with developmental disabilities need to be prepared for employment opportunities that require the skills and abilities associated with modern technology. The result is that there is a new suite of challenges and opportunities for clients and service providers. Knowledge of contemporary job market trends and the specific needs and strengths of the client is important for job matching. Functional areas such as literacy; vision and visual processing; physical, cognitive, and cultural access to work and equipment; and cognitive performance (attention to task, distractibility, left-to-right sequencing, and learning) must be considered in preparing clients for the job market.

A client-centered, comprehensive vocational plan is essential to placing people with developmental disabilities in the modern workplace. An awareness of the particular issues related to modern jobs will greatly increase our clients' chances for success as members of our communities today. As Radabaugh (1988) so eloquently said, "Technology makes things easier for most people. For individuals with disabilities, technology makes things possible" (p. 6). There are limitless opportunities for those who take the challenge.

Acknowledgments

The authors gratefully acknowledge the assistance of Martin Rice, PhD, OTR/L, Medical College of Ohio, for his review and comments on the first edition draft of this chapter; Bob Robertson, OTR/L, Murdoch Center, for his review and comments on sections of the draft; Denise Plachcinski, MEd, Murdoch Center, for her contributions to the chapter's knowledge base through her work and leadership on Project TechWork; and Patricia Keul, United Cerebral Palsy of North Carolina, for her persistent efforts to foster meaningful community employment opportunities, positively affecting the lives of her clients and coworkers.

References

Abbott, M., Franciscus, M., & Weeks, Z. R. (1988). An overview of occupational therapy. *Occupational therapy careers* (pp. 1–11). Lincolnwood, IL: VGM Career Horizons, National Textbook Company.

Adelstein, L. A. (1992). Work-related treatment for youth. *Work, 2*(2), 7–10.

Adults with developmental disabilities. (1995, Fall). *OT Week for Today's Student*, p. 16.

American Occupational Therapy Association. (1992). White Paper: Occupational therapy and the Americans With Disabilities Act. *American Journal of Occupational Therapy, 46*, 470–471.

American Occupational Therapy Association. (2002). Occupational therapy practice framework: Domain and process. *American Journal of Occupational Therapy, 56*, 609–639.

Angelo, J., & Gross, K. (Eds.). (1994). Relationships with colleagues and clients [Special issue]. *Technology Special Interest Section Newsletter, 4*(2), 1–4.

Armstrong, J., & Rennie, J. (1986). We can use computers too: The setting up of a project for mentally handicapped residents. *British Journal of Occupational Therapy, 49*, 297–300.

Barber, M., McInerny, C. A., & Struck, M. (1993). Training for independence: Transition from school to work. *Work Programs Special Interest Section Newsletter, 7*(2), 1–2.

Bellamy, G. T., Rhodes, L. E., Bourbeau, P. E., & Mank, D. M. (1986). Mental retardation services in sheltered workshops and day activity programs: Consumer benefits and policy alternatives. In F. R. Rusch (Ed.), *Competitive employment issues and strategies* (pp. 168–203). Baltimore: Brookes.

Blackwell, T. L, Conrad, A. D., & Weed, R. O. (1992). *Job analysis and the ADA: A step-by-step guide*. Athens, GA: Elliott & Fitzpatrick.

Brollier, C., Shepherd, J., & Markley, K. F. (1994). Transition from school to community living. *American Journal of Occupational Therapy, 48*, 346–353.

Burkhead, E. J., & Sampson, J. P., Jr. (1985). Computer-assisted assessment in support of the rehabilitation process. *Rehabilitation Counseling Bulletin, 28*, 262–273.

Carrasco, R. C. (1993). Work-related programs for children and adolescents: Part I. *Work Programs Special Interest Section Newsletter, 7*(1), 1–4.

Ciner, E. B., Macks, B., & Schanel-Klitsch, E. (1991). A cooperative demonstration project for early intervention vision services. *OT Practice, 3*(1), 42–46.

Cook, A. M., & Hussey, S. M. (1995). *Assistive technologies: Principles and practice*. St. Louis, MO: Mosby/Yearbook.

Costello, C. (1992). School-based supported work/supported employment. *Work, 2*(2), 11–14.

Crist, P. A. H., & Stoffel, V. C. (1992). The Americans With Disabilities Act of 1990 and employees with mental impairments: Personal efficacy and the environment. *American Journal of Occupational Therapy, 46*, 434–443.

Daggett, W. R. (1995). *Technology: What is it?* [Keynote address]. Schenectady, NY: International Center for Leadership in Education.

Dwyre, A. E., & Trach, J. S. (1996). Consumer choice for people with cognitive disabilities: Who makes the choices in the job search process? *Journal of Applied Rehabilitation Counseling, 27*(3), 42–47.

Federal Register. (1984). *Employment of handicapped clients in sheltered workshops*. Chapter V, Part 525, 17509.

Fiedorowicz, C. A. M. (1986). Training of component reading skills. *Annals of Dyslexia, 36*, 318–334.

Gordon, R. E., & Kozol, K. P. (1984). Occupational therapy and rehabilitation engineering: A team approach to helping persons with severe physical disability to upgrade functional independence. *Occupational Therapy in Health Care, 1*(4), 117–129.

Havranek, J. E. (1992). Methods and uses of job analysis: Implications for implementation of the Americans With Disabilities Act of 1990. *NARPPS Journal and News, 7*(3), 113–117.

Hecker, D. E. (2001, November). Occupational employment projections to 2010. *Monthly Labor Review, 124*(11), 57–84.

Hill, M., Hill, J. W., Wehman, P., Revell, G., Dickerson, A., & Noble, J. H. (1987). Supported employment: An interagency funding model for persons with severe disabilities. *Journal of Rehabilitation, 53*(3), 13–21.

Jacobs, K., & Wyrick, J. (1989). Use of Department of Labor references and job analysis. In S. Hertfelder & C. Gwin (Eds.), *Work in progress* (pp. 23–65). Rockville, MD: American Occupational Therapy Association.

Kielhofner, G. (1992). Functional assessment: Toward a dialectical view of person–environment relations. *American Journal of Occupational Therapy, 43*, 248–251.

Kiernan, W. E., McGaughey M. J., & Schalock R. L. (1988). Employment environments and outcome for adults with developmental disabilities. *Mental Retardation, 26*, 279–288.

Kirkland, M., & Robertson, S. C. (Eds.). (1985). *Planning and implementing vocational readiness in occupational therapy.* Rockville, MD: American Occupational Therapy Association.

Kornblau, B. L. (1996). The occupational therapist and vocational evaluation. *Work Programs Special Interest Section Newsletter, 10*(1), 1–4.

Krantz, G. (1971). Critical vocational behaviors. *Journal of Rehabilitation, 36*, 14–16.

Lagomarcino, T. (1986). Community services. In F. Rusch (Ed.), *Competitive employment issues and strategies* (pp. 65–75). Baltimore: Brookes.

Lash, L., & Licenziato, V. (1995). Career transitions for persons with severe physical disabilities: Integrating technological and psychosocial skills and accommodations. *Work, 5*, 85–98.

Links, C., & Frydenberg, H. (1988). Microcomputer skills training program for the physically disabled in long-term rehabilitation. *Physical and Occupational Therapy in Geriatrics, 6*(3–4), 133–140.

Mann, W. C., & Svorai, S. B. (1994). COMPETE: A model for vocational evaluation, training, employment, and community for integration for persons with cognitive impairments. *American Journal of Occupational Therapy, 48*, 446–451.

Metzler, C. A. (1995). Federal legislation and services for persons with developmental disabilities. *Developmental Disabilities Special Interest Section Newsletter, 18*(2), 1–3.

Minkel, J. L. (1995). Assistive technology credentialing: What is RESNA's program and plan? *Technology Special Interest Section Newsletter, 5*(3), 1–2.

Minkel, J. L. (1996). Credentialing in assistive technology: Myths and realities. *RESNA News, 8*(5), 1, 6–7.

Mitchell, M. M. (1985). Values. In M. Kirkland & S. C. Robertson (Eds.), *Planning and implementing vocational readiness in occupational therapy* (pp. 45–47). Bethesda, MD: American Occupational Therapy Association.

Mitchell, M. M., Rourk, J. D., & Schwarz, J. (1989). A team approach to prevocational services. *American Journal of Occupational Therapy, 43*, 378–383.

Murray, B., & Kenny, S. (1990). Telework as an employment option for people with disabilities. *International Journal of Rehabilitation Research, 12*, 205–214.

Neulicht, A., Primlani, S., & Chewning, L. (1995). *Computer utilization training for employment: A program guide.* Raleigh, NC: Council on Developmental Disabilities.

North Carolina Vocational Alternatives Task Force. (1992). *Supported employment in North Carolina.* Raleigh: Author.

Olshansky, S. (1971). Breaking workshop exit barriers. *Rehabilitation Record, 12*(6), 27–30.

Parent, W. S., Hill, M. L., & Wehman, P. (1989). From sheltered to supported employment outcomes: Challenges for rehabilitation facilities. *Journal of Rehabilitation, 55*(4), 51–57.

Peet, W., Saka, T., & Nakasone, D. (1985). *Teaching word processing to young handi-capable adults: A manual for the trainer.* Honolulu: State Planning Council on Developmental Disabilities Computer Training Project.

Plachcinski, D. (2000). *TechWork: The basic computer curriculum.* Butner, NC: Murdoch Center Foundation.

President's Committee on Mental Retardation. (1977). *Mental retardation past and present.* Washington, DC: Author.

Prouty, R., & Lakin, K. C. (Eds.). (1996). *Residential services for persons with developmental disabilities: Status and trends through 1995* (Rep. 48). Minneapolis: University of Minnesota, College of Education and Human Development.

Radabaugh, P. (1988). *Quality indicators applicable to service delivery programs.* Atlanta: Smart Exchange.

Ranii, D. (1994, October 29). Thriving on unusual strategy. *Raleigh News and Observer,* pp. 1D, 6D.

Reed, K. L. (1991). Part I—Developmental disorders. In *Quick reference to occupational therapy* (pp. 1–86). Gaithersburg, MD: Aspen.

Reynolds-Lynch, K. (1985). In M. Kirkland & S. C. Robertson (Eds.), *Planning and implementing vocational readiness in occupational therapy* (pp. 175–178). Bethesda, MD: American Occupational Therapy Association.

Ross, M. (1991). Using computers for vocational training. *OT Week, 5*(10), 6–7.

Ryan, C. P. (1995). Work isn't what it used to be: Implications, recommendations, and strategies for vocational rehabilitation. *Journal of Rehabilitation, 61*(4), 8–15.

Sampson, J. P., Jr., McMahon, B. T., & Burkhead, E. J. (1985). Using computers for career exploration and decision making in vocational rehabilitation. *Rehabilitation Counseling Bulletin, 28,* 242–261.

Sandlin, J., Prouty, R., & Lakin, K.C. (1996). Large state MR/DD facility closures, 1960–2000. In R. Prouty & K. C. Lakin (Eds.), *Residential services for persons with developmental disabilities: Status and trends through 1995* (Rep. 48, pp. 30–41). Minneapolis: University of Minnesota, College of Education and Human Development.

Scheiman, M. (1990). Assessment and management of the exceptional child. In A. A. Rosenblum & M. W. Morgan (Eds.), *Pediatric optometry* (pp. 388–419). Philadelphia: Lippincott.

Scheiman, M. (2002). *Understanding and managing vision deficits: A guide for occupational therapists* (2nd ed.). Thorofare, NJ: Slack.

Schmitt, P., & Growick, B. (1985). Computer technology in rehabilitation counseling. *Rehabilitation Counseling Bulletin, 28,* 233–240.

Shelly, C., Sample, P., & Spencer, K. (1992). The Americans With Disabilities Act of 1990 expands employment opportunities for persons with developmental disabilities. *American Journal of Occupational Therapy, 46,* 457–465.

Spencer, J. E., Emery, L. J., & Schneck, C. M. (2003). Occupational therapy in transitioning adolescents to postsecondary activities. *American Journal of Occupational Therapy, 57,* 435–441.

Spencer, K. C. (1990). Supported employment: The role of occupational therapy at the job site. *OT Practice, 1*(2), 74–82.

Suchoff, I. B., Kapoor, N., Waxman, R., & Ference. W. (1999). The occurrence of ocular and visual dysfunctions in an acquired brain-injured patient sample. *Journal of the American Optometric Association, 70,* 301–308.

U.S. Department of Labor. (1991). *Dictionary of occupational titles.* Washington, DC: U.S. Government Printing Office.

U.S. Department of Labor. (1995). *Occupational outlook handbook.* Washington, DC: U.S. Government Printing Office.

U.S. Department of Labor. (2002). *Occupational outlook handbook.* Washington, DC: U.S. Government Printing Office.

U.S. Department of Labor, Bureau of Labor Statistics. (2001). *BLS releases 2000–2010 employment projections.* Washington, DC: U.S. Government Printing Office.

Velozo, C. A. (1992). Work evaluations: Critique of the state of the art of functional assessment of work. *American Journal of Occupational Therapy, 43,* 203–209.

Ward, K. M. (1996). School-based vocational training. In L. A. Kurtz, P. W. Dowrick, S. E. Levy, & M. L. Batshaw (Eds.), *Handbook of developmental disabilities: Resources for interdisciplinary care* (pp. 237–248). Gaithersburg, MD: Aspen.

Wehman, P. (1986). Competitive employment in Virginia. In F. Rusch (Ed.), *Competitive employment issues and strategies* (pp. 23–33). Baltimore: Brookes.

Wehman, P., & Kregel, J. (n.d.) *At the crossroads: Supported employment ten years later.* Richmond: Virginia Commonwealth University, Rehabilitation Research and Training Center on Supported Employment.

Wehman, P. H., & Moon, M. (1987). Critical values in employment programs for persons with developmental disabilities: A position paper. *Journal of Applied Rehabilitation Counseling, 18*(1), 12–16.

Wood, R. L. (1986). Rehabilitation of patients with disorders of attention. *Journal of Head Trauma Rehabilitation, 1*(3), 43–53.

Appendix 11.A. Resources for the Occupational Therapy Practitioner in Work and Developmental Disabilities

Because of the community-based nature of most developmental disabilities work intervention, the available resources come from a combination of professional and client-related organizations. Many of these organizations have state or local chapters.

American Occupational Therapy Association
    Developmental Disabilities Special Interest Section (SIS)
    Technology SIS
    Work Programs SIS
    P.O. Box 31220
    Bethesda, MD 20824
    (301) 652-2682
    (800) SAY-AOTA (members)
    TTY: (800) 377-8555
    http://www.aota.org

The ARC (Association for Retarded Citizens)
    National Headquarters
    P.O. Box 1047
    Arlington, TX 76004
    (817) 261-6003
    TTY: (817) 277-0553
    http://www.thearc.org

Association for Persons in Supported Employment (APSE)
    1627 Monument Avenue
    Richmond, VA 23220
    (804) 278-9187
    http://www.apse.org

Brain Injury Association Inc. (Formerly National Head Injury Foundation)
    8201 Greensboro Drive, Suite 611
    McLean, VA 22102
    (703) 761-0750
    http://www.biausa.org/Pages/home.html

Closing the Gap, Inc.
    P.O. Box 68
    526 Main Street
    Henderson, MN 56044
    (507) 248-3294
    http://www.closingthegap.com

Down Syndrome Research Foundation
    1409 Sperling Avenue
    Burnaby, BC V5B 4J8
    Canada
    (604) 444-3773
    (888) 464-DSRF (Canada only)
    http://www.dsrf.org

Job Accommodations Network (JAN)
    P.O. Box 6080
    Morgantown, WV 26506
    V/TTY: (800) 526-7234
    http://janweb.icdi.wvu.edu

National Down Syndrome Society
    666 Broadway, 8th Floor
    New York, NY 10012
    (212) 460-9330
    (800) 221-4602
    http://www.ndss.org

National Rehabilitation Association
    633 South Washington Street
    Alexandria, VA 22314
    (703) 836-0850
    http://www.nationalrehab.org

National Rehabilitation Counseling Association (NRCA)
    8807 Sudley Road, Suite 102
    Manassas, VA 22110
    (703) 361-2077
    http://nrca-net.org

National Rehabilitation Information Center (NARIC)
    4200 Forbes Boulevard, Suite 202
    Lanham, MD 20706
    (301) 459-5900
    (800) 346-2742
    http://www.naric.com

Office of Disability Employment Policy
    (Formerly President's Committee on Employment of People With Disabilities)
    U.S. Department of Labor
    Frances Perkins Building
    200 Constitution Avenue, NW
    Washington, DC 20210
    (202) 693-7880
    TTY: (202) 693-7881
    http://www.dol.gov/odep

RESNA (Rehabilitation Engineering and Assistive Technology Society
of North America)
    1700 North Moore Street, Suite 1540
    Arlington, VA 22209
    (703) 524-6686
    TTY: (703) 524-6639
    http://www.resna.org

Trace Research and Development Center
    University of Wisconsin–Madison
    2107 Engineering Centers Building
    1550 Engineering Drive
    Madison, WI 53706
    (608) 262-6966
    TTY: (608) 263-5408
    http://trace.wisc.edu

UCP (United Cerebral Palsy)
    1660 L Street, NW, Suite 700
    Washington, DC 20036
    (800) 872-5827
    (202) 776-0406
    TTY: (202) 973-7197
    http://www.ucpa.org

Rehabilitation Research and Training Center on Workplace Supports (RRTC)
    Virginia Commonwealth University RRTC
    1314 West Main Street
    Richmond, VA 23284
    (804) 828-1851
    TTY: (804) 828-2494
    http://www.worksupport.com

CHAPTER 12

Using Supported-Employment Principles to Develop Self-Employment Opportunities

Carol Estes, BS
David Matheis, BA, ATP

Introduction

Project ASSET (Advancing Supported Self-Employment Techniques) is a model collaborative project of the Kentucky Department of Vocational Rehabilitation and the Kentucky Council on Developmental Disabilities. Over a 2-year period, the project has used supported-employment techniques to help 15 persons with significant developmental disabilities start their own business.

Employment Patterns for People With Disabilities

As a group, people with disabilities are disproportionately underemployed or without jobs altogether. A Harris Poll (Taylor, 1998) for the National Organization on Disability indicated that 69% of working-age Americans with disabilities were unemployed. When the survey was repeated 4 years later, the unemployment rate was even higher—71% (Taylor, 1998). Figures from the 2000 Census show that 76% of noninstitutionalized, nondisabled Kentuckians between ages 21 and 64 were employed; only 46.9% of noninstitutionalized Kentuckians with disabilities in the same age group were working (U.S. Bureau of the Census, 2000b, Table DP.2).

There is also a significant earnings discrepancy between people with and without disabilities. In 2000, nationwide mean earnings for people who did not have disabilities were $30,155 (McNeil, 2000), those with disabilities earned $23,403, and those considered to have significant disabilities earned $18,582.

For people with developmental disabilities, particularly those whose limitations are considered most significant, the lack of employment is a major impediment to full inclusion in the community. Too often they are unable to develop the peer relationships that for others occur naturally on the job. They are deprived of the status and role in the community that accompany salary-earning, tax-paying citizenship. Their income—often limited to government assistance—cannot support the recreational or leisure opportunities available to their nondisabled peers, who benefit from the purchasing power that results from full employment at living wages. In short, employment provides the most important entry point into the life of the community.

Self-employment can be an important vehicle for access to a better standard of living for adults with developmental disabilities, particularly for those who live in rural areas. The flexibility and degree of personal control that self-employment makes possible can help people with developmental disabilities overcome, or at least address, the obstacles to full inclusion in community life that exists in rural areas. "People with disabilities are just as well equipped to run a small business as the next person, as long as support is available and affordable" (Griffin & Hammis, 2003, p. 34).

The lack of employment opportunities generally available in rural communities is especially problematic for people with developmental disabilities, who can have difficulty competing in limited job markets. Rural areas of Kentucky are well known for their lack of employment options, and opportunities are particularly limited in the Appalachian area of Eastern Kentucky. The economy of those areas has long had its base in coal mining, and there has never been effective diversification of the job market. According to the Kentucky Workforce Development Cabinet (2003), the statewide unemployment rate in December 2003 was 5.1%. However, in the coal counties of Eastern Kentucky, the rate was as high as 12.0%, more than twice the state average.

Compounding the high unemployment rates in Appalachian Eastern Kentucky is the high prevalence of disability in the region's population. According to the 2000 Census (U.S. Bureau of the Census, 2000a), many counties in Eastern Kentucky have disability rates in excess of 30%. Those areas also are among the poorest counties in the state.

Benefits of Self-Employment

Self-employment can be a small but important part of the answer to the chronic underemployment and joblessness among people with developmental disabilities. It contains the possibility for someone to invent a job, provided that a service or product that is needed or valued in the community can be identified.

Transportation is another problem endemic to rural communities that greatly hinders people with disabilities in becoming gainfully employed and integrating fully into the life of the community. According to a study performed by the University of Kentucky for the Kentucky Developmental Disabilities Council (Jennings, Hall, Black, & Wade, 2002), transportation options are severely limited in the rural areas of Kentucky, particularly Eastern Kentucky. Two areas of Eastern Kentucky showed the state's lowest ratios of accessible vehicles to individuals with mobility impairments. The same areas had the fewest number of vehicles available overall to transport those with disabilities. Self-employment could serve as a solution to the transportation problem for some people with developmental disabilities by providing flexibility in the range of employment locations. A self-employed person often can locate a business at home or in a place that is accessible to transportation. The self-employment possibilities available through e-commerce can even make transportation an obsolete issue and open a whole new world of community integration to the entrepreneur.

Another persistent problem is the lack of employment-related services for people with developmental disabilities who live in rural communities. Supported-employment providers are particularly scarce in some rural areas of Kentucky, but to people who have the most significant disabilities, their services often can be crucial for identifying work opportunities and maintaining employment. When supported-employment services are combined with self-employment goals, more people will have the capacity to succeed.

Self-employment is ideal for providing natural supports on the job, whether the assistance comes from family members who help with the business, from suppliers or customers who have a stake in the success of the business, or from nondisabled business partners.

Self-employment can offer a unique tool for ending isolation and for facilitating full community inclusion. First, as in all employment, a steady income in itself opens many doors. Purchasing power brings the valued identity of a customer for area businesses. It also opens up increased recreational opportunities with nondisabled peers. Successful owners of small businesses bolster the economy by becoming valuable customers to suppliers and by providing products or services that are valuable to their own customers.

These two roles—customer and entrepreneur—are by their nature accorded respect and status in the community, although they are seldom available to people with developmental disabilities. Successful owners of small businesses often become readily identifiable in their communities, and they are generally known more for contributing to society than for their individual life circumstances. Such respect, status, and identification will naturally bring a degree of community inclusion that people with developmental disabilities often cannot obtain in any other way. The U.S. Department of Labor (2003) has reported that people with disabilities have a higher rate of self-employment than do those without disabilities (12.2% vs. 7.8%), but that few receive assistance for their enterprises from federal or state vocational rehabilitation programs. In 1995 and 1996, the Rehabilitation Services Administration (RSA) (Arnold, 1998) reported that only 2.6% of its consumers who obtained jobs had done so through self-employment. In particular, people with the most significant developmental disabilities are among the least likely to be offered opportunities for self-employment because of the extent of their limitations. This despite the fact that self-employment can be particularly suited to the individual circumstances and interests of people with disabilities, offering as it does increased freedom and flexibility. Self-employment, for example, can allow a person to adjust his or her work schedule to address disability-related barriers such as fatigue or the need for personal assistance.

Project ASSET: Searching for Solutions

The Rehabilitation Act Amendments of 1998 are part of the Workforce Investment Act (P.L. 105-220). The act and its amendments include an emphasis on increasing employment outcomes, specifically in the areas of telecommuting, self-employment, and the establishment of small businesses. In support of these goals, the Kentucky Department of Vocational Rehabilitation (DVR) and the Kentucky Council on Developmental Disabilities together created Project ASSET. The project is funded by the council and DVR, and it uses DVR staff and expertise to increase self-employment options for people with the most significant developmental disabilities.

The project's genesis came in the fall of 2001 at a meeting attended by several members of the council; DVR's supported-employment staff; and Cary Griffin, an expert on self-employment for people with disabilities. At the time, Griffin was employed by the University of Montana's Rural Institute on Disabilities. Griffin is now a principal with Griffin-Hammis Associates. The council had already established as a goal in its 5-year state plan the development of self-employment opportunities for people with developmental disabilities and was investigating ways of reaching the goal. DVR was exploring new methods for developing self-employment options for its consumers as one way to respond to the increased federal emphasis on self-employment, as promoted by RSA.

The needs of the council and DVR were converging. At the meeting, the group decided that the application of supported-employment principles to self-employment might be the best avenue to providing that option to a population often overlooked for inclusion—people with the most significant developmental disabilities. The group also decided that DVR's supported-employment infrastructure would offer the most efficient means of providing the necessary services. DVR had in place a supported-employment service branch that consisted of a director and three regional coordinators who could manage and monitor services.

In most states, supported employment's emergence came in the 1980s and 1990s, and it fostered the inclusion of more first-time workers in the labor force than had any other special federal program for people with disabilities (Wehman, 1998). In 1986, statistics showed that fewer than 10,000 people were in supported employment. By 1998, the number had increased to more than 170,000, and the success of the program established it as a national model (Wehman, 1998). Because funding is insufficient to cover the extended services that provide long-term support, Kentucky and other states must maintain waiting lists of those who wish to become involved in supported-employment programs.

Project Design

The design of the model project owes much to the professional experience and extensive research of Cary Griffin and his associate, Dave Hammis, an expert on Social Security disability issues. Highlights of the design include use of a supported-employment provider to assist each participant in all aspects of business development and the formation of a support team for each enterprise. The supported-employment provider assists with writing the business plan, developing the support team, searching for start-up funding, operating the business in its initial stages, and providing long-term support as needed. The provider applies the proven principles of supported employment to the business start-up: using job matching and job carving, in-depth task analysis, on-site instruction and off-site support, and fostering development of natural long-term supports.

The development of a support team for each enterprise is an integral and innovative aspect of the project. The teams can consist of family, friends, business associates, full business partners (in some cases), volunteers from SCORE (Service Corps of Retired Executives), representatives from small business development centers in the state, and others who might have an interest in the business. The teams advise the business owners and their supported-employment providers at every step in the business development process.

> Staying focused one person at a time reduces the risks to agencies
> and policy makers, slowly builds credibility one success at a time,
> allows time for learning from mistakes, and redirects what should
> be nonthreatening amounts of money a little at a time. (Griffin &
> Hammis, 2003, p. 31)

The first 5 of the project's 15 participants were selected in the spring of 2002. They are a diverse group: Their developmental disabilities include muscular dystrophy, autism, perinatal brain injury, and moderate mental retardation. Two participants live in isolated rural communities in Eastern

Kentucky; one lives in Frankfort, the state capital (population 27,741 according to the 2000 U.S. Census); and two are residents of Lexington, the second largest city in the state (population 260,512). Their business ideas ranged from a NASCAR hobby shop to a greenhouse to a lunch delivery business.

Introducing the Project to Participants

The 5 original participants were invited to attend the first activity of the project, a supported–self-employment summit that was funded by the council and that convened in Lexington, May 22–24, 2002. The summit brought together the professionals, advocates, and potential support team members in the state who might be able to aid the development of the initial enterprises and form a base of support and knowledge for the owners of the new small businesses. The potential business owners were encouraged to bring family members; the supported-employment providers, if already identified, also received invitations. Summit participants included representatives from DVR, the council, the Small Business Development Center at the University of Kentucky, the Interdisciplinary Human Development Institute at the University of Kentucky (the state's Center for Excellence on Developmental Disability), SCORE, and other organizations and agencies. Participants were trained on a variety of topics related to small business development for individuals with disabilities: business plan development; start-up funding; compliance with relevant tax laws; how to coordinate support; and, most important, the implications of self-employment for Social Security recipients. Cary Griffin and Dave Hammis were the main presenters.

After the conference, DVR's supported-employment consultants and staff members of the Interdisciplinary Human Development Institute began to develop the support teams to start planning for the small businesses. They relied on a process that was based on personal futures planning. At the time of this writing, the first five businesses are in various stages of development. In the spring of 2003, five more people were invited to participate, and their support teams have been forming and organizing.

Case Study: Marvin

Marvin is a 28-year-old man with autism. He lives with his mother, father, and an older brother on a family farm near Berea, an Eastern Kentucky community of about 10,000 people. Berea is nationally known for its vibrant arts and crafts industry and for Berea College, a progressive private institution.

Marvin has severe communication limitations and exhibits inappropriate social behaviors. He has been a client of DVR since

1996. Before his involvement with Project ASSET, Marvin had tried several employment-related activities but had not been very successful. He had been given at least one vocational assessment, and he worked briefly in a community rehabilitation facility. With the assistance of Cardinal Employment, the local supported-employment provider, he had tried several jobs in the community, including a number at Wal-Mart. None had worked out, however, chiefly because of his lack of social skills and his high level of social anxiety.

Once Marvin was selected for the project, his support team formed. The team consisted of his parents and an aunt; DVR's supported-employment consultant for the area; his vocational rehabilitation counselor; four staff members from Cardinal Employment; a staff member from Kentucky GROW (Gardening for Recreation or Work), a project of the University of Kentucky; and a representative from Benefits Plus, a project funded by the Social Security Administration to provide information about Social Security benefits to recipients.

Kentucky GROW is a federally funded grant project that provides assistance to individuals with disabilities who are interested in gardening. A representative from the project was asked to join the team because it was envisioned that Marvin's business would be connected with agriculture. This team was facilitated by a staff member from the Interdisciplinary Human Development Institute at the University of Kentucky and employed through a contract with DVR.

As it turned out, the staff members from the local small business development center provided valuable advice and assistance to the development of the enterprise, although none of them ever formally became team members.

The team's first order of business was to give more focus and definition to the ideas for Marvin's self-employment enterprise. With the valuable resource of the family farm available to them, his family had long given some thought to how they might use it to benefit Marvin in terms of employment and activity as he reached adulthood. They had envisioned building a greenhouse so Marvin could grow plants and vegetables to sell. They also could offer the greenhouse and land for use by the surrounding community, which would provide Marvin with a continuing source of social interaction. When he was selected for Project ASSET, the plan was to build on this concept.

When the team started to meet, it soon became apparent that the original concept of a greenhouse would not be appropriate for Marvin. Using the principles of person-centered job selection or vocational profiling, the team began to better understand the features of employment that would be a good fit for Marvin and to identify those features that would not match well with his interests and abilities. He had a low tolerance for heat and humidity and, as a result, would probably not do well working in the greenhouse for any length of time. Marvin also did not particularly like being around groups of people.

The team began to look for other self-employment opportunities for Marvin that would still take advantage of his family's land. The Kentucky GROW representative was familiar with the development of several agricultural microenterprises in the state that involved nontraditional products. He suggested mushroom production as a possible avenue for Marvin's business. Shiitake mushrooms have gained popularity as a commodity crop, particularly in several counties surrounding Marvin's home. The mushrooms are relatively easy to grow in cool places, so Marvin could work mostly at his own pace in an environment he prefers.

Building on that suggestion, the team attended a shiitake mushroom workshop where all of the members received hands-on experience in mushroom farming. The team members came away from the workshop encouraged. They also came away with 30 starter logs, inoculated with mushroom spores, to launch Marvin's enterprise. With luck and proper care, the logs would produce Marvin's first mushrooms in about 6 months.

With assistance from the small business development center and Kentucky GROW, the team developed a business plan. Tools and equipment were purchased, including hand drills to inoculate the logs, 300-gallon tubs to soak the logs in water, and tarpaulins to cover the logs while the mushrooms grow. With weekly assistance from his supported-employment provider, Marvin proved capable of performing the necessary tasks for developing the mushrooms. Although 30 logs was a very small start, the team believed that scale would give Marvin an opportunity to see whether the enterprise suited him.

Initially, he will sell his produce to local restaurants and residents. More logs will be added as he masters the increased workload. The team has plans to renovate a small, unoccupied cabin on the property for Marvin to use for his business. At the time of this writing, Marvin was preparing to harvest his first crop.

Case Study: Tim

Tim is a 23-year-old man with muscular dystrophy. He lives in Pikeville, a community of about 6,000 nestled deep in Appalachia in the very far eastern part of the state. Pikeville's economy traditionally has been based on coal mining, but it has not diversified in recent years. Employment opportunities are severely limited in the area, particularly for people with the most significant disabilities. Tim uses a wheelchair. He has no use of his legs and very limited use of his arms. He became a DVR client in December 1999. Because of his very significant physical limitations and the limited local employment, finding a job that matched his skills and interests has been difficult. With assistance from the local supported-employment provider, Mountain Comprehensive Care Center, Tim went to work for a computer technical support company in the summer of 2000, but the company was not able to fully accommodate Tim, and the job was short-lived. Tim's prospects for further employment did not look promising.

Like many Americans, Tim is a passionate follower of NASCAR; his interest is well known to his family and friends. When the creation of Project ASSET was formally announced and the search for prospective owners began, DVR's supported-employment consultant for that area of the state remembered Tim's strong interest. In the past, she had worked with Tim and his job coach to identify possible jobs. Immediately, she thought of Tim as a Project ASSET candidate in a business built around his interest in NASCAR.

A support team was formed that included Tim's mother and an aunt, his vocational rehabilitation counselor, a representative from Benefits Plus, and his supported-employment specialist from the local service provider. That person's involvement would prove crucial to the creation of the business. A staff member from the Interdisciplinary Human Development Institute at the University of Kentucky also facilitated this team. The team met formally three times, but smaller meetings of various team members were convened as well. A representative from the local small business development center provided technical assistance.

The team set out to develop a business plan for a NASCAR-focused retail operation. Most of the plan's writing fell to Tim's aunt, but the supported-employment specialist helped to gauge the viability of such a business in the community and to identify a prospective site—an empty storefront just outside Pikeville on busy

U.S. Highway 23. That road is the main route through the region to Bristol, Tennessee, where two major NASCAR events take place each year. The location seemed ideal because so many fans would pass by on the way to Bristol. The supported-employment specialist spent some time at the location during the writing of the plan, monitoring traffic to estimate the potential number of customers.

Once the business plan was completed, the real work of turning the business into a reality began. Tim first had to obtain the proper business licenses. He also had to become certified by NASCAR as a dealer, and that involved a detailed application process. Starting the business also required a significant investment. The building itself had to be made accessible for Tim, and he needed computer equipment and a cash register to run the business. DVR agreed to finance the necessary renovations and to supply the equipment. DVR also agreed to pay operating expenses for the first 6 months after the business opened. This still left the purchase of a starting inventory. The representative from the small business development center was instrumental in helping Tim apply for a small business loan from a local bank. His loan for $20,000 is guaranteed by the Small Business Administration.

After many delays in the purchasing of equipment, Tim was ready to open Speedway Hobbies. Although not totally prepared, the business opened its doors on December 2, 2002, in an effort capture at least some portion of holiday sales. The formal grand opening was April 25, 2003, amid much local fanfare and press coverage. Today, the business continues to grow, and by the fall of 2003, Tim was expecting to break even.

In Tim's case, the importance of the assistance provided by the supported-employment provider cannot be overstated. He has aided Tim in every facet of business development, from feasibility research to plan writing to actual business management. Tim recently admitted he has learned a lot about retail sales and about NASCAR in the process. Family member involvement also was critical to the successful beginning of Speedway Hobbies. Tim's aunt was the author of the business plan, and his mother, who retired from state government when Tim opened his business, works in the store with him every day.

Program Evaluation

Although Project ASSET is still relatively new, DVR has identified several preliminary conclusions as it has examined the achievements of the project to date. First, much has been learned about the business-planning process. Those who benefit from this experience include DVR staff, consumers, families, case managers, staff members of Supports for Community Living (Kentucky's Medicaid waiver program), and members of the individual planning teams. Patience and persistence were valuable assets to the team members, as each learned their roles and responsibilities. Developing a business plan, if done well, requires a significant investment of team members' time. Although one person often takes the lead in developing that document, every member influences the content.

Person-centered planning tools are valuable in the development of small businesses, and person-centered planning facilitators are critical to the work of the support groups, keeping them focused and providing leadership to ensure that the business model fits the person and that all services and supports are in place.

When applied to self-employment, the principles of supported employment ensure that the business owner has the interest, the capacity for participation, and the support required to ensure success. Each team spent many hours making sure that the businesses were not simply created "around" the owners without the principals' active participation. Valued roles in the businesses for the owners with the disabilities are priorities. With each business, the owner will have varying degrees of involvement and support.

Because of funding limitations, modified strategies were needed to pay for the services, supports, and business needs of each participant. Existing policies for purchasing were often cumbersome and caused delays in business start-up. Project ASSET values the principles of self-determination and anticipates a positive effect for supported self-employment from Kentucky House Bill 501, the Kevin Webb and Kim Brown Self-Determination Act, which was signed by Governor Paul Patton in March 2003. The act calls for the development of model projects that implement self-determination principles and individualized budgets. The project personnel recognize the benefits those concepts can bring to supported self-employment.

The income from self-owned businesses can affect participant benefits such as Social Security benefits and disability insurance eligibility, Medicaid, and Medicare. Potential and existing small business owners who receive Social Security cash benefits must understand and plan for the effect of self-employment earnings on their benefits (Griffin & Hammis, 2003). Planning that aims at minimizing profits to prevent a loss of benefits is not in keeping with the objectives of supported employment, nor is it in the best interest of the person with the disability. Every effort is being given to fully elucidate Kentucky's policies and regulations regarding work incentives. If changes in regulations that will remove disincentives to employment are identified, we will propose them and advocate for their passage. The confusion surrounding these issues in Kentucky has created some delays in moving forward for four of the teams whose business owners receive Medicaid benefits.

We have been disappointed to learn that our original schedules for business plan development were unrealistic. In retrospect, considering the significance of the disabilities involved, this should have come as neither a surprise nor a disappointment. For various reasons, each team took longer than we expected to complete the business plan. Participant illnesses; questions, concerns, and the need to conduct research into the effects of earnings on benefits; the need for other rehabilitation services; family issues; supported-employment personnel issues; and funding delays all contributed to the delay.

Analyzed separately, however, each team made significant progress. None of the business owners has given up or abandoned a business start-up, even though at least two participants have changed or modified their original ideas.

The importance of sharing information cannot be underestimated. In the spring of 2003, the first five business owners and their teams came together to report on and hear about the work of their counterparts. They also received assistance, support, and feedback from Griffin and Hammis and from DVR personnel involved in Project ASSET. Each team prepared excellent presentations and summations of their progress, and the meeting received high evaluations from all who attended. A similar meeting is scheduled for the second group of participants in the spring of 2004.

Throughout project development, the technical assistance from Griffin and Hammis has proven invaluable. They have provided small- and large-group training and offered regular support and technical assistance by e-mail and telephone.

Conclusion

Project ASSET has made significant progress toward its goals and objectives. Ten persons are in varying stages of business development, and three of the businesses were in active operation as of December 31, 2003. We are pleased that as a result of our efforts, business opportunities are being designed to fit the unique circumstances of each Project ASSET participant.

The experiences of two persons in particular illustrate that self-employment can be a viable option for individuals with the most significant developmental disabilities, so long as the business is crafted around particular strengths, abilities, and interests. Their experiences also illustrate how forming a support team around the person and applying the principles of supported employment and planning for the individual's future can be instrumental to success. Although there is much work to be done in both businesses highlighted here—and, for that matter, in all five of the original self-employment enterprises—the preliminary results are encouraging.

Project ASSET has already begun to have replication impact, as a few people whose disabilities do not meet the definition of "developmental disabilities" are still able to work with DVR in developing self-owned businesses based on experience and knowledge gained from this project. In one case in Western Kentucky, the business owner was able to obtain DVR and other state funding, and he received technical assistance from his local small business development center as recommended by the Project ASSET advisory team when we could not include him in the project. DVR is so encouraged by these preliminary results that it plans to use its own financial resources to begin a similar project with five persons who have been diagnosed with mental illnesses.

References

Arnold, N. (1998). *Self-employment: Improving policy and practice.* Missoula: University of Montana Rural Institute.

Griffin, C., & Hammis, D. (2003). *Making self-employment work for people with disabilities.* Baltimore: Brookes.

Jennings, E. T., Jr., Hall, J., Black, T., & Wade, A. (2002). *Meeting the transportation needs of Kentuckians with disabilities: Public policy solutions* (Report prepared for the Kentucky Developmental Disabilities Council). Lexington: University of Kentucky, School of Public Policy and Administration.

Kentucky Workforce Development Cabinet. (2003). *Statistics from the Kentucky Department of Employment Services.* Retrieved December 28, 2003, from www.workforcekentucky.ky.gov/cgi/datanalysis/AreaSelection.asp?TableNews=Labforce.

McNeil, J. (2000, June/July). *Employment, earnings, and disability.* Paper prepared for the 75th Annual Conference of the Western Economic Association International, Vancouver, British Columbia, Canada.

Taylor, H. (1998). Americans with disabilities still pervasively disadvantaged on a broad range of key indicators. (Harris Poll 56). Retrieved December 7, 2003, from http://www.harrisinteractive.com/harris_poll/index.asp?PID=152.

U.S. Bureau of the Census. (2000a). *State and county QuickFacts.* Retrieved November 24, 2003, from http://quickfacts.census.gov/qfd/states/21000.htm.

U.S. Bureau of the Census (2000b, July). *Statistics from the 2000 United States Census: DP-2. Profile of selected social characteristics: 2000. Geographic area: Kentucky.* Retrieved November 24, 2003, from http://www.census.gov/data/KY/04021.pdf.

U.S. Department of Labor. (2003). *Small business and self-employment for people with disabilities.* Office of Disability Employment Policy, http://www.dol.gov/odep.

Wehman, P. (1998, Fall) Supported employment: How are we doing? *Supported Employment Consortium Newsletter.* Richmond: Virginia Commonwealth University.

CHAPTER 13

Adaptive Driver Evaluation and Training

Deena Garrison Jones, OTR, CDRS

Introduction

As a clinician you might have inherited a driver training program or started your own driver rehabilitation program and now wonder, "What do I do?" This chapter discusses clinical and the on-the-road assessments for drivers with disabilities, medical clearance, insurance issues, funding, passenger transportation safety, and special considerations. Appendixes 13.A–13.E contain a list of abbreviations, a checklist for driver training, a sample consent form, several case studies, and a listing of resources.

The ability to drive increases the independence of people with disabilities; it enables them to obtain employment and participate in community life. To many, operating a motor vehicle is a rite of passage. However, driving requires responsible action from the operator of the vehicle, and driving is not a right but a privilege that must be earned. Some people with physical, cognitive, perceptual, or emotional disabilities are able to legally operate a motor vehicle safely and efficiently once they have been evaluated and trained with the appropriate techniques and adaptive equipment (Garrison Jones, 1997). However, not all those who are evaluated for the ability to drive or receive driver training will obtain an operator's license. Therefore, it is imperative to also understand other transportation options.

Brief History

Driver rehabilitation is not a new field. Modified vehicles have been in use at least since World War II, when many disabled veterans modified their cars with curtain rods, canes, or even coat hangers. Since that time, the industry has grown to include manufacturers and vendors who design and market equipment that allows people with disabilities to operate many types of motor vehicles.

The use of that equipment requires training by professionals. Driving is not only a matter of accelerating, braking, and steering; "driving an automobile consists of taking skilled and properly-timed actions under varying road and traffic conditions based on decisions which are dependent upon: sound judgment, realistic perception, and learned information" (American Automobile Association, 1993). Before the development of the specialty field, commercial driving instructors taught people with disabilities how to drive. As the need continued and the task became more complex, the driver educators and on-the-road driving instructors worked with occupational therapists, physical therapists, and kinesiology therapists to better understand disabilities and better serve the clients. Those groups created the Association of Driver Educators for the Disabled (ADED) in 1977. ADED recognized that the field of driver training for people with disabilities needed to include specialists in equipment modification as well, and it changed its name and became incorporated as the Association for Driver Rehabilitation Specialists. Information about ADED and its programs is available on the Internet: http://www.driver-ed.org. ADED works to support professionals in the fields of driver education, driver training, and transportation equipment modifications for people with disabilities (Association for Driver Rehabilitation Specialists, n.d.).

ADED is an international nonprofit association dedicated to enhancing the lives of individuals with disabilities and impairments by providing services that help clients attain the skills that will enable them to operate motor vehicles safely and efficiently. To do so may require use of adaptive equipment and modified vehicles. ADED is the primary professional association in this specialized area, and it offers its members educational conferences and resource support. ADED also encourages equipment development to maximize transportation and driving options for people with disabilities. ADED works collaboratively with members of its sister organization—the National Mobility Equipment Dealers Association (NMEDA)—to ensure the highest quality and compliance with safety standards for equipment development and prescription.

Members of ADED commit to a code of ethics and comply with the organization's standards of practice (go to "Code of Ethics/Standards of Practice" on the ADED Web site). Certified driver rehabilitation specialists are likewise committed to such compliance. The standards of practice set forth minimal requirements that govern professional behavior in the provision of driver rehabilitation services. The ADED code of ethics is a set of principles that guides the professional conduct of the driver rehabilitation specialist.

Training for people with disabilities should be provided by a certified driving instructor or by a driver rehabilitation specialist who provides rehabilitation services for this population. The trainer is expected to follow and interpret all applicable federal, state, and local laws and policies. Instructors come from a variety of backgrounds—rehabilitation, education, health, safety, therapy, or a related profession. Many hospitals and private facilities employ driver specialists to instruct their clients in the use of adaptive equipment. The clinician should be well informed of state rules and regulations and seek training through workshops, seminars, and other forms of education pertinent to the driver rehabilitation field.

It is also strongly suggested that the clinician take the ADED certification exam, which is an entry-level test that sets forth the minimum competency in the core knowledge areas pertaining to the specialty of driver rehabilitation. A certified driver rehabilitation specialist (CDRS) "plans, develops, coordinates and implements driver rehabilitation services for individuals with disabilities" (Association for Driver Rehabilitation Specialists, n.d.). The ADED certification process protects the public by providing a measurement of a standard of current knowledge desirable for individuals practicing driver rehabilitation; encouraging individual growth and study, thereby promoting professionalism among driver rehabilitation specialists; and formally recognizing driver rehabilitation specialists who fulfill the requirement for certification. As of fall 2003, ADED had 488 members, including 305 who currently hold the CDRS credential.

Evaluating and training in the field of adaptive driving is not a one-time thing. No one can complete a study for driver evaluation and an on-the-road assessment in a day. The driving evaluator who performs on-the-road assessments must be familiar with people with disabilities. The clinician who has experience with clinical assessments should seek continuing education to become a certified driver educator. State certification requirements vary, but preparation usually entails 6–9 credit hours of safety and highway safety training. This education helps inform the occupational therapist, physical therapist, and kinesiology therapist of the true goals of driver education and training. The objectives involve more than evaluating clients or teaching them how to use adaptive equipment. The broader goal is to help drivers become competent and responsible users of the highway transportation system. If specialized training is not possible, the clinician should follow up with a local commercial driving school to have driver educators who are familiar with the field of driver rehabilitation perform behind-the-wheel training and testing.

Medical Clearance

A driver evaluation, including clinical and on-the-road assessment, usually lasts 4–5 hours. Depending on the facility involved, medical statements, doctors' orders, and medical records should be obtained and reviewed for clients who have disabilities before the driver evaluation begins. During the clinical (or in-house) evaluation, there should be an examination of such client-specific issues as sensory loss and how the driver can be expected to operate the vehicle in an emergency. It is also important to note any medication a client uses regularly. Each state's medical advisory board sets guidelines for how often people who use specific medications need to be seen. For example, antispasticity, antidepressant, anticonvulsant, antihistamine, antipsychotic, cold and asthma, and tranquilizing medications could be listed with the client's medical information sent to the state's department of motor vehicles. Some clients will be subject to an annual review by the department's medical board. Dilantin and Tegretol are examples of medications that must be kept at therapeutic dosages and listed on the client's medical report.

The motor vehicles department must be informed when there is any question that driving capabilities could be affected by cognitive, emotional, physical, or psychiatric impairments. Medical statements are almost always needed when adaptive equipment is required. Medical statements are needed with the following diagnoses: spinal cord injury, cerebral palsy, uncontrolled hypertension, cerebrovascular accident, heart disease, traumatic or congenital brain damage or other cognitive deficits, amputation, visual deficit, and orthopedic problem. The medical review board of the state licensing agency may require the driver to resubmit information yearly to maintain a valid license. Periodic reviews usually are required for people with such progressive disorders as multiple sclerosis, muscular dystrophy, and psychiatric impairment; seizures, epilepsy, and a history of blackouts or dizzy spells; or a history of alcohol or drug abuse. Typically, a driver must be seizure-, drug-, or alcohol-free for a minimum of 6 months, but some states mandate that drivers in those groups meet a 1-year requirement.

Each state has different requirements for driver education and minimum age to obtain a permit. It is best for all first-time drivers to receive classroom training through a high school, a local driving school, a driver educator, or a CDRS. This training will prepare them for the basics of driving: how to identify road signs and road markings and how to maintain the vehicle, for example. It also can expose them to the Smith System, a driver training program that teaches eye–mind coordination to prevent collisions before they happen (Smith System, n.d.).

Smith System training can help drivers to see, think, and act their way through a multitude of driving environments. Total awareness, perceptive anticipation, accurate forecasting, early detection, and deliberate reaction are the primary features of the technique. By emphasizing greater visibility and maintaining more space surrounding the vehicle, the Smith System teaches a driver how to create more time to react to driving challenges. The CDRS must teach clients to look ahead and understand the big picture. Doing so requires that drivers keep their eyes moving at all times to alert the brain to any danger along the path ahead.

Clinical Evaluation

When looking for a CDRS, a prospective driver needs assurance that the instructor can and will complete the clinical evaluation before beginning on-the-road driver's training. The clinical evaluation consists of assessing the client's visual, perceptual, cognitive, and physical function. It is important to understand that if the clinician does not feel comfortable evaluating the above-mentioned areas, the client needs to be referred to the appropriate professional.

An initial interview with the client seeks important information: Has the client ever driven before? What are the client's concerns about driving? Where will the client be driving? How often will the client drive? The CDRS must ascertain whether the client is someone who fatigues easily, note what medications the client takes and how often the client reports taking them, review medical records and ask whether there is any drug or alcohol abuse, and identify diabetes or the presence of a progressive disorder. The local department of motor vehicles should have information about whether the client already holds a valid license and what restrictions if any have been placed on that license.

Visual Evaluation

It is crucial that clients' vision be tested thoroughly. Other sensory systems, such as the vestibular system and the auditory system, react to motion and sound, but the visual system allows one to anticipate what may happen. Therefore, we need a good working visual system to allow safe driving.

The clinical visual assessment evaluates visual acuity, peripheral field of vision, alignment of the eyes, range of motion of the eyes, convergence, saccades (rapid eye movement), pursuits, and scanning. Visual acuity is the ability to look at close and distant objects. It is imperative to note clients' visual acuity, and the evaluation should be done with and without corrective lenses if they are used by the client. Visual acuity can be measured by using the Bernell or Snellen visual charts, an American Automobile Association tester, Porto-Clinic, or the Optic 2000 (Stereo Optical Company). In most states, the licensing agencies set restrictions for distance acuity only. It is very important to know that each state differs, so CDRSs must learn local requirements.

The CDRS must evaluate oculomotor skills for each eye: range of motion, saccades, visual fixation, and visual scanning. It should be noted whether the eyes work together or separately from one another—a condition that is not unusual for people with some developmental disabilities. Visual tracking and visual scanning might not be intact. Depth perception and color perception also should be evaluated during the clinical visual assessment. The alignment of the eyes can be tested with the alternate cover test. If a client's eyes are not aligned, the neuroplasticity of the brain can allow the suppression of one eye or the other. This, too, would need to be evaluated during the clinical visual assessment. The Keystone Telebinocular System and the Optic 2000 are used to test for suppression. People with some disabilities, such as cerebral palsy, sometimes exhibit visual deficits early on in their lives with maybe a ptosis of eyelids or misalignment of the eyes. Saccades are very important. Clients with saccades deficits have difficulty looking from the rearview mirror to the side mirrors, back to the front of the vehicle, down to the dashboard, and again back to the rearview mirror. Convergence of the eyes is central to the ability to check a speedometer rapidly and then look up through the windshield, for example. Clients who have deficits with tracking and scanning often have problems maintaining lane position. Remember that the visual system needs to accomplish tracking and scanning in a very accurate, adequate, and quick manner. It is important to note whether drivers maintain fixation on an object in front of them while confronted with other objects in their peripheral fields.

Every state has minimal standards for peripheral field of vision in drivers for daytime or nighttime driving. If a state allows bioptic telescopic driving (for people with macular degeneration, albinism, or retinitis pigmentosa), other visual guidelines apply. Most states do not specify peripheral fields as inferior, superior, nasal, and temporal. The state guidelines are concerned with the complete horizontal field of vision. On occasion, a client is unable to make use of a full horizontal field, and the CDRS might involve a behavioral optometrist in the driver training program. The behavioral optometrist might prescribe prism glasses to expand the driver's functional visual field.

As part of the visual evaluation, the CDRS might find that the driver would benefit from referral to an ophthalmologist or an optometrist. Ophthalmologists are licensed physicians who evaluate and diagnose visual deficits and eye diseases. They offer medical and surgical treatment. Optometrists are licensed health care professionals who examine the structure of the eyes, diagnose visual problems and eye disease, and prescribe corrective lenses. Some optometrists also provide developmental visual enhancement therapy (K. Clark, personal communication, May 1993).

The Neuro-Optometric Rehabilitation Association (NORA) is a group of behavioral optometrists concerned with vision and how it relates to a person's functional ability. Behavioral optometrists work with people who have blurred vision (diplopia), double vision (diploria), field loss (hemianopsia), altered spatial awareness, undiagnosed headaches, reduced reading skills, poor tracking skills, eye turnout or lag (strabismus), and poor hand–eye coordination. Optometrists sometimes use compensatory and training devices to improve the client's functional vision (NORA, n.d.).

Intervention from a behavioral optometrist can be useful, for example, in the case of a driver who mentions that he or she is having trouble distinguishing between two identical cars that appear in the rearview mirror. It would be important in that case to rule out ocular movement dysfunction. The behavioral optometrist can work on eye muscle exercises, which can help the client see only one object and see the objects more clearly. If treated successfully, the client could return to driver training. One-eyed drivers or people who have lateral hemianopsia in some cases can be trained to drive safely and efficiently with the adaptive techniques.

Perceptual Evaluation

The perceptual system allows the brain to understand or interpret what the eyes see. Therefore, it is imperative to have a good visual assessment. If the information is not getting into the brain correctly, the brain will be unable to process the information correctly. Visual perception then is more complex than visual function, because it requires the brain to search and receive the data correctly.

Perceptual skills can be measured through the Motor Free Visual Perceptual Test (MVPT), which assesses the visual figure–ground, or the ability to separate an object from the background by correctly placing it on the foreground, such as "the white towel on the white bedspread." People with figure–ground deficits would not be able to recognize this. It is imperative that drivers have adequate visual figure–ground ability so that they can distinguish one sign from a group of signs of similar size, shape, or color— for example, the ability to identify the sign pointing to Interstate 64 when there are numerous road signs surrounding it. Another figure–ground deficit can be noted when a driver pulls up to a busy intersection where there are two or three lanes with separate signal lights. If the driver can distinguish one from another, the driver is more likely to proceed safely through the intersection.

The MVPT also assesses visual memory and visual recall, which are important skills. If a client passed a construction site, he or she would need to remember to slow down and then accelerate to the regular posted speed limit. It is necessary in that case to be able to recall what the posted limit was. Visual closure is the ability to close off the objects in our mind. A client might have difficulty writing such letters as O, P, B, or D. However, with driving, visual closure will present the following: If a stop sign is partially blocked by a tree, the driver may not recognize it as a complete stop sign and thus fail to stop. In this case, the client does not recognize the whole picture. When, for example, the driver is passed by an ambulance that has its lights flashing and the driver does not understand that there could be an accident scene ahead, the driver might not release the accelerator and cover the brake in anticipation of a stop. A driver who has a deficit in the area of visual discrimination might mistake the object in front of the mailbox and learn too late that what looks like a ball is actually a dog that could run into the street in front of the vehicle. The MVPT also allows the CDRS to judge the client's visual-perceptual-processing time.

No single test can indicate whether a person can operate a motor vehicle safely. That is determined only with the on-the-road test drive. There are clients who will do extremely well on paper but will not be able to do well in the environment of driving. It is also true that clients who have done extremely poorly on the written tests have done well with the on-the-road driver's training. This is especially true for clients returning to driving after a disability or for clients who grew up in an environment where they drove tractors and lawn mowers. The clinical evaluations are not for passing or failing the client. The clinical evaluation gives the CDRS an idea of what to look for and what to anticipate on the road. The CDRS is then better able to identify the client's deficits, making appropriate accommodations for the client when training him or her to operate the motor vehicle. The state's visual requirement is the only one each client must meet to obtain a valid driver's license.

Cognition

Any of the routine modalities used for cross-training, including those for using full body movements and sensory integration to improve the client's tracking and scanning skills, also will be helpful for the beginning of driver training. However, it is imperative to note that, even with improvement in areas of visual, perceptual, or cognitive skills, the client still might not be able to do everything in an organized fashion. In that case, it is not safe for that client to operate a motor vehicle.

When making recommendations for driving, look at your test analyses, treatment plans, and goal setting. You may be doing more harm to the clients by building up false hopes. The clients may increase their working knowledge of rural roads and their awareness of the functions needed for driving, but when they put the fast-moving vehicle into an unpredictable environment, they may not be able to safely search, identify, predict, and decide fast enough to avoid a collision.

Searching is the ability to scan the environment with visual, auditory, and tactile techniques. The identifying phase of driving requires the ability to locate specific clues in the environment around the vehicle—road features and condition, traffic controls, other vehicles, and pedestrians. The predicting phase requires the ability to predict what others are going to do and anticipate the appropriate range of reactions. The decision phase requires the ability to recall and organize the data to take appropriate necessary actions (Edds, 2002). Does the client know to steer to the left while changing speed and using turn signals or the horn?

The ability to carry out a decision is the executing phase: "I need to make a lane change because the car in front of me is slowing down, so I need to check my rearview mirror, give my signal, do a head check, and pull over into the lane." Can the clients execute that decision appropriately?

Cognition requires the ability to interpret and comprehend a situation in its entirety by attending to the visually presented parts of the situation. It also requires the ability to distinguish essential from nonessential information. Cognition skills include sequential analysis (ability to comprehend the ordering of events) and problem solving (ability to seek relevant information and set goals in response). Self-monitoring (ability to observe and track one's own behavior and thought processes) is an important part of cognitive skill, as is the ability to choose and initiate responses swiftly. Cognitive skills also require the ability to inhibit responses, plan (devise, organize, and carry out steps necessary to achieve a goal), and maintain the same enactment of the plan over time. Cognitive skills require flexibility (the ability to shift responses in accord with new information). Therefore, cognition assessment is an imperative part of the driver's evaluation.

Cognitive evaluation can be done as preclinical testing, with an instrument such as the neurobehavioral cognitive status exam (NCSE) or with the trial-making A and B subtests. The CDRS can assess the way a client pulls out a chair and sits down, puts on his or her coat, and follows two- and three-step instructions. Cognitive information also should be obtained on the road.

Physical Evaluation

Another important assessment involves the driver's physical strength and endurance. There are guidelines that have been used for the exact dynamometer strength, and goniometer measurements can be used to assess range of motion, although the use of these tests has not been standardized for driving. Therefore, the CDRS needs to assess the client's ability to perform evasive maneuvers—controlled braking, off-road recovery, steering around corners—without physical intervention from the examiner. If the client cannot brake successfully, the cause is either decreased processing time or insufficient strength to apply the brake, and reduced-effort braking could be needed.

Garrison Jones (1997) discusses the physical evaluation:

The CDRS must look at the client's physical status. Are there any hearing limitations? What is the stability of the client when seated? Are there any limitations to the neck rotation to the right or to the left? The CDRS must also look for spasticity of both the upper and lower extremities. The following [range of motion] should be evaluated: the shoulder flexion, shoulder extension, shoulder horizontal movement, elbow and wrist flexion and extension, hip abduction and adduction, knee flexion and extension, and dorsiflexion and plantar flexion of the ankle. The individual's overall endurance and coordination should be assessed. Simple coordination tests such as bringing the index fingers to the nose, or even performing rapid alternating movement (diadochokinesia) can be used. Sensation, position sense, and stimulus location may also be evaluated. A seating evaluation may also be needed, depending upon the individual's trunk stability. (pp. 641–642)

At the end of all of the above evaluations, it is likely that rapport will have been established with the client. The CDRS should be comfortable with taking the client out on the road for the driver assessment.

Test Drive

All vehicles that are licensed through a commercial driving school for driver training are to be marked with "student driver" signs on both sides of the vehicle and to the rear. Depending on the state, a "student driver" sign on top of the vehicle also can be required. It is strongly suggested that all vehicles that are used for driver training have an instructor's brake installed. The road evaluation should begin in a very simple environment and progress to residential, highway, city, and interstate traffic. This part is the evaluation and not driver training. Therefore, if at all possible, the CDRS should have determined a standard route, so that all clients perform the same maneuvers. The CDRS needs to develop a road course for the test drive (this is the preferred method for driver training as well). The standardization allows the CDRS to state objectively what all drivers should do and how each driver actually performs. It also shows that all clients are subjected to the same degree of difficulty in training and testing.

A task analysis should be performed, including exact requirements, before the route is determined. This analysis allows the CDRS to have specific checklist items: Client stops at traffic light limit line, gives correct signal, maintains lane position. Checklists should always be used for objective documentation, and there must be a consistent standard for all clients.

It might be determined that the client has the potential to operate a motor vehicle and could be reevaluated after 6 months or a year. During that time, the client might be directed to increase hand–eye control. Sometimes people buy steering wheels from auto parts dealers and then mount the wheels on two-by-fours for use in practicing steering, increasing strength, and building and increasing range of motion. If the CDRS can break down driving into discrete tasks, the client can have a list of skills to improve that can be incorporated into a treatment plan.

Alternatively, the CDRS could determine that a client will never be able to successfully operate a motor vehicle. The client must know that and be offered alternatives modes of transportation. People whose physical limitations require automobile modification systems that are too costly might consider purchasing a van modified for their transportation and hiring drivers. (The cost for passenger transportation or driving a van from a wheelchair typically averages $40,000 using low-tech primary controls and can run as high as $80,000 to $90,000 when using high-tech primary control options.)

Case Examples

A 28-year-old man diagnosed with cerebral palsy and learning disabilities was referred to the driving instructor. Because the evaluation showed that he could not be an independent driver, he purchased a custom-modified van and hired a coworker to drive him to and from work.

Another client was diagnosed with mild retardation and physical limitations and had never worked before. At age 32 he completed driver training with a modified van and was able to work out of his home as a Web-page designer. Because he was able to drive, he was able to purchase office supplies and services and visit his customers. After a year of working, he was a taxpayer who no longer required government assistance. He also stated that he was able to buy Christmas presents because he could go shopping.

A client with mild cerebral palsy and C5 tetraplegia was able to find employment after driver training. "I would again pay the $92,000 for me to drive," he reported. "I can finally take my mom to McDonald's. She was the one who always tied my shoes for me and got me dressed."

Driver Training

There are instances when the professional will determine that a client can drive with adaptive equipment and training. That driver's training should incorporate residential, highway, city, and interstate traffic. The client should be given the opportunity to train at night. Training to go to a drive-through window at a bank or fast-food restaurant is imperative. Off-road recovery is very important, especially for new drivers. Clients need to learn the eight colors and eight shapes of road signs. They need to know there is decreased visibility on hills and curves. They must understand that as speed increases, the driver's peripheral field decreases. Sharing the road with big trucks, which can weigh more than 40 times what a car weighs, requires understanding that trucks cannot stop quickly. It is important for drivers to understand the causes of hydroplaning and why tire inflation and condition are important aspects of safety. It is also important to remind drivers to inspect their cars— including the tires—at least once a week. Clients must understand that they can control only the space that is in front of them, so it is important to have a "cushion" around them, or a "gap acceptance" to the front and the rear of the vehicle at all times.

There is other useful information: It takes 48 seconds to clear an intersection from a stop. Drivers must keep their eyes moving constantly (scanning) and concentrate on the intended path of travel. Drivers who have decreased vision at night will need to drive more slowly than in the daylight, and they need to remember not to override their headlights (high beams show 350–500 feet, low beams show at 100 feet) (Thiel, Gaines, & Taylor, 1987). The CDRS must remember to put books, clothing, and other loose objects into the trunk of the vehicle, because those objects can become projectiles in case of a sudden stop or an accident.

It is important to use "commentary driving," that is, the driver giving short appraisals of what he or she is doing, where he or she is going, and how to accomplish that. Commentary driving is really a method of checking out whether the driver is able to identify the highway and the cues that should direct the driver's response to conditions. It consists of making comments about the current traffic scene (Stockton & Macy, 1989). Anything that can affect the path of travel should be described, including what is visible ahead, to both sides, and in the rearview mirror. The method helps the client identify things quickly and gives the CDRS a better idea of what the client is seeing.

As a client progresses, the CDRS could even teach defensive driving, through reaction and serpentine courses. This method will help identify the client's indecision on approach of even the first cone. The CDRS might find that the client fails to maintain proper speed or uses improper hand position. A client might also oversteer, causing greater weight change and spinout of the vehicle. On the reaction course, a client might exhibit jerky movements, wrong reaction, or a failure to anticipate a signal.

The CDRS must be able to complete the serpentine and reaction courses as well, to ensure the instructor's ability to deal with an emergency should the client make an inappropriate turn. Some state highway administrations offer defensive-driver training. In one case, the state police allowed the therapists who were in training to be driver educators and trainers to participate in a program on the same road course and offering the same evasive training that state troopers complete. An experience of that kind can greatly increase the ability of a trainer to cope with unexpected situations.

The CDRS should use a daily checklist to show progress or lack of progress for each client. Students should not listen to the radio during training sessions until the end of the course. At that time, the CDRS should use CD players, cell phones, and radios to test for distractibility. Clients will need to know how to use radios and cell phones safely. Clients should be instructed that cell phones are for emergency use only and that every driver should pull safely to the side of the road before making a phone call.

The minimum that a CDRS should accept for a client is an average level of driving skill. This standard is for the protection of the client as well as for the protection of other drivers. The most common reasons for client failure to pass road tests administered by CDRSs are anxiousness, lack of judgment skills, inability to complete multiple steps, lack of recall for the rules learned, poor decision-making skills, failure of the state's written test, lack of concentration, inconsistent class attendance, and a lack of control of emotions. At a 1-year follow-up with clients with mental retardation/learning disabilities who had been trained through driver education at a local vocational rehabilitation center, many clients had stopped driving either because family members would not allow them to continue or because they did not have enough money to buy and register a vehicle.

Liability Issues

Liability issues vary by state, and state and federal laws change. CDRSs must continue to keep up with the regulations and know that they are responsible for a release of information. A major issue for people who have suspended licenses is that the CDRS releases confidential information. However, anyone can release information to the motor vehicle administration if he or she feels that the public is in danger because of a driver's disability. (Some states even grant anonymity to physicians and family members who report such information to the motor vehicle administration.) A rising issue is the 1:1 ratio of driver to evaluator in the vehicle. Drivers have stated that the evaluator/trainer has used inappropriate comments or gestures. Some trainers have chosen to install auditory or video equipment on their training vehicles.

Insurance Issues

Drivers with disabilities should obtain insurance for all assistive devices installed on their vehicle. This insurance is in addition to insurance on the vehicles themselves. Clients must inform the insurance agent about the adaptive equipment of the vehicle. They may need to pay higher premiums because they would be listed as new drivers. Clients should not have any difficulty obtaining insurance coverage. The Americans With Disabilities Act does not allow insurance companies to discriminate because of disabilities.

Funding

Typically, the cost of drivers' evaluations is not reimbursed through third parties such as Medicare, Medicaid, or private medical insurance carriers because it is considered a medical luxury. Some clinicians will use certain status codes to get reimbursement through functional mobility. This is not recommended. Reimbursement is also available through new Medicare guidelines. However, the clinician may need to go through many appeals processes before payment is received. Most reimbursement and funding come through state Workers' Compensation and vocational rehabilitation programs. If the client is school age, P.L. 94–142 (the Education for All Handicapped Children Act) may help with partial payment for the driver assessment.

Vehicle Selection

One goal of the CDRS is to give independence through mobility. In some cases it will be useful to modify or adapt a vehicle to accommodate a driver who has disabilities. One of the first things to examine is how the client gets in and out of the vehicle. It is typically recommended that people who are planning to load their own wheelchairs purchase a two-door car. (However, a four-door car with a bench-style seat can also be used.) Power windows, door locks, and mirrors are also suggested. All vehicles that are to be modified with hand controls must have power brakes, power steering, and automatic transmission.

Vehicular modifications might also be needed for people who are transported rather than who drive themselves. The required adaptations depend on the client's height, wheelchair measurements, and family needs. If the person will be driving, the CDRS will prescribe the appropriate height to sit behind the steering wheel, the appropriate strength, and needed modifications (see the end of the chapter for how to match equipment to client needs).

Remember that driving is an independent task. It is one activity of daily living that cannot be at a minimum-assist level. A driver must be fully independent. During the past several years,

> Manufacturers of vehicles [have been] getting serious about answering the call for help for persons with disabilities by increasing leg room, making entry easier, use of friendly control panels, and much more. The goal is to keep persons behind the wheel longer, and making it safer for them to operate the motor vehicle. Making the car more ergonomic, by making the internal controls' size and shape to conform to one's natural movement, is becoming more common. (Dimartino, 2002, pp. 47–49)

The following features can be useful for people who need to modify vehicles to accommodate their disabilities:

- Auto-dimming rearview mirrors help dampen bright lights.

- Heated outside mirrors dissipate condensation and eliminate the need to reach out and clean them.
- Heated seats can reduce stiffness and pain.
- Higher seats reduce the amount of bending and stooping for entering and exiting, resulting in less strain on the back, legs, and torso.
- Quick-launch and seamless gearshifts do not require the driver to push or pull with the arms and hands.
- The memory driver's seat eliminates the need to exert effort to reset the driver's seat when entering the car. The seat automatically returns to the seat conformations on demand.
- Power-tilt and telescoping steering wheels move the steering wheel up or down, in or out from the column to allow the maximum amount of space when entering and exiting the vehicle.
- Eight-way power driver's seats offer more options for positioning and allow drivers to change position to relieve pressure during long drives.
- Remote keyless entry allows drivers to enter the vehicle without unlocking the door, thus reducing stress on the hands and fingers.
- Shorter wheelbases are easier to turn and manipulate in tight parking spaces.
- Side third rear access door columns allow fuller access to the back seat for loading and unloading, with less physical effort.
- Left-to-right dash-mounted ignition switches reduce the motion needed to activate the steering column.
- Adjustable pedals are controlled with a dashboard button that allows the driver to move accelerator and brake pedals toward or away from the driver. This feature eliminates stress and pressure on the legs, ankles, and feet. It coordinates with the power seats to allow a driver to customize driving position.
- Adaptive cruise control eliminates the need to keep the foot on the accelerator, automatically adjusting the vehicle speed to maintain a safe following distance from the car ahead, thereby reducing the need to use the brake pedal.

There are several features that clients have noted that make driving a possiblity (Dimartino, 2002):

- Adjustable seats allow drivers to move easily to their favorite position.
- Door handles that are at right angles allow for easier grasp.
- Leather seats allow sliding in and out more freely.
- Push-button starters remove the need to turn an ignition key.
- Straight-back seats keep posture aligned.
- Padded door handles and steering wheels are more comfortable to use.

It is important to test drive a car before purchase to ensure that the driver will be comfortable during driving. Purchasers should note pressure on the limbs, neck, head, or torso. Check to be sure that the trunk and doors are easily opened and closed. Remember that the preceding are only guidelines; people with disabilities all function differently, and they should be fully evaluated by the CDRS before learning to operate (or returning to operating) a motor vehicle. The CDRS also should be aware of all the equipment needs and the type of basic equipment available. The following sections describe some of the modifications that can be made to vehicles for people with disabilities.

Wheelchair Loaders

Four basic wheelchair carriers are available, some of them for people who cannot load their own chairs:

- Pickup carriers automatically fold and load wheelchairs into the back of pickup trucks.
- Bumper-mounted carriers require that someone fold and place a wheelchair on the carrier.
- Hitch-mounted carriers automatically fold a wheelchair and hold it in place on the back of the vehicle or inside a vehicle's trunk.
- Car-top carriers automatically fold and load a wheelchair onto the top of the car.

Pedal Extensions

Pedal extensions are available for people whose legs are not long enough to operate the existing acceleration and braking controls. Some units provide a quick release, and some units fold down to move the pedals out of the way for a driver who does not have disabilities.

Left-Foot Accelerator

Like pedal extensions, when not in use, the unit can be removed from its base or folded down toward the floor to allow a person without disability to operate the motor vehicle.

Hand Controls

When operating vehicles by hand controls, drivers should steer with their stronger arm. Hand controls can be placed on the right or the left side and should be adapted with horn and dimmer switch as needed. Hand controls will fall into one of four categories:

- Standard right-angle hand controls, the most common type, are operated by pulling the handle toward the floor to accelerate and pushing back toward the dashboard to brake. They typically are mounted on the left-hand side of the dashboard.

- Push–pull controls are operated by being pulled toward the driver to accelerate and pushed back toward the dashboard to brake. Push–pull hand controls can be used with reduced-effort gas and brake systems.
- Push–twist controls work by twisting the throttle to accelerate (like a motorcycle throttle) and pushing back toward the dashboard to brake.
- Floor-mounted push–pull controls extend upward from the floor and allow the client full active range of motion. They can be used by drivers who cannot use column-mounted mechanical devices, such as some people with C6–C7 tetraplegia.

Steering Devices

Drivers who use hand controls will have only one hand to steer the vehicle and therefore will need an adaptive device for steering. It is suggested that a steering device be placed between the 4 and 5 o'clock positions on the steering wheel for use with the right upper extremity and between the 7 and 8 o'clock positions for use with the left upper extremity, so that it is located below the airbag. There are several types of steering device:

- Spinner knobs are the most common type. They require a functional grasp and intact active range of motion in the limb.
- Amputee rings are used by people who steer with prostheses.
- U-grips require minimal grasp efficiency; they generally are used by drivers who have a loss of finger function but typically have wrist motion.
- Tri-pin spinner knobs consist of series of three posts arranged in a triangle; the bottom two posts support the wrist and each side, and the third fits in the palm of the hand with the thumb wrapping around the top post. They are used to stabilize the hand and the wrist.

Van Modification

It is important to shop carefully for a full-size van that is to be converted for transportation or for use by a driver who uses a wheelchair. Some vans can be ordered from the manufacturer already modified with floors that are lowered by 9 inches. For people who want to use a van with a floor that is lowered only by 4 or 6 inches, or with a raised roof, the following are the suggested options:

- V-8 engine or equivalent
- Long wheel base
- Automatic transmission
- Power steering
- Power brakes

- Heavy-duty battery
- Heavy-duty alternator
- Privacy glass
- Swinging, as opposed to sliding, doors
- Super engine cooling package, to include heavy-duty radiator, transmission cooling
- Tilt steering wheel
- Power windows and door locks.

Typically, an interior height of at least 2 ½ inches above the client's sitting height is recommended. Lowering the floor or raising the roof of the vehicle can create the desired interior height. When a lowered floor is chosen, the floor must meet National Mobility Equipment Dealers Association (NMEDA) and Society of Automotive Engineers (SAE) standards. The dropped floor should extend up into the driver area if the person is to be driving from a wheelchair. It is then typically recommended that the dropped floor be undercoated, rustproofed, primed, and painted. Floor lowering is usually attempted only for vans that have a separate body and chassis (such as the Ford van). If a raised roof is chosen or added, additional structural supports (roll bars) are recommended for client safety in the event of a rollover collision (Garrison Jones, 1997).

Van Entry

The first thing to consider for entry and exit is exterior-mounted controls, most often accomplished through remote control or magnetic keyless entry. After the doors are open, the client can choose from a lift or a ramp to independently get in and out of the van. Drivers who use this type of vehicle need to have fully automatic lifts with outside door contols, internal- and external-mounted controls, and manual backup systems.

There are three basic types of lift: the platform lift (which can be semi- or fully automatic), the rotary lift, and the under-the-vehicle lift. Each has advantages and disadvantages that should be evaluated depending on the type of vehicle, the type of wheelchair, and the client's preference. This is very important if the client has family members who will be transported; the front passenger's seat might need to be in a fully upright position for correct lift placement. If such a position presents a problem for the person who is to use the front passenger seat, the client might want to purchase an under-the-vehicle lift. It is imperative to ascertain client preferences during the interview and to determine how a vehicle is to be used to specify the appropriate modifications.

Safety Equipment

Drivers with disabilities must be able to operate seatbelts without assistance, and seatbelt systems must meet federal safety standards. The Grandmar Torso-Support Positioning Belt is designed for drivers with poor upper-body strength. The Grandmar prevents unwanted forward and lateral movement and maintains the torso in proper mid-line position while sitting. The dual-strap composition ensures secure torso position without restricting breathing (International Medical Equipment Corporation, n.d.). The CDRS might order a belt custom-fit to the client's measurements or one that is adjustable for use during driver evaluations. The recommended chest strap material is 4-inch-wide soft-loop fabric. That belt is only an upper-torso support device designed for postural support to keep a client in the desired position; it is not intended to provide occupant restraint during vehicle impact.

It is also recommended that a passenger wheelchair restraint system be mounted in the rear of the van in case of emergency. This restraint system must be forward facing because side-facing systems provide inadequate protection in a crash. The passenger wheelchair restraint also must include lap and shoulder belts that are separate from the wheelchair. If the person is driving from a wheelchair, a power wheelchair lockdown in the driver area with separate lap and shoulder belt mechanisms must be installed.

Even if a client will not be driving, a thorough evaluation is needed to obtain the same kinds of information just detailed. How tall does the client sit in his or her wheelchair? How wide is the wheelchair? What is the length of the individual from the tip of the wheelie bars to the tip of the toes? The occupational therapist also will need to consider the type of lift that is preferred and whether a lowered floor or raised roof is required. If the roof is raised, the client's height in the wheelchair also will dictate whether the size of the door opening will require modification. Passengers who use wheelchairs need to be in forward-facing, four-point tie-down systems as well. Because all people with disabilities have unique circumstances, caregivers might not use appropriate tie-down techniques, and it is strongly suggested that power lockdown systems be installed, even for passenger transportation. The van prescription also might need to address safety issues for a person who is ventilator dependent and for someone who uses assistive communication (lapboard).

Primary Driving Devices

Some drivers with disabilities will have general muscle weakness and require special adaptation for steering and braking. People who cannot operate standard power-steering systems can obtain modifications to the steering column and steering resistance by having reduced- or low-effort steering devices added to the vehicle. Although most steering reductions are achieved by modifying the existing steering column, digital and hydraulic–electric auxiliary systems are available that allow more flexibility in placement. A backup system should be installed for safety in the event of a system failure (Nead, 1997). A backup system allows the driver to safely pull the vehicle to the side of the road and out of the way of traffic until help arrives.

The following assistive devices can be added to some vehicles (Garrison Jones, 1997):

- Reduced- or low-effort steering is for those people who have limited use of the upper extremities. The effort required to steer the vehicle is reduced by 30%–40%.
- Zero-effort steering reduces the effort required by 60%–70%.
- Horizontal steering wheels are placed horizontal to the client's lap, therefore decreasing the need for full range of motion in the upper extremities.
- Electronic steering and electronic gas and braking systems and combination hydraulic–electric equipment allow people with even the most limited strength, endurance, and range of motion to operate motor vehicles safely.
- Joystick controls are similar to those used for electric-powered wheelchairs; they require the use of only one extremity for steering, braking, and acceleration of the vehicle.

Accessory Switches and Console Operations

After the primary driving modifications have been determined, it is still necessary to determine whether accessory switches are needed for secondary controls. Some drivers will require modifications that allow them to use the vehicle's horn, lights, directional signals, and windshield wipers. When choosing a console system, you must see what features work best with the client. Note how the client will use the ignition, gear shift, turn signals, wipers, cruise control, horn, dimmer, heating, ventilation, air conditioning, parking brake, front and rear fans, windows, door locks, wheelchair restraints, and dome light.

The features differ for many consoles. Individuals who use joystick systems for driving and who have the use of just one extremity often require touch buttons to operate such essential functions as left and right turn signals, horn, dimmer, windshield wipers, and cruise control. Some drivers also will require powered headrests. In some cases, it is possible to install voice-activated systems that allow the driver to operate vehicle functions with speech.

It is important to note that standard vehicle types change every year. NMEDA and SAE have set standards of practice and safety for the vehicle modification industry. Installation of all adaptive equipment should be done by NMEDA-certified dealers. In general, vehicle modifications should allow modified vehicles to be used by people who do not have disabilities.

Disabilities

It could be necessary for a driver with disabilities to use cushions or power seats to adjust for adequate height to be able to see over the steering wheel.

It is important to remember that the client's head height should not be higher than the rearview mirror. There are cases in which the CDRS will need to work with a rehabilitation engineer to fabricate a seating system that is safe for the individual client. The following is a brief overview of disabilities and how they can affect driving.

Learning Disabilities and Attention Deficit Hyperactivity Disorder

Attention deficit hyperactivity disorder (ADHD) is known to consist of developmental deficiencies in the regulation and maintenance of behaviors. Those deficiencies give rise to problems with inhibiting, initiating, or sustaining responses to a task and with adhering to rules and instructions. The major components of ADHD are inattention, impulsivity, and overactivity. ADHD is broken down into subgroups as well. There are 14 diagnostic criteria for ADHD, including the following: has difficulty following through on instructions, does not seem to listen to what is being said, has difficulty sustaining attention to a task, often engages in physically dangerous activity, and performance is uneven. People with ADHD make careless mistakes. ADHD is considered an "output" problem as opposed to an "input" problem. Often those with ADHD are not persistent in applying effort. Those with ADHD usually have diminished ability to regulate their behavior, inability to organize and plan behavior over time, and a diminished social effectiveness and adaptability (Chritie, 1995).

Clients with ADHD typically engage in physically dangerous tasks, they do not always recognize cause and effect, they tend to be impulsive and inattentive, and they can experience side effects of medication. It is important to give an extended road test to anyone who has a learning disability, especially ADHD. The question of whether the person with ADHD can drive must be carefully examined. Driving involves more than accelerating, braking, and steering; it consists of taking skilled and properly timed actions under varying road conditions, based on decisions that depend on sound judgment, realistic perception, and learned information. The fact that people with ADHD usually are 5 to 6 years behind their peer group in maturity could account for some proportion of their involvement with traffic accidents (Chritie, 1995).

In my experience, drivers with ADHD are involved in significantly more accidents, particularly "fender benders," than are non-ADHD drivers. Many of these collisions occur at traffic lights and are the result of starting too quickly or not stopping quickly enough. A significant number of violations occur for failing to observe "no turn on red" signs. Sometimes ADHD drivers back up but forget to check the rearview mirror, or their impulsivity leads them to get out of the car without putting it into park. It is imperative that ADHD drivers be tested thoroughly on the road because they typically do well in the prescreening evaluation.

Typically, clients with learning or emotional disabilities do not perform consistently from day to day, so an extended period of road training is recommended. Precise checklists of the client's action on test drives also can be a good indicator of progress. Appendix 13.B is a checklist for driver training and evaluation. The CDRS should collect data for at least 5 days and average the results. If a client cannot go 3 consecutive days without a lower score, or without the need for spoken cues of some sort, the client probably should not drive. The CDRS should be sure to have an objective way to measure and document the client's behind-the-wheel performance.

Cerebral Palsy

Cerebral palsy refers to several disorders of movement that result from damage to the brain. The symptoms depend on the location of the damage, and they can cause significant impairment in speech, sensation, perception, and intellectual development. They also can cause seizure disorders, emotional problems, and involuntary muscle movement. The extent of visual-perceptual, cognitive, and muscle tone impairment determine ability to drive. The presence of spasticity can require push–pull hand controls. As with all disabilities, it is necessary for drivers with cerebral palsy to be able to enter and exit the vehicle appropriately, fasten seat belts, and load necessary ambulatory or assistive devices.

Spina Bifida

Spina bifida is a birth anomaly that is caused by the prenatal failure of the vertebral canal to close normally around the posterior end of the spinal cord. The effects can include weakness or paralysis of the lower extremities, visual-perceptual deficits, and abnormal sensation in the lower legs and back. Depending on the extent of disability, the person with spina bifida might be unable to reach and operate the accelerator or brake pedal. The person also might have difficulty getting into and out of the seated position. The need for vehicular modification will depend on the parts of the body that are affected and on any deficits in strength and joint mobility. Some clients may require hand controls, spinner knobs, and transfer boards; others might require wheelchair-accessible vans. There is a universal legal requirement for drivers to use lap and shoulder belts, and difficulty can arise because of those devices' interference with colostomy bags (Sabo & Shipp, 1980).

Spinal Cord Injury

People with spinal cord injuries have disabilities that can range from mild to severe. Specially modified vans are required for people who are unable to enter or exit a vehicle or wheelchair unassisted. The clinician should determine whether the client has muscle spasms; whether that condition will interfere with the operation of a vehicle; and whether the spasms are controlled through medication, positioning, or restraint.

Brain Injury

A person who experienced a traumatic brain injury at or near birth, or who has an acquired brain injury, often can have numerous deficits, muscle loss, and loss of sensation. Speech and perceptual skills also can be affected, as can cognitive skills such as problem solving, judgment, memory, and attention span. Mood and personality changes also can occur. Because the symptoms resulting from traumatic brain injury vary, significant time will need to be devoted to the preclinical assessment, and even more time should be devoted to the on-the-road assessment. Assessment can include extended test drives and the evaluation of skills over a period of days.

Dwarfism

Disproportional short stature, occurring primarily in the trunk or limbs, cannot in and of itself be considered a disability. However, depending on the type of dwarfism, joint stiffness, hand deformity, hip dislocation, spinal curvature, and hand–eye coordination problems may occur. Proper seating can present the greatest difficulty. In some cases, a driver with dwarfism might need no more than a set of pedal extensions; in others, a modified van will be required (Sabo & Shipp, 1980).

Other Disabilities

The lists that follow are the common modifications required, by disabling condition, for motor vehicles (Garrison Jones, 1997).

Right Hemiplegia
- Left-foot accelerator
- Left spinner knob
- Automatic transmission
- Optional gear selector extension
- Hand-operated dimmer switch.

Left Hemiplegia
- Regular gas and brake pedals
- Right spinner knob
- Automatic transmission
- Right directional signal cross-over
- Hand-operated dimmer switch on the right side.

Paraplegia
- Hand controls for braking and acceleration with dimmer switch and horn button

- Automatic transmission
- Emergency brake pedal extension
- Steering device.

Tetraplegia

- Hand controls for brake and acceleration, with dimmer switch and horn button
- Automatic transmission
- Emergency brake extension
- Torso support device that allows for anterior and posterior stability and lateral positioning
- Steering device (U-grip, Tri-pin).

Some people with tetraplegia (C5 and above) might require the use of computer-assisted devices described earlier in this chapter.

Bilateral Lower Extremity–Limb Amputee

- Hand-controlled brake and accelerator, with dimmer switch and horn button
- Steering device
- Automatic transmission
- Emergency brake extension
- Torso support device
- Directional signal adapter.

Bilateral Upper Extremity–Limb Amputee

- One or two rings for steering
- Gear lever extension
- Extensions for dashboard accessory controls (lights, fans, windows)
- Foot steering.

In the case of a person with arthrogryposis, where there might be no limb present, foot steering would be an option, and secondary controls for the lights, horn, and fan, for example, would be mounted on the floor.

Right Lower Extremity–Limb Amputee

- Left-foot accelerator
- Automatic transmission.

Left Lower Extremity–Limb Amputee

- Automatic transmission.

Dwarfism, Congenital Smallness, Growth Disorders

- Adjusted seat
- Pedal extensions
- Switch extensions
- Dashboard and ignition control extensions.

Cerebral Palsy
- Hand controls for accelerating and braking, with horn and dimmer switch (push–pull hand controls typically are recommended for people with cerebral palsy to compensate for spasticity)
- Automatic transmission
- Parking brake extension
- Steering device.

Conclusion

It is important to remember that driving is significant for most people and that, with the continuing improvement in technology, even more adaptive driving equipment will become available to people with disabilities. The appendixes to this chapter detail a list of organizations and terminology (Appendix 13.A), a checklist for driver evaluation and training (Appendix 13.B), a sample consent form (Appendix 13.C), case studies for three drivers with disabilities (Appendix 13.D), and a noninclusive list of resources and suppliers (Appendix 13.E). No endorsement of suppliers or vendors listed in Appendix 13.E should be inferred. Appendix 13.D can be used as a template for driving instructors who are in need of evaluation and training reports.

References

American Automobile Association. (1993). *How to drive.* Heathrow, FL: Author.

Association for Driver Rehabilitation Specialists. (n.d.). Retrieved December 15, 2003, from http://www.driver-ed.org.

Chritie, L. (1995, February). *Attention deficits in children and adults.* Conference presented by Professional Development Resources, Jacksonville, FL.

Dimartino, C. (2002). Freedom on four wheels. *Arthritis Today, 16*(2), 44–53.

Edds, J. (2002). *Driver rehabilitation—Gateway to independence.* St Louis, MO: Author.

Garrison Jones, D. (1997). Assistive devices for driving. In B. Goldberg & J. Hsu (Eds.), *Atlas of arthoses and assistive devices* (3rd ed., pp. 641–654). St. Louis, MO: Mosby.

International Medical Equipment Corporation. (n.d.). Retrieved December 15, 2003, from http://www.imec-online.com.

Nead, R. (1997). Behind-the-wheel driver training. In B. Bain & D. Leger (Eds.), *Assistive technology—An interdisciplinary approach* (pp. 209–221). New York: Churchill Livingstone.

Neuro-Optometric Rehabilitation Association. (n.d). Retrieved December 15, 2003, from http://www.nora.cc.

Sabo, S., & Shipp, M. (1980, March). *Disabilities and their implications for driving.* (Unpublished grant information). Ruston: Louisiana Techical University, Center for Rehabilitation Science and Biomedical Engineering.

Smith System. (n.d.). Retrieved December 15, 2003, from http://www.smith-system.com.

Stockton, E., & Macy, R. (1989, June). *Various driving techniques to enhance driver training.* Workshop presented for In-Car Instructors Driver Education, State Police Academy, Richmond, VA.

Thiel, R., Gaines, J., & Taylor, K. (1987). *Drive right—A responsible approach* (8th ed.). Glenview, IL: Scott, Foresman.

Suggested Reading

American Automobile Association. (1986). *Managing time, space, visibility.* Falls Church, VA: Author.

Appendix 13.A. Organizations and Terms

AAA	American Automobile Association
AAMVA	American Association of Motor Vehicle Administrations
AARP	American Association of Retired Persons
ADED	Association of Driver Rehabilitation Specialists
ADTSEA	American Driver and Traffic Safety Education Association
CDRS	certified driver rehabilitation specialist
DOT	Department of Transportation
DSAA	Driver Schools Association of America
DRS	Department of Rehabilitation Services
FMVSS	Federal Motor Vehicle Safety Standards
Gap acceptance	Safe interaction of a vehicle with other road users to the front, sides, and rear
HTS	Highway Transportation System (traffic safety)
Limit line	The ability to stop a vehicle safely and completely at a given point
MVPT	Motor-Free Visual Perceptual Test
NDR	National Driver Records
NHTSA	National Highway Traffic Safety Administration
NMEDA	National Mobility Equipment Dealers Association
NORA	Neuro-Optometric Rehabilitation Association
OEM	original equipment manufacturer
ROM	range of motion
SAE	Society of Automotive Engineers
Travel path	Keeping the vehicle in a straight line within the lane
VA	Veterans Administration
VADETS	Virginia Driver Education Training Society (each state has its own driving school association)

Appendix 13.B. Driver Evaluation/Driver Training Checklist

- *Preparation to drive:* Does the driver adjust the seatbelt, mirror, and seat and check placement and operation of secondary controls?
- *Basic maneuvers:* Does the driver accelerate and brake smoothly? Is braking controlled? Are turning, driving straight forward, driving in reverse, and maintaining the appropriate distance between vehicles executed correctly?
- *Minimal traffic:* Is speed control appropriate? Is lane placement with right turns correct? When making left turns, does the driver maintain correct lane placement and speed, check both ways at intersections, give signals at least 100 feet before turns, make full stops, and control speed curves and hills?
- *Moderate to heavy traffic:* The areas to consider are the same as those for minimal traffic. Look more closely at eye checks: Does the client do blind-spot checks? Does the driver merge appropriately, adjust speed when passing appropriately, and adjust speed for different road surfaces?
- *Defensive driving:* Does the driver yield to other drivers, identify potential hazards, and determine and execute appropriate action?

Additional Comments

Note whether any physical assistance was needed with steering, accelerating, or braking throughout the driver's training. Note how often physical assistance and spoken cues were needed to maintain the correct position and appropriate speed.

Driving instructors can arrange their own checklists to include any of the items above and note with either a 1-to-5 rating scale or a scale of "Satisfactory," "Unsatisfactory," "Needs Improvement," or "Cues Needed."

Appendix 13.C. Sample Consent Form

I AUTHORIZE RELEASE OF ANY MEDICAL, PSYCHOLOGICAL, VISUAL, OR OTHER PERTINENT INFORMATION THAT WOULD ASSIST IN DETERMINING MY ABILITY TO OPERATE A MOTOR VEHICLE TO *NAME OF COMPANY.*

I REALIZE THAT DRIVER EVALUATION, DRIVER TRAINING, AND VEHICLE MODIFICATION MAY PRESENT CERTAIN RISKS TO ME, AND I VOLUNTARILY ASSUME SUCH RISKS IN ORDER TO PARTICIPATE IN THIS PROGRAM. I ALSO UNDERSTAND THAT PARTICIPATION IN THE ABOVE-MENTIONED SERVICES DEPENDS ON THE CONSENT OF MY PHYSICIAN AND THE DEPARTMENT OF MOTOR VEHICLES FOR FINAL DETERMINATION OF MY ELIGIBILITY TO HOLD A VALID DRIVER'S LICENSE.

CONSENT IS VALID UNTIL REVOKED IN WRITING. I UNDERSTAND THAT IF I AM FOUND INELIGIBLE TO OPERATE A MOTOR VEHICLE SAFELY THAT THE DMV WILL BE NOTIFIED OF THIS EVALUATION. A FINAL REPORT OF MY EVALUATION WILL BE SENT TO ME AND MY PHYSICIAN UPON MY REQUEST.

THIS FORM HAS BEEN FULLY EXPLAINED TO ME, AND I UNDERSTAND ITS FULL MEANING.

Client's Signature (Parent or Legal Guardian If Under 18)
Date
Witness
Client Social Security Number
Client Date of Birth

Appendix 13.D. Case Studies With Evaluation Reports

Driver Evaluation Report 1: Mr. Driver

Mr. Driver is a pleasant, well-educated, 31-year-old man with a diagnosis of muscular dystrophy and possibly attention deficit disorder. He was seen and this report was prepared today (1/1/04) for a driver evaluation and an on-the-road test drive at Mr. Company. Mr. Driver presents with partially functional upper extremities and nonfunctional lower extremities for operating a motor vehicle.

There is no stated history of drug or alcohol abuse, diabetes, or seizures. Mr. Driver has a Virginia driver's license, which will expire on xxxxx. (It is worth noting that there are no restrictions to hand controls on this permit.) He reports that he is on no medications at this time. Mr. Driver brought a completed Med 2-DMV Customer Medical Report to today's evaluation (completed by Dr. xxxxx). This form was faxed to DMV Medical Review Board on today's date. Because Mr. Driver's diagnosis is a progressive disorder, he will have periodic reviews by the DMV.

A brief ocular motor screening on today's date revealed that range of motion, visual pursuits, visual scanning, and saccades were intact. He reports that he has not been seen by an eye health care specialist and that his last eye exam was completed by his family physician who "looked only at visual acuities."

According to the Optic 2000 (Stereo Optical Driver Rehabilitation Vision Tester), he scored with his eyes working separately for simultaneous vision. He scored below normal limits for stereo depth at far vision. He scored within normal limits (WNL) for lateral phoria "far," vertical phoria "far," and fusion "far." He also scored WNL for color perception and peripheral fields. He identified 12/12 road signs and scored 20/20 usable vision right eye, 20/20 usable vision left eye, and 20/20 usable vision both eyes together for near and distance vision. The above test was administered without glasses.

The Motor-Free Visual Perception Test was administered and indicated that visual perception was WNL (36/36 accuracy). Visual perceptual processing time was also WNL.

Mr. Driver ambulated with a straight cane but was not able to walk up curbs. He plans to purchase a Permobil Chairman 2K Corpus (power wheelchair). He was able to obtain the wheelchair from the vendor for today's evaluation.

An on-the-road test drive using the client's vehicle (GMC Sonoma pickup) demonstrated Mr. Driver is an appropriate candidate for learning to operate a motor vehicle. The extended test drive revealed that Mr. Driver centered his car in the lane, steered around corners, parked between vehicles (perpendicular), and identified road signs. Mr. Driver was evaluated in residential and highway traffic. He drove his vehicle with his right lower extremity. Because he is not able to move his lower extremities, he has a straight cane tied to his brake, and he uses the cane to brake for the vehicle. Mr. Driver was informed that this approach is not safe and that he needs to be cleared by his physician and DMV to operate a motor vehicle. He was able to get in and out of the vehicle, with minimal assistance needed to get out of the minivans (both Braun Entervan conversions—Pontiac Montana and the Ford Windstar). He manipulated all secondary functions (heater and fan switches, ignition switch, window up–down, vehicle lights on–off, signals, horn, dimmer, and windshield wipers). He donned and doffed the seatbelt independently. The test drive using push–pull hand controls demonstrated that Mr. Driver was not successful with this equipment because of decreased strength and range of motion in his upper extremities. Mr. Driver was not able to demonstrate adequate brake reaction, completion, or steering times without the use of adaptive equipment. He required physical intervention during the test drive when using push–pull hand controls mounted on the left, and therefore reduced-effort equipment is being recommended.

Once van modifications are completed, Mr. Driver will need to be instructed in evasive maneuvers such as controlled braking and off-road recovery. He will need training with grading pressure on the accelerator and brake. He will need training in city and interstate traffic. He will also need to demonstrate smooth and controlled starts and stops, a good ability to change lanes by checking traffic and blind spots, appropriate body position with backing, and awareness of surrounding traffic through the use of commentary driving. Training also should take place at night, and Mr. Driver should practice purchasing gasoline for the vehicle and going through a drive-through bank teller.

Recommendations

- Schedule an eye health exam with an eye care professional because he has never had one in the past.
- Have vehicle modified with the below-mentioned equipment.
- Have a final fitting with vendor and evaluator at the time of completion of the van work to change van modifications according to any changes in Mr. Driver's functional ability.
- Complete driver training with adaptive equipment to address the above-mentioned areas.
- Return to DMV to have license revalidated with the adaptive equipment.

Van Modifications

Mr. Driver's diagnosis is progressive, so he will become more dependent in transfers. A transfer to a car will become increasingly more difficult and time-consuming, and loading his wheelchair will become impossible. Therefore, he will need to drive a specially adapted van for maximum safety, efficiency, and independence. The following modifications would best meet his needs. (At the time of this evaluation, Mr. Driver had not yet decided whether to purchase an already modified full-size van or a van that he would have modified.)

- Fire extinguisher and cellular phone for emergency use. Cellular phone to be ordered after van is received to enable Mr. Driver to choose a unit he can operate independently. It is suggested that a hands-free, voice-activated model be installed.
- Norcal Max with 9-inch lowered floor.*
- Fully automatic wheelchair lift with automatic door opener–closer to include inside–outside mounted control (with a third station on the dashboard). Must include manual override system. Client prefers UVL.
- Remote control with magnetic keyless entry as backup.
- Mobility Product and Design 3700 hand controls mounted on the right.
- Mobility Product and Design accelerator–brake guard.
- Reduced-effort steering with backup.
- Spinner knob paced at 9 o'clock on the steering wheel.
- Power wheelchair lockdown in driver's area (E-Z Lock). Client also prefers a separate lockdown system in the front passenger area if available.

If Mr. Driver decides not to purchase the Norcal Max (modified van), the following van modifications will be necessary:

- An interior vehicle height at least 2 inches taller than Mr. Driver when he sits in his wheelchair needs to be created. This can be done by lowering the floor of the vehicle 7 inches and raising the roof of the vehicle. When a lowered floor is chosen, the drop floor must be extending into the driver's area. The drop floor must be undercoated, rust-proofed, primed, and painted. The floor is to be fully leveled and covered with client's preference of floor covering. The additions of the raised roof *must* include structural support (roll bars).
- Passenger wheelchair restraint system mounted in the rear of the van *must* be forward facing; side facing will *not* be tolerated for safety reasons. *Must* include lap and shoulder restraint *separate* from the wheelchair. Kinedyne or Q-Straint is recommended.

- Removable captain's driver seat, quick disconnects on casters to facilitate use by nondisabled drivers.
- Rear lockdown for removable captain's chair.
- At this time, Mr. Driver is able to manipulate secondary functions of the vehicle. He understands that additional modifications could be needed later to the ignition, gear selector, seat belt, lights, heater, fan, and so on.

Elimination of *any* of the above equipment will jeopardize the safety of the driver and passengers of this vehicle. If there are any changes to this prescription, Ms. CDRS *must* be notified (555-555-5555) and written approval obtained before changes are acted upon. Any alteration to or deviation from the prescribed modifications written above shall make this prescription invalid and release Mr. Company and its evaluator of all liability.

Note: Hand controls must be VA accepted and installed according to VA specifications. All vehicles to be equipped with hand controls must have automatic transmission, power steering, and power brakes.

Material regarding the manufacturers and vendors of the above equipment was issued to and discussed with the client.

Equipment should meet or exceed the requirements established by the NMEDA and VA. Recommendations made as a result of this driver evaluation should be considered valid for one year from the date of evaluation. Beyond that time, a reevaluation of the client may be necessary.

Driver Evaluation Report 2: Mr. Wonder

Mr. Boy Wonder is a 24-year-old man with "possible autism." He is under psychiatric care for medication management of mood swings. He takes the following medications: Effexor, Haladol, Ditrapan, Baclafin, lithium, and Pamelor.

Mr. Wonder presents with partially functional left upper and left lower extremities and nonfunctional right upper and right lower extremities for driving. He has had numerous learners' permits from the time he "left high school." A DL-13 form completed by Dr. Goodwill was returned to the physician. The DL-13 form is generated from the motor vehicle administration in Pennsylvania under the category of Customers Medical Reports. It is signed by the client and physician and states the client's disabilities, limitations, and adaptive equipment needs. This author believes that it is necessary to ensure the DMV and the physician both know about the intended evaluation. There have been situations in which a person with a fully loaded van (from the VA) could not drive because the doctor felt he was not medically stable. Similarly, the DMV might also indicate that there are too many outstanding fines and that payment must be made in full before obtaining a license.

Mr. Wonder was seen on 3/21/03 at Mr. Company for a driver's evaluation and an on-the-road test drive. He was seated in a Quickie II manual wheelchair with Jay back and Jay cushion with the following measurements: 26 inches wide, 44 inches long, and 55 inches high. Visual assessments on this date demonstrated that visual pursuits, saccades (rapid eye movement), and convergence were within normal limits (WNL). The MVPT was administered and indicated that visual-perceptual skills were WNL, as was visual-perceptual processing time. The King Devick was completed and suggested a decreased ability with visual scanning. Visual acuities and peripheral fields were not obtained because Mr. Wonder had recently visited an optometrist.

An on-the-road test drive was completed using a 2000 Chrysler minivan (kneel car conversion) with rear entry and driver transfer seat. Mr. Wonder also used a left-foot accelerator and left spinner knob. Mr. Wonder required moderate to maximum assistance with transfers to and from the driver's seat. Such transfers are time-consuming and inefficient, so Mr. Wonder would need to drive from a *power* wheelchair. Mr. Wonder was tried with rear and side entries and was unable to negotiate ramps into the vans without assistance. However, in a power wheelchair Mr. Wonder could enter and exit the vehicle independently. Mr. Wonder was able to start the vehicle and change gears without assistance.

During the test drive, Mr. Wonder was unable to grade the pressure on the accelerator or brake. He was unable to maintain constant speed and demonstrated inadequate brake completion and steering times even after a two-day test drive. On three occasions, his left hand came off the spinner knob, causing a loss of steering control. This was due in part to decreased coordination of the left upper extremity. Mr. Wonder became extremely angry when the examiner made suggestions about maintaining lane position. Mr. Wonder did not maintain lane position in straight paths or around curves. He consistently drove too far to the right, and on several occasions physical intervention from the evaluator was required to brake the vehicle before hitting road signs to the right. Mr. Wonder again became angry, cursing at the examiner and stating that "he would have stopped in time." On two occasions, Mr. Wonder spat at the examiner.

Mr. Wonder is not an appropriate candidate for successful and safe operation of a motor vehicle. Mr. Wonder is able to improve in coordination of operating the vehicle, but this would not improve his ability to the extent that he could handle the vehicle in all areas on residential, highway, or city roads—and especially not in emergency situations. This concern was discussed at length with Mr. Wonder and his case manager, who attended today's evaluation.

Driver Training Report: Mr. Goodfellow

Mr. Goodfellow is a 26-year-old man with a diagnosis of "trainable mental retardation," as reported by Mr. Goodfellow. He presents with functional upper and lower extremities for driving. He has no prior driver training.

Mr. Goodfellow was seen at Mr. Company for a driver's evaluation and an on-the-road test drive and driver training. He ambulates without assistance. He reports that he lives alone with an attendant for 4–5 hours at night. Visual assessments on this date demonstrated that visual pursuits, saccades (rapid eye movement), and convergence were within normal limits. The MVPT as administered indicated that visual-perceptual skills were below normal limits, as was visual-perceptual-processing time. The King Devick was completed, but it is not believed that this test was reliable, as Mr. Goodfellow reported that he "did not recognize his numbers that well." He did not remember the last time he saw an eye doctor, but he reported that he wore glasses when he went to school.

An on-the-road test drive was completed using a Dodge Aspen. Mr. Goodfellow reports that he owns the car, but the car does not have valid registration or tags. Mr. Goodfellow stated that he did not have any insurance because he did not know he needed it.

Mr. Goodfellow stated that he could drive if given the opportunity. Driver training began on 1/2/03. Mr. Goodfellow was trained in getting in and out of the vehicle safely, locking the doors, adjusting his mirrors, and using the seatbelt. After the first week of training, Mr. Goodfellow would still become angry that there was no "B" on the gearshift—"B is for backing up," he would state angrily when the driver educator suggested putting the car in reverse. Mr. Goodfellow would drive over speed bumps at 20 mph, stating that he needed to maintain a consistent speed.

Mr. Goodfellow could state the rules of the road but did not follow the road signs or road markings. Throughout his training, he continued to improve in small areas. Initially he drove with speeds under 10 mph, advancing to 35–40 mph. Training was in residential and highway traffic only; he never successfully completed the goals set for highway driving to move toward interstate or city traffic. He needed seven physical assists in 1 hour when moving at speeds of 40 mph. He continually needed spoken cues to look ahead and to the sides and not have "tunnel vision." Mr. Goodfellow made unsafe errors in judgment: not looking both ways when pulling out in front of traffic, not maintaining lane position, and missing road signs. He was trained in perpendicular and angular parking and reversing for three days but still required physical assistance when moving the vehicle in reverse. He would constantly look forward even though he was moving the car in reverse. After three weeks of training, Mr. Goodfellow could steer the car in a familiar environment near his home, but he could not add secondary switches, such as the lights and signals, even in residential traffic.

Mr. Goodfellow is not able to safely operate a motor vehicle. Mr. Goodfellow has a list of the two buses he uses to go to and from his place of employment. (He works cleaning stables near his home.) No recommendation is made for continued driver training at this time.

Appendix 13.E. Resources and Suppliers

Access Unlimited
    570 Hance Road
    Binghamton, NY 13903
    (800) 849-2143
    Power-lift chairs for cars and trucks
Accessible Vans of America
    (888) AVA-VANS (888-282-8267)
    http://www.accessiblevans.com
    Van rental (new and used)
Adaptive Driving Alliance
    (623) 434-0722
Advance Driving Skills Institute
    (800) 327-6781
    http://www.advdrivskills.com
American Automobile Association (AAA)
    http://www.aaa.com
    Traffic Safety Division
    Digest of motor vehicle laws, by state
    Contact any local AAA office for information on instructional equipment and
    training supplies
American Occupational Therapy Association (AOTA)
    (301) 652-2682
    http://www.aota.org
    Professional membership organization
Americans With Disabilities Act
    Transportation Guidelines
    (202) 366-9306
    Request accessible formats
Association for Driver Rehabilitation Specialists (ADED)
    (800) 290-2344
    Fax: (318) 255-4175
    http://www.aded.net
B and D Independence Company, Inc.
    (800) 292-7117
    Power seat bases
Braun Corporation
    (800) THE LIFT (843-5438)
    Chair lifts for vans, cars, and trucks
Bruno Independent Living Aids, Inc.
    (800) 882-8183
    http://www.bruno.com
    Scooter and wheelchair lifts
CCI (Creative Controls, Inc.)
    (248) 577-9800
    http://www.creativecontrolsinc.com
    Low-effort brakes, scooter lockdown
Crescent Industries
    (207) 777-3500
    http://www.crescentindustries.com
    Adaptive vehicle control products

Doron Precision Systems
  P.O. Box 400
  Binghamton, NY 13902
  (607) 792-1610
  Driving simulators, rehabilitation, and assessment
Drive-Master
  (973) 808-9709
  http://www.drivemaster.net
  Driving aids, home and van conversions
DSI (Driving Systems, Inc.)
  (818) 782-6793
  e-mail: dsi2@mail.idt.net
EZ Lock Wheel Restraint Systems
  (225) 926-2403
  http://www.ezlock.net
  e-mail: info@ezlock.net
  Driver and passenger wheelchair restraints
DADC (Driving Aids Development Corporation)
  (800) 767-6435
  http://www.drivingaids.com
  Assisted hand controls
Daimler Chrysler Motors Corporation
  (or local dealers)
  http://www.automobility.daimlerchrysler.com/
  Rebate assistance, credit, and vehicle purchase
Driver Performance Test
  Advanced Driving Skills Institute
  (727) 669-8308
  Fax: (727) 799-2874
  Video of driving situations
Driver Rehabilitation Associates
  1300 South Maple Street
  Ruston, LA 71270
  (318) 255-7567
  Publications, Louisiana Tech University
  Mike Shipp, Anne Havard
EMC, Electronic Mobility Controls
  (225) 927-5558
  http://www.emc-digi.com
  Primary, secondary electronic controls
Ford Motor Company
  Mobility Motoring Program
  (800) 952-2248
  http://www.mobilitymotoringprogram.com
  Rebate assistance, Ford credit
General Motors Mobility Assistance Program
  (800) 323-9935
  http://www.gm.com/vehicles/us/mobility
  Rebate assistance, credit, and vehicle purchase
Gresham Driving Aids, Inc.
  (800) 521-8930
  Controls, seating, lifts, and chair storage

Handicapped Driver Services, Inc.
    e-mail: handicapdriver@mindspring.com
    Installation, evaluations, and training in vans
IDS (Independent Driving Systems)
    (713) 864-1460
    http://www.intellidrive.com
    Steering systems and secondary control pads
IMS (Independence Mobility Systems)
    (800) IMS-VANS (800-467-8267)
    http://www.imsvans.com
    Ramp vans, wheelchair restraint systems
International Medical Equipment Corporation (IMEC)
    (800) 547-9514
    http://www.imec-online.com
    Grandmar Torso Support Device
Kinedyne Securement and Restraint Systems
    Contact: Lift Aids, Inc.
    (817) 834-3881
    Restraints for adaptive uses
Life Science Associates
    (516) 472-2111
    Cognitive rehabilitative services
    e-mail: Cogrehab@pipeline.com
    Testing programs
Mobility Products and Design
    (800) 488-7688
    http://www.mobilityproductsdesign.com
MPS (Manufacturing and Product Services Corporation)
    (760) 796-4300
    Spinner knobs, tri-pins, and left-foot accelerator
MVPT Testing Copyright
    Academic Therapy Publications
    20 Communications Boulevard
    Novato, CA 94949
    Motor-Free Visual Perception Test
National Highway Traffic Safety Administration
    http://www.nhtsa.dot.gov
    Federal standards and practices, adaptive criteria
National Mobility Equipment Dealers Association
    (800) 833-0427
    http://www.nmeda.org
    Dealers, vendors of adaptive vans
Neuro-Optometric Rehabilitation Association (NORA)
    (866) 222-3887
    http://www.nora.cc
Ohio Safe-T-Brake, Inc.
    (800) 773-4104
    http://www.OhioSafeTBrake.com
    Instructor's brake
Q'Straint
    (819) 472-4111
    Wheelchair and driver–rider restraint system

RESNA (Rehab Engineering and Assistive Technology Society of North America)
(703) 524-6686
http://www.resna.org
Advancement of modification technology, certification
RICON Corporation
(800) 322-2884
http://www.riconcorp.com
Wheelchair lifts, lowered-floor minivans, and seat bases
Safety Products
York, PA 17402
(888) 480-1419
http://www.YP.prod.com
Reaction timers, night sight testing, and dual brakes
Simulator Systems International, Inc.
(918) 250-4500
Measures cognitive, perceptual, and behavioral skills
Smith System
(800) 777-7648
http://www.smith-system.com
Society of Automotive Engineers
(412) 776-4891
Stereo Optical Co., Inc.
(800) 344-9550
http://www.steroptical.com
Visual testing equipment
Sure Grip
Howell Ventures, Ltd.
(506) 363-5289
e-mail: suregrip@nbnet.nb.ca
Hand control system
Tip Top Mobility
(800) 735-5958
Car-top wheelchair carriers
Wells-Engbert
(800) 642-3628
e-mail: wellseng@aol.com
Hand controls

Index

A

Access to places of public accommodation
ADA requirements, 11–13
advocacy for, 13
in rural communities, 331
Accountability
managed care and, 166, 167
quality of life framework for, 24
Acquired immune deficiency syndrome, 117
Activities of daily living
assistance for client with profound disability, 60
vision problems affecting, 120, 135–139
Adult foster care, 5
Advocacy for individuals with disability, 266
Developmental Disabilities Act and, 15–16
disability community, 4
ethical issues in, 18
historical development, 3–6
in physical access, 13
quality of life issues, 21, 35
rules of, 15–18
as therapist role, 4, 14–18
understanding of, by individuals with disability, 282
Alzheimer's disease, 43
Amblyopia, 115
American Association on Mental Retardation, 42
American Hippotherapy Association, Inc., 154
Americans with Disabilities Act (1990), 4, 305, 306
access requirements, 11–13
employment issues, 9–10
Title III, 11
Amygdala, 269
Arousal management, 270–271
Assessment
clinical reasoning, 180–181
craniosacral structures and functioning, 216–217
for driving rehabilitation and training, 344–345, 346, 352
for employment, 292–293, 305, 306–307
for equine-assisted therapy, 162–163
functional capacity evaluation, 302
movement, 218
muscle energy, 212
nonstandardized approach, 171
participant-observation methodology, 179–180
patterns of deficits and strengths, 183
prevocational, 301–302
profound disability, 42, 45–51
Assessment (*continued*)
quality of life framework for, 24, 25, 32–33
for sensory intervention, 71–75
sensory processing, 95–100
standardized instruments, 170–171
strain and counterstrain, 212
for structurally-based manual therapy, 219–221, 228–231
vision problems, 119–126
vocational, 302–303
See also Let's Do Lunch assessment tool
Assisted movement, 59–60
Assistive technology, 304–305, 306, 321
Association for Driver Rehabilitation Specialists, 343
Association of Driver Educators for the Disabled, 343
Attentional problems, 97–98
driver training for client with, 362
Autonomic nervous system, 269

B

Behavioral interventions, 104
clients with profound disability, 76–78
sensory approach and, 81
Biomechanical functioning
assessment, 212

concept of dysfunction in manual
        medicine, 206, 207–208
Brain stem sensation, 86–88, 269

C
Centre for Health Promotion approach,
        20, 35–36
    applications, 31
    for assessment, 32–33
    conceptual basis, 26–27
    conceptual development, 26, 36
    information collection for, 31–32
    for policy evaluation, 35
    for program evaluation, 34
    for program planning, 33–34
    quality of life definition and
        domains in, 27–31
    for research, 35
Cerebral palsy, driver with, 363, 366
Civil rights movement, 4, 9
    human rights declarations, 13–14
Cleland, Max, 13
Clinical practice
    quality of life framework, 25
Committee on Employment of the Physi-
    cally Handicapped and Mentally
    Retarded, 3
Communication
    difficulties related to vision prob-
        lems, 138–139
    group processes, 276, 278,
        281–282, 285
    at mealtimes, 176
    neurophysiology of group processes,
        269–270
    during structurally-based manual
        therapy, 226–227
Community rehabilitation facility, 295
Community residential programs
    origins of, 4–5
    resistance to, 5–8
Competency. See Guardianship/
    conservatorship
Computer technology occupations
    job market trends, 308–309
    opportunities for persons with
        disability, 309, 310, 314–315,
        321
    skills requirements, 309
    training and preparation for,
        310–314, 315–320
Confrontation testing of visual field
    deficits, 122–123

Conservatorship. See Guardianship/
    conservatorship
Craniosacral osteopathy, 210, 216–218
Craniosacral therapy, 210, 216–218,
    245–246

D
Declaration of Rights of Mentally
    Retarded Persons, 14
Definitional issues
    developmental disability, 6
    quality of life, 22–23, 27–28
Deinstitutionalization movement, 4,
    41–42, 292
Dementia, 43
Department of Housing and Urban
    Development, 16
Developmental Disabilities Act, 15–16
Diabetic retinopathy, 119
Diet and nutrition
    difficulties related to vision prob-
        lems, 135–136, 137–138
Diet and nutrition (continued)
    sociocultural and clinical signifi-
        cance of food-related behaviors,
        172–177
    See also Let's Do Lunch assessment
        tool
Differential reinforcement, 65
Discrimination
    in employment, 9–10, 306
    in housing access, 6–7
    in physical access, 11–13
Documentation, 17
Down syndrome, 43
    visual problems in, 115
Driver training and rehabilitation
    amputee drivers, 365
    checklist, 342
    client with attentional problems, 362
    client with brain injury, 364
    client with cerebral palsy, 363, 366
    client with dwarfism, 364
    client with hemiplegia, 364, 365
    client with learning problems, 363
    client with paraplegia, 364–365
    client with spina bifida, 363
    client with spinal cord injury,
        363–364
    client with tetraplegia, 364–365
    clinician qualifications and certifica-
        tion for, 343–344
    consent form, 342

cost and reimbursement, 355
driver cognitive capacity for,
349–350
driver evaluation, 344–345,
346–352
driver physical abilities for, 350–351
driver vision requirements, 346–349
elements of instruction, 352–354
goals, 343, 344
historical development, 342–343
insurance issues, 354
liability issues, 354
resources, 342, 343 366
seatbelt systems, 359–360
Smith System, 345–346
test drive, 351–352
van design, 358–361
vehicle controls, 357–358, 360–361
vehicle selection and modification,
354–361
Dura mater, 216

E
Education and training of practitioners
driver rehabilitation specialists,
343–344
for equine-assisted therapy, 156,
162, 163–164
for sensory intervention, 108
special education teachers, 3
Education for All Handicapped Children
Act, 298
Employment
assessment issues, 292–293,
301–303, 305, 306–307
assistive technologies for, 304–305,
306, 321
case example of assessment and
intervention, 293–294, 306–308
challenges in rural areas, 330, 331
developmental disability and, as a
research and practice topic,
291–292
earnings trends, 329
environmental conditions, 303–304
historical development of clinical
approach, 294–295
individual program plans, 300–301
intervention in residential settings,
299
job coach role, 297
job market trends, 308–309
legal protections, 8–10

minimum wage laws, 8–9
practice framework, 293
prevocational interventions, 301–302
psychosocial significance, 291, 320,
330
school-to-work transition, 297–299
scope of developmental disability
issues in, 292–294, 300
settings for occupation-based interventions, 295–301
sheltered workshops, 295
supplemental interventions, 305
supported employment concept,
295–297, 331, 332–333
therapist role in service delivery,
320–321
types of interventions, 301
unemployment rate, 298, 329
vocational interventions, 302–304
vocational team, 301
See also Computer technology occupations; Self-employment
Empowerment, 4
Enclave employment, 296
Epidemiology, 41–42, 43
visual problems, 114
Equal Employment Opportunity
Commission, 16
Equine-assisted therapy
application, 156–158
assessment for, 162–163
benefits, 164–165
billing and reimbursement, 156
clinical features, 153–154
equine-facilitated mental health,
158–160
hippotherapy, 157–158
rationale, 153
resources, 163–164
safety considerations, 162–163
therapeutic horseback riding, 153,
160–161
therapist role, 154–156
vocational and pre-vocational
opportunities, 161–162
Ethical practice in advocacy, 18
Ethnicity, 175
Eye charts, 121

F
Fair Housing Amendments Act (1988), 5,
6, 7
Fair Labor Standards Act (1938), 8

Fascial restrictions and release, 209, 214–216
  craniosacral, 216–218
  systemic effects, 218–219
Five-Stage Model
  advantages, 264–266
  bilateral motor coordination activities, 261–262
  closure stage, 257–258
  cognition stage, 256–257
  cognitive skills focus, 262–263
  effectiveness, 264
  group processes, 250–251, 274, 284
  movement stage, 252–253
  neuromusculoskeletal focus, 259–261
  orientation stage, 252
  psychosocial skills focus, 263
  role of activities, 251, 254
  sensorimotor focus, 258–259
  stages, 250
  techniques, 251
  treatment goals, 251
  visual motor perceptual activities stage, 253–256
Frame of reference
  behavioral, 76–78
  clinical application, 92
  developing new, 75, 79–81
  Ready Approach, 75, 89–96
  sensory, 71, 75, 79, 80, 81
Functional capacity evaluation, 302

G
Glaucoma, 118, 120
Government programs
  employment-based interventions, 298, 300, 305, 306
  historical development, 3
  school-to-community transition, 300
  school-to-work transition, 298, 300–301
  See also Legislation
Gratings tests, 121–122
Group experiences, 268
  arousal management in, 270–271
  benefits of, 268–269, 271–273, 282–286
  communication styles in, 276, 278, 281–282, 285
  control issues, 279
  differences in diagnoses within group, 276–277
  Five-Stage Model, 250–251, 274, 284
  Goodwill Industries therapeutic groups, 273–274
  neurophysiology of learning, 269–270
  peer interactions, 274, 275–276, 279–280, 283, 284
  rhythm of, 277–278
  role development, 276, 279
  therapist role, 278–281
  types of groups, 283
  types of therapeutic experiences, 274–275
Group homes, 5, 6–8
  design for residents with profound disability, 66–68
  occupation-based interventions in, 299
Guardianship/conservatorship, 14
Guided movement therapy, 57–59

H
Handicap, defined, 6
Hippotherapy, 157–158
Histoplasmosis, 117
Horseback riding. See Equine-assisted therapy
Housing, 4–8, 16
Human rights, 13–14
Hypothalamus, 269

I
Immune function, 269–270
Individual program plans, 300–301
Informed consent, guardianship responsibilities, 14
Institutionalization, 4
  current trends, 91–92
  historical development of clinical approach, 294–295
  long-term, 44–45
  occupation-based intervention and, 299
  See also Deinstitutionalization movement
Insurance for automobile operators, 354
Intensive Care Facilities, 224
International Society of Crippled Children, 3
Isometric contractions, 212

J

Joint problems, 209–210

L

Lea Symbols chart, 121, 122
Learning, neurophysiology of, 269–270
Legal action
    alternatives to, 17–18
    documentary evidence for, 17
Legislation, 4
    education-to-work transition, 298
    employment issues, 8–10, 305, 306,
        332
    housing, 4–8
    human rights guarantees, 13–14
    regulation and, 16, 17–18
    therapist knowledge of, 15–16
Let's Do Lunch assessment tool, 166,
    177–178
    advantages, 199–200
    application in other activities, 199
    case examples, 183–199
    conceptual basis, 171–172, 178–179
    goals, 177
    implementation, 179–181
    outcome measurement, 168, 169
    rationale, 172–177, 179
    scoring, 181–183
Life history approach, 266
Low birth-weight babies, 43

M

Macular degeneration, 118, 120
Magnifying glasses and devices, 129–134
Managed care, 21, 265
    accountability and, 166, 167
    definition and characteristics,
        166–167
    outcomes research and, 167
Manual therapy, 206
    functional techniques, 210–212, 222
    therapeutic goals, 207, 208
    See also Structurally-based manual
        therapy
Memory processes, 83
Mental retardation
    clinical conceptualization, 43, 206
    prospects for improved information
        processing, 271
    structurally-based manual therapy
        rationale, 222–224
    See also Profound disability
Minimum wage, 8–9

Mobility

    specialists, 142
    vision problems and, 140–141
Model of Human Occupation, 79
Muscle energy protocol, 209–210, 212
Muscle spasms, 209–210, 212, 218, 219
Muscle strain and tenderness, 212–214
Myofascial release, 209, 214

N

Narrative techniques, 266
Neurofascial release, 209, 215
Neurophysiology, 81
    arousal management, 270–271
    brain stem sensation, 86–88
    concept of dysfunction in manual
        medicine, 207
    fight-or-flight response, 286
    frame of reference, 79
    learning in social interaction,
        269–270
    memory processes, 83
    muscle strain, 212–214
Neurophysiology (*continued*)
    neural plasticity, 85, 271
    psychoneuroimmunology, 269–270
    of Ready Approach, 89–90
    sensory processing, 82–88, 105
North American Riding for the Handi-
    capped Association, 154, 163

O

Orientation and mobility specialists, 142
Outcomes measurement
    behavioral frame of reference, 78
    client perspective in, 169–170
    managed care and, 166
    occupational therapy outcomes,
        168–169
    process factors and, 167
    in profound disability, 170
    quality of life measures in, 21,
        24–25, 34
    selecting, 168
    standardized instruments for,
        170–171

P

Pain, referred, 210
Peer relations in group processes, 274,
    275–276, 279–280, 283, 284
Pelli-Robson test, 121, 122
Perimetry testing, 123

Person-centered approach, 4
Policy making, quality of life approach in, 35
Posture assessment, 229–230
Profound disability
    activities of daily living assistance, 60
    assessment and categorization, 45–51
    assisted movement techniques, 59–60
    behavioral interventions, 76–78
    benefits of early intervention, 45
    clinical conceptualization, 42
    clinical features, 43–44, 75–76
    comorbid conditions, 43
    deinstitutionalization movement and, 41–42
    effects of long-term institutionalization, 44–45
    environmental considerations, 66–68
    epidemiology, 41–42
    etiology, 43
    guided movement therapy, 57–59
    intervention rationale, 45
    outcomes measurement, 164
    positioning problems, 56–57
    program planning, 51–56
    Ready Approach intervention, 89–92
    Self-abuse and self-stimulation behaviors, 62–66
    sensory interventions, 62–66, 67–68
    therapeutic use of switches, 61–62
    therapeutic use of toys, 61
    therapist role, 68–69
    therapy resource assessment, 45–46
    treatment team, 68
Project ASSET, 329, 332–341
Psychoneuroimmunology, 269
Public opinion and understanding, resistance to community residential programs, 5–6, 8

Q
Quality of life, 20
    client perceptions, 26
    conceptual development in occupational therapy, 21–22
    definition, 22–23, 27–28
    as framework for practice, 24–26
    mealtime experiences, 176–177

outcomes measurement, 21, 24–25, 169
    significance of, in occupational therapy, 23–24
    See also Centre for Health Promotion approach

R
Ready Approach, 75, 89–96, 100–102, 105–109
Reasonable accommodation, 7, 9–10
    in physical access, 11–13
    in workplace, 306
Recreational activities, 4
Rehabilitation Act (1973), 4, 9–10, 306, 332
Rehabilitation Engineering and Assistive Technology Society of North America, 304
Retinitis pigmentosa, 115
Rural communities, 330, 331

S
Saccades, 125
School system interventions
    school-to-community transition, 300
    school-to-work transition, 297–299, 300–301
Scotoma, 116
Self-employment
    benefits, 330–333
    business plan development, 338–339
    current extent, 331–332
    disincentives, 339–340
    model program for promoting, 332–341
Self-injurious/self-stimulating behaviors
    clinical conceptualization, 62–64
    sensory interventions, 64–66, 71–75
Sensory interventions
    assessment and intervention planning, 71–75
    behavioral interventions and, 81
    challenges in, 217
    client sensory defensiveness, 84–85, 96–97
    client with profound disability, 62–66, 67–68
    frame of reference approach, 71, 75, 79, 80, 81
    implementation, 80–81, 88–89, 107–108
    neurobiological basis, 82–88, 105

Ready Approach, 89–96, 100–102, 105–109
  therapeutic approach, 102–105
  transdisciplinary therapy team, 100–101
  types of sensory processing problems, 96–99, 106
Settings for service delivery
  occupation-based interventions in, 295–301
  residential/institutional, 299
  structurally-based manual therapy, 224–225
  See also School system interventions
Sheltered workshop, 295
Smith System training, 345–346
Snellen fraction, 120
Somatoemotional release, 218
Somatosensory stimulation, 65
Spina bifida, driver with, 363
Strabismus, 124
Strain and counterstrain manual therapy, 210, 212–214
Structurally-based manual therapy
  assessment for, 228–231
  case histories, 233–245
  communication during, 226–227
  concept of dysfunction in, 206–208
  conceptual basis, 207
  craniosacral therapy/osteopathy, 210, 216–218, 245–246
  manifestation of effects, 227–228
  muscle energy protocol, 209–210, 212
  myofascial release, 209, 214
  neurofascial release, 209, 215
  rationale, 212–214
  strain and counterstrain technique, 210, 212–214
  systemic effects, 218–221
  techniques, 208–212
  therapeutic relationship in, 225
  treatment environment, 224–225
  treatment goals, 218, 231, 245
  treatment protocol, 231–233
  treatment schedule, 224
  treatment session, 224–227
  visceral manipulation, 209, 215–216
  working with adults with mental retardation, 245–247
  zero balancing technique, 210, 218
Subclavian vein compression, 207

Supported employment, 295–297, 331, 332–333

T
Technology-Related Assistance for Individuals with Disabilities Act (1988), 305
Telescopes, 134
Therapist role
  advocacy, 4, 14–18
  in community residential programs, 5, 8
  in driver training and rehabilitation, 343, 344
  in ensuring physical access, 13
  equine-assisted therapy, 154–156
  as group facilitator, 270–271, 278–281
  historical development of, 4
  in managing vision problems, 115–116
Therapist role (*continued*)
  in participant-observation assessment, 179–180
  quality of life issues, 23–24
  in work-based interventions, 300
  in working with client with profound disability, 68
  in workplace, 10
Therapist–client relationship
  in manual therapy, 225
  in occupational counseling, 293
Therapy planning
  for clients with profound disability, 45–56
  frame of reference for, 71
  quality of life goals, 25, 33–34
  structurally-based manual therapy, 231–233
  vision problems, 127
Tilt-in-space wheelchair, 56–57
Toxoplasmosis, 117
Transitional employment, 296
Truman, Harry S., 3

U
Universal Declaration of Human Rights, 14

V
Visceral manipulation, 209, 215–216
Vision problems, 114
  activities of daily living and, 120, 135–139

adaptation deficits, 125–126
assessment, 119–126
causes, 114–115, 116, 117–119
communication problems related to,
    138–139
compensatory visual skills, 134–135
distance viewing, 139
driver evaluation for, 346–348
early intervention, 115
eating difficulties related to,
    135–136
environmental changes to improve
    coping with, 127–129
epidemiology, 114
mobility problems related to,
    140–141
pattern recognition, 129
physiology, 116
preferred retinal locus, 134–135

professional resources, 141–142
therapist role, 115–116
treatment goals, 126
treatment outcome factors, 126
treatment planning, 127
types of, 114
use of magnifying devices, 129–134
visual field loss, 122–123, 135

W
Wheelchair, tilt-in-space, 56–57
Wheelchair loaders and carriers, 357,
    359
Workforce Investment Act, 333

Z
Zero balancing technique, 210, 218
Zoning ordinances, 7

About the Editors

Susan Bachner, MA, OTR/L, FAOTA, CEAC, owner and president of Susan Bachner Consulting, LLC, has almost 40 years of clinical practice with individuals who have developmental disabilities. Susan's numerous articles and book chapters appear in both professional and lay publications. Her universally designed cookbook, *Picture This—An Illustrated Guide to Complete Dinners,* is used extensively by people of all abilities. Evidence of her graduate degree in sociology and anthropology is especially evident in her chapter "Let's Do Lunch," in which she discusses the symbolism of food as it conveys culture, customs, attitudes, and values. Susan became certified as an environmental access consultant in 1999 and now guides the transformation of inaccessible or unsafe residences into supportive environments. In 2003, Susan was awarded Occupational Therapist of the Year 2002–2003 by the Kentucky Occupational Therapy Association.

Mildred Ross, OTR/L, FAOTA, has practiced as an occupational therapist since her graduation from Columbia University in 1951. Having been engaged in private practice since 1984, she served people with developmental disabilities; worked in home care with dual diagnoses; and held per diem contracts in school settings, in mental health settings, and with nursing facilities. She has provided more than 100 presentations on the Five-Stage Group Model and included this subject, as well as others, in many articles and six books. She is the recipient of several service awards. Her emphasis at present is on the value of movement in the lives of those with and without disabilities.